OVERWEIGHT AND THE METABOLIC SYNDROME:

FROM BENCH TO BEDSIDE

ENDOCRINE UPDATES
Shlomo Melmed, M.D., Series Editor

J.A. Fagin (ed.): Thyroid Cancer. 1998. ISBN: 0-7923-8326-5
J.S. Adams and B.P. Lukert (eds.): Osteoporosis: Genetics,
Prevention and Treatment. 1998. ISBN: 0-7923-8366-4.
B.-Å. Bengtsson (ed.): Growth Hormone. 1999. ISBN: 0-7923-8478-4
C. Wang (ed.): Male Reproductive Function. 1999. ISBN: 0-7923-8520-9
B. Rapoport and S.M. McLachlan (eds.): Graves' Disease:
Pathogenesis and Treatment. 2000. ISBN: 0-7923-7790-7.
W.W. de Herder (ed.): Functional and Morphological Imaging
of the Endocrine System. 2000. ISBN 0-7923-7923-9
H.G. Burger (ed.): Sex Hormone Replacement Therapy. 2001.
ISBN 0-7923-7965-9
A. Giustina (ed.): Growth Hormone and the Heart. 2001.
ISBN 0-7923-7212-3
W.L. Lowe, Jr. (ed.): Genetics of Diabetes Mellitus. 2001.
ISBN 0-7923-7252-2
J.F. Habener and M.A. Hussain (eds.): Molecular Basis of Pancreas
Development and Function. 2001. ISBN 0-7923-7271-9
N. Horseman (ed.): Prolactin. 2001. ISBN 0-7923-7290-5
M. Castro (ed.): Transgenic Models in Endocrinology. 2001
ISBN 0-7923-7344-8
R. Bahn (ed.): Thyroid Eye Disease. 2001. ISBN 0-7923-7380-4
M.D. Bronstein (ed.): Pituitary Tumors in Pregnancy
ISBN 0-7923-7442-8
K. Sandberg and S.E. Mulroney (eds.): RNA Binding Proteins:
New Concepts in Gene Regulation. 2001. ISBN 0-7923-7612-9
V. Goffin and P.A. Kelly (eds.): Hormone Signaling. 2002
ISBN 0-7923-7660-9
M.C. Sheppard and P.M. Stewart (eds.): Pituitary Disease. 2002
ISBN 1-4020-7122-1
N. Chattopadhyay and E.M. Brown (eds.): Calcium-Sensing Receptor.
2002. ISBN 1-4020-7314-3
H. Vaudry and A. Arimura (eds.): Pituitary Adenylate Cyclase-
Activating Polypeptide. 2002. ISBN 1-4020-7306-2
R.C. Gaillard (ed.): The ACTH AXIS: Pathogenesis, Diagnosis
and Treatment. 2003. ISBN 1-4020-7563-4
P. Beck-Peccoz (ed.): Syndromes of Hormone Resistance on the Hypothalamic-
Pituitary-Thyroid Axis. 2004. ISBN 1-4020-7807-2
E. Ghigo (ed.): Ghrelin. 2004. ISBN 1-4020-7770-X
C.B. Srikant (ed.): Somatostatin. 2004. ISBN 1-4020-7799-8
V.D. Castracane and M.C. Henson (eds.): Leptin. 2006. ISBN 0-387-31415-6
G.A. Bray and D.H. Ryan (eds.): Overweight and the Metabolic Syndrome. 2006.
ISBN 0-387-32163-2

OVERWEIGHT AND THE METABOLIC SYNDROME:

FROM BENCH TO BEDSIDE

Edited by

George A. Bray, MD
Pennington Biomedical Research Center
Louisiana State University System
Baton Rouge, Louisiana, USA

Donna H. Ryan, MD
Pennington Biomedical Research Center
Louisiana State University System
Baton Rouge, Louisiana, USA

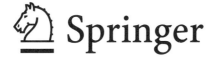 Springer

George A. Bray, MD
Pennington Biomedical Research Center
Louisiana State University
6400 Perkins Road
Baton Rouge, LA, USA

Donna H. Ryan, MD
Pennington Biomedical Research Center
Louisiana State University
6400 Perkins Road
Baton Rouge, LA, USA

OVERWEIGHT AND THE METABOLIC SYNDROME:
FROM BENCH TO BEDSIDE

Library of Congress Control Number: 2006922024

ISBN-10: 0-387-32163-2 e-ISBN-10: 0-387-32164-0
ISBN-13: 978-0387-32163-9 e-ISBN-13: 978-0387-32164-6

Printed on acid-free paper.

Printed in the United States of America.

9 8 7 6 5 4 3 2 1

springer.com

Contents

Chapter 5: Etiology of Obesity: The Problem of Maintaining Energy Balance

Chapter 6: Current Views of the Fat Cell as an Endocrine Cell: Lipotoxicity

Chapter 7: Ectopic Fat and the Metabolic Syndrome

Chapter 8: Abdominal Obesity and the Metabolic Syndrome

Chapter 9: The Problems of Childhood Obesity and the Metabolic Syndrome
Sonia Caprio and Ram Weiss   153

Chapter 10: Evaluation of the Overweight and Obese Patient
George A. Bray and Donna H. Ryan   169

Chapter 17: Surgical Treatment of the Overweight Patient
George A. Bray

Preface

The field of obesity and the metabolic syndrome continues to advance on all fronts. This book is an effort to bring together a series of chapters that cover many of the newer facets of the problem. We have tried to capture the goal of this book in the subtitle "from bench to bedside". Fundamentally, as human biologists, we are interested in understanding the problem of obesity and the metabolic syndrome and then applying this new knowledge to easing the burden of people afflicted in this disease state. We begin with the laboratory findings. Butler and his colleagues begin the process with an illuminating discussion of the factors that control the termination of meals. After a brief review of the neuroendocrine control system, they provide a detailed look at the gastrointestinal and pancreatic factors that can stimulate or inhibit food intake. They then look at the long-term control affected by leptin and insulin. In the next chapter, Dr. Chumlea discusses the various methods for measuring "obesity". Dual-energy absorptiometry (DXA) has the ability to provide estimates of fat mass, lean mass and bone mass making it quite versatile. However, from a practical perspective, weight, waist circumference and the body mass index (body weight in kg divided by the square of height in meters) are the most useful. The body mass index (BMI) has been the most widely used index in the assessment of the current changes in prevalence of obesity, providing a good picture of the increasing epidemic of obesity. The progress of this epidemic has been well characterized by Dr. Mokdad from the Centers for Disease Control and Prevention, the U.S. Governmental agency charged with tracking this epidemic. Genetic factors are clearly behind the susceptibility to obesity that characterizes this epidemic. Dr. Comuzzie, who has contributed important information to this problem, focuses on the advances that we have experienced in understanding the relations of nature and nurture. In a well written and timely chapter, Drs. Levin and Clegg argue the case of a "set-point" or a defended body weight. They begin with the historical and anatomic data and the move to discussing the intricacies of the mechanisms that control this process. Fat is the site for storage of extra energy. When the fat cells reach their maximum storage capacity, new fat cells may be recruited, but fat may also be stored ectopically in other organs. Tchkonia, Corkey, Kirkland explore this important new concept in a chapter dealing with lipotoxicity. The conditions for lipotoxicity occur when net capacity to store and utilize lipids is exceeded in diseases such as diabetes, obesity, the metabolic syndrome, indexmetabolic syndrome lipodystrophies, aging, and other conditions. The chapter by Toledo and Kelley extends this concept of lipotoxicity to the issues associated with visceral adipose tissue. This ectopic storage of fat is associated with insulin resistance. This group has coined the term "metabolic inflexibility" to describe the setting in which an infusion of insulin fails to enhance carbohydrate metabolism in muscle. They develop the "portal hypothesis" which suggests that visceral adipose tissue provides fatty acids to the liver than lead to accumulation of lipid there and in the intramyocellular compartment. Fatty-acyl-CoAs, diacylglycerol and ceramides are important candidates for these metabolic changes. As demonstrated by several groups, this effect is associated with changes in mitochondrial genes and their enzymes that are involved in oxidative phosphorylation. Finally, they discuss the lipodystropic states where loss of fat is associated with increased insulin resistance. Recent studies show that replacing leptin, a product of the fat cell, to individuals with too little fat can ameliorate most of the metabolic features of lipodystrophy. Drs. Lemieux and Despres, leaders in the field of studying visceral adipose tissue and the metabolic syndrome provide a succinct summary of the advances in this area. Children who become overweight bear the stigma associated with obesity, and at the same time experience the detrimental health benefits that are often seen. Caprio and Weiss, who have been leaders in establishing criteria for the metabolic syndrome in adolescents, review their data and the types of changes that characterize this condition in the adolescents in their clinic. From the laboratory side of the problem, we now turn to translating these findings into the evaluation and treatment of obesity and the metabolic syndrome. Evaluating any patient is the first step in deciding how serious the problem may be and what steps to take in correcting it. Ryan and Bray provide the introductory steps in this process with a chapter dealing with evaluation of the patient with obesity and the metabolic syndrome. It is now clear that measurement of waist circumference along with the BMI provide the first steps. For establishing the metabolic syndrome other measurements such as blood pressure, a lipid panel and glucose are needed. If two of these are abnormal and there is an enlarged waist one can diagnose the metabolic syndrome. Once the diagnosis is made, treatment is in order. Since all of the components of this syndrome will respond positively to weight loss, strategies to help people lose weight are the first steps. However, when the lipid, blood pressure or glucose abnormalities remain abnormal, they should be treated with one of the appropriate therapies. Lifestyle strategies are the first line of approach. Diet, exercise and behavioral therapy make up the 3 components of these lifestyle approaches. Diet is the first line of attack and the chapter by Foster and Makris introduces us to this problem. Their chapter provides a nice review of the low carbohydrate diets in comparison with other diets. Foster and Makris first review the low and moderate fat diets and the turn to the low carbohydrate diets and provide us a feeling for the value that each of these groups of diets have in the treatment of overweight. Diets reduce energy intake and thus require overweight individuals to draw fat from their fat stores. Exercise, reviewed by Jakicic and Otto, works by increasing the utilization of energy through physical exertion. They begin by convincing us that those who are more active have improved health benefits and longevity. They then review the literature on weight loss studies and show that exercise alone is not a very effective strategy. However, for maintaining weight loss, becoming and remaining more active clearly plays a central role. The third arm of lifestyle is behavior therapy whose role is reviewed in a chapter by Williamson, Stewart and Martin. They provide an historical background and then describe the many features that come under this category. The use of portion controlled foods and the use of the internet are two of the more recent advances, each of which offers the hope of extending the scope and success of this approach. Obviously we would prefer to prevent overweight than to have to treat it. Kumanyika and Daniels take us through the literature on studies that have attempted to prevent the progression of overweight. Two broad kinds of approaches have been taken—population wide approaches and targeted approaches. In spite of much work, the authors correctly note that at present we have no definitive studies to guide a clear approach to the problem. Where prevention fails, therapy is needed. Two drugs are currently approved by the U.S. Food and Drug Administration for treatment of obesity. Dr. Wyatt discusses the use of these two drugs, sibutramine and orlistat. Although both are effective in producing weight loss, the loss is moderate and often frustrating to the participant who is taking the drug. Although only 2 drugs are currently approved, Greenway and Bray review the burgeoning new drug armentarium. Several drugs approved for use in diabetes, like metformin, pramlintide and exenatide produce weight loss. Rimonabant, an antagonist to the cannabinoid CB1 receptors in the brain is a promising new agent that will soon be evaluated by the FDA for approval and clinical use. There is cautious optimism that it may change the landscape of treatment for those individuals whose overweight has not been prevented. The final chapter deals with surgical interventions for overweight patients. Since laparscopic techniques for this procedure became wide spread, its performance and safety have both changed significantly. Over 100,000 operations were performed last year, and the number continues to rise. With this final chapter, we complete our tour from laboratory to clinic. We hope it meets the needs for which it was put together—a survey of new strategies to bring the laboratory to the clinic for treatment of obesity and the metabolic syndrome.

George A. Bray, M.D.

Contributors

1. Natalie Alméras
   Laval Hospital Research Center, Laval Hospital, Ste-Foy, Québec, Canada
2. Raul A. Bastarrachea
   Department of Genetics, Southwest Foundation for Biomedical Research, San Antonio, TX, USA
3. George A. Bray
   Pennington Biomedical Research Center, Baton Rouge, LA, USA
4. Andrew A. Butler
   Pennington Biomedical Research Center, Louisiana State University System, Baton Rouge, LA, USA
5. Guowen Cai
   Department of Genetics, Southwest Foundation for Biomedical Research, San Antonio, TX, USA
6. Sonia Caprio
   Department of Pediatrics and the Children's General Clinical Research Center, Yale University School of Medicine, New Haven, CT, USA
7. Wm. Cameron Chumlea
   Departments of Community Health and Pediatrics, Lifespan Health Research Center, Wright State University School of Medicine, Dayton, OH, USA
8. Deborah J. Clegg
   Department of Psychiatry, Genome Research Institute, Cincinnati, OH, USA
9. Shelley A. Cole
   Department of Genetics, Southwest Foundation for Biomedical Research, San Antonio, TX, USA
10. Anthony G. Comuzzie
    Department of Genetics, Southwest Foundation for Biomedical Research, San Antonio, TX, USA
11. Barbara E. Corkey
    Obesity Center, Evans Department of Medicine, Boston University, Boston, MA, USA

12. Stephen R. Daniels
    Departments of Pediatrics and Environmental Health, Cincinnati Children's Hospital Medical Center and the University of Cincinnati College of Medicine, Cincinnati, OH, USA

13. Jean-Pierre Després
    Québec Heart Institute, Laval Hospital Research Center, Laval Hospital, Ste-Foy, Québec, Canada and
    Department of Social and Preventive Medicine, Laval University, Ste-Foy, Québec, Canada

14. Earl S. Ford
    Centers for Desease Control and Prevention, Atlanta, GA, USA

15. Gary D. Foster
    University of Pennsylvania School of Medicine, Philadelphia, PA, USA

16. Frank Greenway
    Pennington Biomedical Research Center, Louisiana State University System, Baton Rouge, LA, USA

17. John M. Jakicic
    Department of Health and Physical Activity, Physical Activity and Weight Management Research Center, University of Pittsburgh, Pittsburgh, PA, USA

18. David E. Kelley
    Division of Endocrinology and Metabolism, Department of Medicine, University of Pittsburgh, School of Medicine, Pittsburgh, PA, USA

19. Jack W. Kent Jr.
    Department of Genetics, Southwest Foundation for Biomedical Research, San Antonio, TX, USA

20. James L. Kirkland
    Obesity Center, Evans Department of Medicine, Boston University, Boston, MA, USA

21. Shiriki K. Kumanyika
    Department of Biostatistics and Epidemiology, Department of Pediatrics, and Graduate Program in Public Health Studies, University of Pennsylvania School of Medicine, Philadelphia, PA, USA

22. Isabelle Lemieux
    Québec Heart Institute, Laval Hospital Research Center, Laval Hospital, Ste-Foy, Québec, Canada

23. Barry E. Levin
    Department of Neurology and Neurosciences, New Jersey Medical School, University of Medicine and Dentistry of New Jersey, Newark, NJ, USA and Neurology Service, VA Medical Center, NJ, USA

24. Angela P. Makris
    University of Pennsylvania School of Medicine, Philadelphia, PA, USA

25. Corby K. Martin
    Pennington Biomedical Research Center, Baton Rouge, LA, USA
26. Ali H. Mokdad
    Centers for Desease Control and Prevention, Atlanta, GA, USA
27. Christopher D. Morrison
    Pennington Biomedical Research Center, Louisiana State University System, Baton Rouge, LA, USA
28. Amy D. Otto
    Department of Health and Physical Activity, Physical Activity and Weight Management Research Center, University of Pittsburgh, Pittsburgh, PA, USA
29. Donna H. Ryan
    Pennington Biomedical Research Center, Baton Rouge, LA, USA
30. Tiffany M. Stewart
    Pennington Biomedical Research Center, Baton Rouge, LA, USA
31. Tamara Tchkonia
    Obesity Center, Evans Department of Medicine, Boston University, Boston, MA, USA
32. Frederico G.S. Toledo
    Division of Endocrinology and Metabolism, Department of Medicine, University of Pittsburgh, School of Medicine, Pittsburgh, PA, USA
33. James L. Trevaskis
    Pennington Biomedical Research Center, Louisiana State University System, Baton Rouge, LA, USA
34. Ram Weiss
    Department of Pediatrics and the Children's General Clinical Research Center, Yale University School of Medicine, New Haven, CT, USA
35. Jeff T. Williams
    Southwest National Primate Research Center, San Antonio, TX, USA
36. Donald A. Williamson
    Pennington Biomedical Research Center, Baton Rouge, LA, USA
37. Holly Wyatt
    University of Colorado at Denver and Health Sciences Center, Denver, CO, USA

Chapter 1

Neuroendocrine Control of Food Intake

Andrew A. Butler, James L. Trevaskis and Christopher D. Morrison

*Pennington Biomedical Research Center, Louisiana State University System,
6400 Perkins Road, Baton Rouge, LA 70808, USA*

1. INTRODUCTION

Most organisms function in environments with marked seasonal and, on a less predictable basis, climactic changes in nutrient availability. Species survival is dependent on systems that are remarkably adept at balancing food intake with the fluctuations in energy expenditure and with the amount of energy stored as triacylglycerol (TAG) in adipocytes. Neural and endocrine regulatory systems affecting feeding behavior must respond to short-term cues, such as the ability to sense and respond to stomach contents, along with signals concerning the long-term status of energy balance over periods of days. Feeding behavior is also linked to the circadian cycle, with the circadian rhythms of feeding behavior recently suggested to be critical for maintaining normal body weight [1].

The problem currently facing the global community is that, faced with an abundance of calories and diminished requirements for physical activity, a significant portion of the population are unable to maintain energy balance, leading to increased fat mass. Investigation of experimental rodent models strongly suggests that excess consumption of calories, especially associated with high-fat diets, is a significant factor causing obesity and insulin resistance [2, 3]. The latter is the defining feature of the insulin resistance syndrome, formerly called syndrome X or the metabolic syndrome, and comprises a cluster of diseases including type 2 diabetes, hypertension, and cardiovascular disease [4]. In the face of an epidemic of obesity and insulin resistance syndrome, there is enormous interest by pharmaceutical and academic groups to elucidate mechanisms that regulate food intake as a means to develop effective therapies against obesity and insulin resistance. This chapter describes the current models for the regulation of food intake by neuroendocrine factors, which integrate signals of long-term energy balance, involving primarily the adipokine leptin and leptin receptors expressed in the central nervous system (CNS), with factors secreted from the gut. Most of these factors have similar effects on energy balance whether administered peripherally or directly into areas of the CNS known to regulate feeding behavior. This chapter therefore begins with a brief introduction to the CNS centers that control feeding behavior.

2.   CENTRAL NERVOUS SYSTEM REGULATION OF FEEDING BEHAVIOR

Feeding is a complex behavior, involving the integration of a number of reward (hedonic) behaviors with the homeostatic systems that sense energy balance [5]. Within the CNS, areas distributed throughout the forebrain and caudal brain stem appear to be important for regulating feeding behavior [6, 7]. One area that appears to be particularly significant is the hypothalamus. Neurons in this area integrate sensory and endocrine signals into outputs that influence fluid and food intake; normal function of the hypothalamus is critical for energy homeostasis [8]. Hypothalamic neurons respond to several of the gut and adipocyte secreted factors known to affect food intake, with hypothalamic lesions sometimes severely abrogating the feeding response. While a comprehensive description of the hypothalamic neuronal circuitry involved in energy homeostasis is beyond the scope of this chapter, a list of some of the hypothalamic neurons identified as being important for the regulation of feeding behavior is provided in Table 1. Several excellent reviews of this topic have also recently been published [5, 6, 14–16].

The caudal brain stem is also an important site in regulating feeding behavior. Neurons within the nucleus tractus solitarius (NTS) and dorsal motor nucleus of the vagus (DMV) in the brain stem receive, and integrate, sensory inputs from vagal nerves involved in sensing the accumulation of nutrients in the stomach and duodenum tract through mechanical and chemical stimuli that include distension, changes in the gastrointestinal nutrient concentration, and changes in pH and osmolarity in the gut lumen [17]. The brain stem is also highly interconnected with the hypothalamus, communicating through ascending projections to regulate the response to fasting [7]. Conversely, descending projections from the hypothalamus to the brain stem may modulate the effectiveness of short-term satiety signals, such as cholecystokinin (CCK), in meal termination [18].

3.   NEUROENDOCRINE FACTORS SECRETED FROM THE GUT

In addition to the mechanosensory inputs received by vagal afferents, the gut releases at least 10 circulating factors, some of which may act as satiety signals to the CNS [19]. Some of these gut factors are described in the following section. For some of these peptides, evidence for suppression of food

Table 1. Neurons that have been identified as critical for the normal regulation of energy homeostasis

Neuropeptides expressed	Location	Effect on feeding	Responds to	References
Proopiomelanocortin/cocaine and amphetamine-regulate transcript (POMC/CART)	Arcuate nucleus	Inhibitory	(+)-leptin, PYY_{3-36}, 5-HT, insulin, glucose, (−)-ghrelin	44, 46, 47, 49, 133–139
POMC	Nucleus tractus solitarius	Inhibitory	(+)-cholecystokinin (CCK)	140–142
Agouti-related peptide/neuropeptide Y (AgRP/NPY)	Arcuate nucleus	Stimulatory	(−)-leptin, PYY_{3-36}, insulin, (+)-ghrelin	44, 47, 133 143
Melanin-concentrating hormone (MCH)	Lateral hypothalamic area	Stimulatory	(−)-leptin	144–148
Orexin	Lateral hypothalamic area	Stimulatory	(−)-leptin, glucose, ghrelin	12, 149

Orexin neurons innervate and regulate AgRP/NPY and POMC/CART neurons in the arcuate nucleus, indicating that these neurons might affect feeding behavior through regulating the hypothalamic melanocortin system [9, 10]. However, deletion of the *Orexin* gene, or ablation of orexin neurons, causes narcolepsy [11]. Orexin may primarily affect food intake by coordinating arousal with feeding [12, 13].

intake has only recently been described (e.g., amylin, glucagon-like peptide 1 [GLP-1], oxyntomodulin, peptide YY [PYY]), and for the case of PYY is still a matter of debate [20]. The administration of GLP-1 and PYY has been associated with the induction of illness-induced behavior, demonstrated by the induction of conditioned taste aversion in rodents [21–24]. These factors may therefore function not only as satiety signals, but possibly also as part of the stress response to visceral illness.

3.1. Cholecystokinin

Of all gut-derived satiety signals, the hormone cholecystokinin (CCK) is perhaps the most well-described hormone mediating satiety [25–27]. The role of CCK in meal termination was first demonstrated by Gibbs et al. in 1973 [28], and many subsequent studies have demonstrated that administration of CCK dose-dependently suppresses food intake. CCK is produced primarily by the enteroendocrine cells of the duodenal and jejunal mucosa, although CCK is also produced by both the enteric system and CNS [29]. These enteroendocrine cells are well positioned to sense the presence of nutrients within the gut, and indeed the secretion of CCK is stimulated by nutrient ingestion, with the presence of fat or protein within the gut being the primary stimulus for CCK secretion [30]. CCK secretion is both rapid and short-lived, peaking within 30 minutes of meal ingestion, and in some species even more rapidly. This increase of CCK after nutrient ingestion serves two main purposes. The first is to act locally within the gut to enhance nutrient absorption, with CCK stimulating gallbladder contraction and also inhibiting gastric emptying [31, 32]. However, nutrient-induced secretion of CCK also acts to terminate individual meals, and this effect has been shown in many species including humans. CCK dose-dependently reduces food intake [28], but it is not a long-term regulator of body weight. Prolonged CCK administration does not effectively reduce body weight, and most individuals treated chronically with CCK compensate for the reduction in individual meal size with an increase is the number or frequency of meals [33], such that overall food intake is not altered. In rodents, exogenous administration of CCK also engages a complete behavioral satiety sequence, accompanied by periods of grooming and sleep [34]. Taken together, these observations clearly implicate CCK as a prototypical satiety signal, with meal-induced CCK secretion being a central event in the termination of individual meals.

The suppression of food intake by CCK is mediated primarily by the brain, although its effects on gastric emptying also contribute to its satiating effects. CCK receptors are expressed within multiple brain regions, and thus a direct effect of gut-derived CCK on the brain is one possible mechanism for CCK action. However, CCK receptors are also expressed on vagal afferents that project from the gut to the caudal brain stem. These vagal fibers are directly stimulated by CCK [35], and vagotomy significantly attenuates CCK-induced satiety indexCCK-induced satiety [36]. The NTS is a key target for vagal sensory input, and exogenous CCK administration robustly activates c-Fos within NTS neurons [37, 38], as well as within other brain areas controlling food intake. In the brain stem, melanocortin neurons appear to be critical for the suppression of food intake by CCK, with activation of melanocortin-4 receptors (MC4R) required for the reduction of food intake [39]. These data therefore support a model in which CCK produced by the gut acts locally on vagal afferents, with these afferents then transmitting this satiety signal to key areas within the brain, and in particular the NTS. In summary, it is evident that CCK satisfies many of the requirements for a circulating satiety signal: it is produced by the gut in response to nutrient ingestion, suppresses meal size, acts rapidly but is short-lived, and does not induce illness or taste aversion. CCK consequently has become a prototypical satiety signal, and has provided a valuable benchmark by which to evaluate the many other proteins and gut hormones subsequently found to impact feeding behavior.

3.2. Peptide YY

Peptide YY (PYY), a member of the pancreatic polypeptide (PP) family which includes neuropeptide Y (NPY) and PP, is a 36-residue peptide with carboxy- and amino-terminal tyrosines (Y) that was isolated from porcine small intestine extracts in 1980 [40]. PYY is secreted from L cells of the gastrointestinal tract, with hydrolysis by the enzyme dipeptidyl peptidase-IV (DPP-IV) at the Pro^2-Ile^3 bond, producing PYY_{3-36} [41]. Full-length PYY_{1-36} is an agonist for at least three receptor subtypes (Y1, Y2, and Y5), with removal of the two amino terminus residues resulting in increased selectivity for the Y2 receptor [42, 43]. The Y2 receptor is widely expressed in the CNS, including the hypothalamus and brain stem. In the hypothalamus, Y2 mRNA is expressed on most NPY-positive neurons, with selective Y2 agonists acting to suppress the secretion of the potent orexigen NPY in hypothalamic slices [44]. Conversely, a selective Y2 antagonist stimulates NPY release, and also increases the release of an anorexigen, alpha-melanocyte stimulating hormone (α-MSH), in hypothalamic slices [44]. Overall, it has been proposed that the regulation of food intake by PYY_{3-36} involves the suppression of hypothalamic NPY/AgRP neurons, which are orexigenic, and stimulation of hypothalamic POMC/CART neurons, which are anorexigenic (Table 1). One group reported that mice lacking functional MC4R, which are the primary receptor involved in the regulation of food intake by α-MSH [45], do not respond to PYY_{3-36} [44, 46, 47]. However, a subsequent study reported that PYY_{3-36} reduced food intake in MC4R-deficient mice [48], while prohormone proopiomelanocortin (POMC) mice that lack α-MSH also respond to PYY_{3-36} [49], suggesting melanocortin-independent pathways for the regulation of feeding behavior by PYY_{3-36}.

The regulation of PYY secretion from the gut, and the regulation of the ratio of PYY_{1-36} to PYY_{3-36} in serum, by nutrient consumption, is consistent with this peptide acting as a satiety signal. PYY levels increase following a meal, peaking approximately 90 minutes after ingestion [50]. The ratio of PYY_{1-36} to PYY_{3-36} in human sera is also dependent on fed state, with PYY_{3-36} dominating postprandially [51]. Furthermore, in some experiments the administration of PYY_{3-36} reduces food intake in mice, and reduces meal size in humans [21, 44, 46, 48, 49].

It should be noted, however, that the role of PYY_{3-36} as a satiety signal has been the subject of controversy, with some groups having difficulty in demonstrating a significant suppression of food intake [20]. Moreover, PYY_{3-36} has also recently been reported to induce a vagal nerve dependent conditioned taste aversion, suggesting that the reduction of food intake in mice might be due to an illness-related behavioral response as opposed to a "satiety" signal [21].

3.3.   Ghrelin

Ghrelin is distinguished from other gut peptides in that it is not a satiety factor, and is the first gut-secreted peptide described that, when infused chronically either intracerebroventricularly or peripherally, causes hyperphagia and weight gain. Two groups simultaneously reported the discovery of a transcript encoding a secreted peptide and expressed in the stomach. Kojima et al. identified a 28-residue protein while screening for ligands of the growth hormone secretagogue receptor (GHS-R), an orphan G-protein-coupled receptor. The full sequence encoding a 117-amino-acid protein was cloned from a rat stomach cDNA library, with the first 23 residues encoding a signal peptide and the 28-residue ghrelin sequence beginning at Gly24 [52]. Kojima et al. also reported that *O-n*-octanoylation of the peptide at Ser3 is essential for inducing a response of Chinese hamster ovary (CHO) cells expressing GHS-R. Given that the peptide is a potent GH secretagogue, Kojima et al. designated the peptide as "ghrelin," based on the Proto-Indo-European root of the word "grow" [52].

Tomasetto et al. reported a transcript encoding a 117-amino-acid protein, identified in a screen for cDNAs expressed in the stomach [53]. This group designated the putative protein encoded by the transcript as motilin-related peptide (MRP), based on a weak homology with motilin, a peptide hormone that regulates smooth muscle contraction in the gastrointestinal tract. Tomasetto et al. were unable to show a biologic effect, owing to the use of a non-*O-n*-octanoylated, and hence biologically inactive peptide. Using Northern blot analysis, both groups demonstrated that ghrelin mRNA expression is highest in stomach, in enteroendocrine cells, with lower levels observed in the duodenum [52, 53]. Ghrelin immunoreactivity and mRNA have been reported in the hypothalamus, suggesting a possible role as an orexigenic neuropeptide [47, 52]. However, analysis of ghrelin knockout mice, in which the coding sequence is replaced by a *LacZ* reporter gene, failed to identify significant ghrelin-specific immunoreactivity, or β-galactosidase staining, in the hypothalamus [54].

Several observations suggest that ghrelin, in addition to regulating GH secretion, might regulate metabolism. GHS-R mRNA expression had earlier been reported in the hypothalamus and brain stem, while the GH secretagogue GHRP-6 stimulates c-Fos mRNA expression in arcuate nucleus NPY neurons, suggesting stimulation of a potent orexigenic neuropeptide [55–57]. Peripherally administered ghrelin affects energy balance by dose-dependently stimulating food intake and weight gain in rats and mice [58, 59]. In mice, the stimulation of food intake by ghrelin is dependent on two orexigenic peptides expressed in the hypothalamus, NPY and agouti-related protein (AgRP) [60, 61].

In humans, ghrelin acutely increases meal size, and can attenuate loss of appetite associated with cancer [62–64]. Ghrelin levels in the circulation exhibit an ultradian rhythm that is also consistent with this peptide stimulating food intake. In marked contrast to other gut peptides, whose secretion peaks postprandially, ghrelin levels in the circulation peak in anticipation of meal ingestion [65], and decline thereafter in correlation with caloric load [66]. These results suggest that ghrelin might function to initiate meals, or as a signal of negative energy balance. Ghrelin knockout mice do not, however, exhibit differences in total 24-hour food intake and have normal body weight [67].

3.4.   Amylin

Amylin, or islet amyloid polypeptide (IAPP), is a 37-amino-acid peptide that was purified from islets of individuals with type 2 diabetics [68]. Amylin is cosecreted with insulin from pancreatic β-cells [69, 70]. Many studies have shown that amylin is a short-term satiety peptide. Amylin levels indexamylin levels in the circulation increase postprandially while administration of the peptide, or analogues thereof, suppresses food intake in rodents and can cause weight loss when administered chronically (reviewed in [71–73]). In humans with type 2 diabetes, pramlintide, an amylin analogue, improves insulin sensitivity and causes weight loss, with a recent study suggesting that pramlintide enhances satiety and reduces food intake [74]. Amylin may therefore have a role in the treatment of obesity by reducing food intake. The regulation of feeding behavior by amylin involves both CNS and peripheral mechanisms [71–73]. Neurons in the area postrema, a circumventricular organ located in the brain stem, are required for the inhibition of food intake by amylin, while the hypothalamus also contains amylin binding activity. In the periphery, amylin may also affect food intake by inhibiting gastric emptying.

Several receptors that interact with amylin have been recently identified [75]. They commonly share the calcitonin receptor domain at their core and are associated with different receptor activity-modifying proteins (RAMPS) that differentially affect amylin binding [76]. The specific distribution of these receptors and the nature of their roles in transducing amylins effects on energy balance remain to be elucidated.

3.5.   Enterostatin

Enterostatin is a pentapeptide cleaved from the amino-terminus of pancreatic procolipase by trypsin. Proteolytic cleavage of enterostatin from procolipase activates colipase, a cofactor for pancreatic lipase, promoting fat digestion [77–79]. In rats, experiments examining the effects of peripheral or intracerebroventricular administration of enterostatin indicate that this peptide selectively inhibits fat consumption [78, 79]. Further, the postprandial increase in enterostatin levels in the circulation of rats following a meal correlates with dietary fat content [80]. Together, these observations indicate that enterostatin might function as a specific regulator of fat consumption. However, while the levels of immunoreactivity for one isoform of enterostatin also increase in humans postprandially [81], in a phase II trial intravenous administration of enterostatin did not significantly affect meal size in humans [82].

The mechanisms and receptors involved in the regulation of feeding behavior by enterostatin are unclear. Crude binding studies using brain lysates indicate two binding sites, one of low affinity ($K_d = 170$ nM) and one of high affinity ($K_d = 0.5$ nM). The low-affinity site might be the F1-ATPase β-subunit, which binds enterostatin with an affinity of 150 nM [83]. The suppression of food intake, and stimulation of c-Fos immunoreactivity in the NTS and parabrachial, paraventricular, and supraoptic nuclei in the brain is inhibited by vagotomy, suggesting that enterostatin interacts with the vagal system to regulate feeding behavior [84].

3.6.   Glucagon-like Peptide

Glucagon-like peptide (GLP-1) is an intestinal peptide released by specialized endocrine cells in the gut (K-cells) in response to the ingestion of glucose or lipids [88]. GLP-1 is produced by the posttranslational processing of proglucagon (Figure 1), which contains several proglucagon-derived peptides (PGDP) [85]. GLP-1 suppresses food intake by acting peripherally to inhibit gastric emptying, and also acting centrally to reduce food intake in the short term, but not long term [88]. Centrally administered GLP-1 elicits a conditioned aversion, while GLP-1R antagonists inhibit the aversive response to the toxin lithium chloride [22–24]. GLP-1 may thus function as a satiety factor, but also appears to be involved in mediating the behavioral and stress response to visceral illness.

Exenatide, or exendin-4, is a GLP-1 synthetic mimetic that stimulates the release of insulin from pancreatic beta cells. Diabetic subjects treated with exenatide showed significantly improved diabetic status and weight loss, with minimal gastrointestinal distress [86], and has recently been approved by the FDA as adjunctive therapy for patients with type 2 diabetes marketed as the drug Byetta (Amylin/Lilly). GLP-1 mimetics such as exenatide may be better tolerated and therefore more useful as therapies for diabetes or energy balance disorders.

3.7.   Bombesin Family: Bombesin, Gastrin-releasing Peptide and Neuromedin B

Bombesin was initially isolated from amphibian skin [87], and is expressed mainly in the brain and gastrointestinal tract. The two most well characterized mammalian homologues of bombesin, gastrin-releasing peptide (GRP) and neuromedin B (NMB), are also expressed in gut and brain, and can inhibit food intake when systemically administered in a number of mammalian

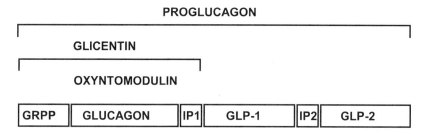

Figure 1. Structure of proglucagon, and a description of the proglucagon-derived peptides (PDRP) [85].

species, including humans [88, 89]. The effects of GRP and NMB are mediated through their respective receptors, GRP-R and NMB-R, although both peptides can bind both receptors. GRP-R is expressed throughout the brain including the hypothalamus whereas NMB-R is expressed in a more restricted fashion, particularly in the olfactory and thalamic areas [90]. More recently another receptor showing homology to GRP-R and NMB-R was cloned and designated bombesin-like peptide receptor subtype-3 (BRS-3) [91]. Expression of BRS-3 was limited to the hypothalamus and hindbrain. Both GRP and NMB have poor binding affinity for BRS-3, suggesting that the endogenous ligand for this receptor remains to be found. Mice deficient for either GRP-R or NMB-R exhibit no differences in food consumption and body weight compared to wild-type mice [92–94], although GRP-R may mediate some of the food intake inhibiting effects of bombesin and GRP [95]. BRS-3 knockout mice, however, are mildly obese, glucose intolerant, and leptin and insulin resistant [96], suggesting that BRS-3 may be a more important member of the hypothalamic appetite-regulatory network.

3.8.   Oxyntomodulin

Oxyntomodulin, like GLP-1, is derived from enzymatic processing of the proglucagon gene (Figure 1), and is released from the small intestine after ingestion of food. Oxyntomodulin is a satiety signal and inhibits food intake in rodents when administered either centrally or peripherally [97], and has also been shown to have anorectic effects when given to human subjects [98], as well as to promote weight loss [99]. Oxyntomodulin treatment in humans reduces plasma ghrelin [98] and leptin levels, while increasing circulating levels of adiponectin [99]. The fact that oxyntomodulin interacts with the GLP-1R, albeit with significantly less affinity than GLP-1, suggest that its effects may be mediated by this receptor, although the existence of an oxyntomodulin-specific receptor remains a possibility.

3.9.   Leptin

Leptin, encoded by the *ob* gene, is thought to be one of the most important hormones involved in energy homeostasis. Primarily secreted by adipocytes in response to positive energy balance, it circulates to areas of the brain, particularly the hypothalamus, and induces negative feedback responses. The wide range of functions and mode of action of leptin are described in more detail later. Leptin, however, is also produced in the stomach in response to feeding, as well as CCK treatment [100]. When leptin is administered via the celiac artery, which perfuses the upper gastrointestinal tract, it dose-dependently reduces meal size in normal, but not in vagotomized, rats [101]. In addition, leptin has also been shown to enhance the food-reducing effects of bombesin as well as CCK [101, 102]. The role of leptin in the modulation of gut-acting satiety peptides remains to be thoroughly understood.

4.   NEUROENDOCRINE INDICATORS OF LONG-TERM ENERGY BALANCE: LEPTIN AND INSULIN

Abnormal metabolism of adipose tissue appears to be an important factor in the development of insulin resistance [103]. Increased adipose mass, and in particular abdominal obesity, increases risk for developing insulin resistance and associated comorbidities, such as cardiovascular disease. On the other hand, insufficient capacity or a failure of adipocytes to proliferate and store excess calories has been suggested to cause excess accumulation of TAG and fatty acids in tissues such as the liver and skeletal muscle, leading to insulin resistance [104]. Abnormal secretion and/or function of the adipokine leptin from adipose tissue is an important factor in the etiology of insulin resistance [103]. In relation to the neuroendocrine control of food intake, leptin is considered one of, if not the, primary neuroendocrine signal of long-term energy balance [105]. Loss of function mutations in the leptin (*Lep*) or leptin receptor (*Lepr*) genes are associated with severe obesity and hyperphagia in mice and in a small number of humans who are homozygous for *Lep* or *Lepr* mutations [106]. Leptin resistance could therefore be an important factor in disorders of energy intake and expenditure causing obesity and insulin resistance [105]. This hypothesis is supported by the observation that the inactivation of genes that inhibit LEPR signal transduction in mice is associated with increased leptin sensitivity, and protection from the development of obesity and leptin resistance in obesogenic environments [107, 108].

In both humans and animals, physiological mechanisms monitor body adipose mass and react to changes in energy balance by altering ingestive behavior and energy expenditure to buffer against drastic changes in body adiposity and restore body weight and adiposity once the nutritional challenge dissipates [109–111]. This process of maintaining a relatively constant level of energy stores over time is known as energy homeostasis, and neuronal circuits within the brain, and in particular the hypothalamus, are critically involved in this process [109–111]. These circuits are sensitive to changes in a variety of circulating nutritional cues, and two hormones that are critical for the homeostatic regulation of body weight are the adiposity signals insulin and leptin.

In 1953, Kennedy first articulated the hypothesis that circulating signals produced by or in proportion to adipose mass act within the brain to reduce food intake [112]. These signals would decrease in response to reductions in body adiposity and conversely increase as body fat mass increases, and would thus represent a negative feedback signal for adiposity. The brain would then "sense" changes in these adiposity signals and regulate food intake and energy expenditure to normalize body adiposity. This initial hypothesis for a functional adipostat was supported by Coleman, who extended this hypothesis by demonstrating that the mouse obesity mutations *ob* (obese, now *Lep^{ob}*) and *db* (diabetic, now *Lepr^{db}*) represented mutations in what was likely a circulating cue and its corresponding receptor, such that the lack of either this putative hormone or its receptor resulted in massive obesity [113]. In 1994 Zhang and colleagues first cloned the obesity (*ob*) gene [114], and it was soon demonstrated that its protein product leptin was indeed a circulating hormone that acted within the brain to suppress feeding [115–122]. Leptin satisfies many of the requirements of an adiposity signal, being produced and secreted by adipocytes via mechanisms that are sensitive to both the chronic level of body adipose mass as well as current metabolic status. Circulating leptin levels increase in response to increases in adipose mass and glucose flux into adipocytes, while levels rapidly fall during periods of negative energy balance. Thus circulating leptin levels are a relatively accurate marker of the nutritional and metabolic status of the organism. While leptin does have clear effects on peripheral tissues, its profound effects on feeding and energy homeostasis are primarily mediated by the brain, where leptin acts to suppress food intake; stimulate energy expenditure; and also influence reproduction, glucose homeostasis, and a number of additional physiological systems. In addition, leptin or leptin receptor deficiency in both humans and animal models results in a profound obesity phenotype, marked by hyperphagia, diabetes, and infertility. Thus appropriate leptin signaling within the brain is necessary for energy homeostasis, and this work collectively supports the role of leptin as an adipostatic signal to the brain.

Other neuroendocrine signals also appear to satisfy the criteria of an adiposity signal. Much of the work focusing on leptin as an adiposity signal was preceded by a series of studies suggesting that insulin functions as an adiposity signal [123]. Although serum insulin levels fluctuate acutely relative to nutrient intake and serum glucose, average or basal insulin levels (such as fasting insulin) are closely coupled to total body adipose mass [124], such that insulin levels increase with increasing adipose mass and are conversely low in response to nutrient deprivation. In addition, insulin rapidly enters the brain and acts within the hypothalamus to suppress food intake and body weight [125]. Recent genetic work supports this role of insulin in the regulation of energy balance, as the loss of neuronal insulin receptors leads to a hyperphagic, obesity-prone phenotype that is in many ways similar to leptin deficiency [126, 127].

In addition to having similar effects on feeding and energy homeostasis, it is increasingly evident that insulin and leptin act on common populations of neurons within the brain, and in particular within the arcuate nucleus of the hypothalamus (Table 1). The ARC contains at least two distinct populations of neurons that are sensitive to leptin and insulin. One population produces the orexigenic peptides NPY and AgRP, and signaling from the NPY/AgRP neuron promotes increased food intake and body weight gain [6]. NPY/AgRP neurons express leptin and insulin receptors, and are negatively regulated by these hormones. An adjacent population of neurons expresses the POMC. POMC neurons also express leptin and insulin receptors, but in contrast to NPY/AgRP neurons, these neurons are stimulated by leptin and insulin and act to inhibit food intake [6, 15]. POMC is a precursor protein that is processed into a variety of neuropeptides, and the melanocortin α-MSH is one POMC-derived neuropeptide that is a particularly well-described regulator of feeding behavior [128]. α-MSH is a ligand for MC4R, and central administration of α-MSH or other MC4R agonists inhibits food intake. Taken together, these observations suggest that these adjacent orexigenic and anorexigenic neuronal populations represent first-order neurons within a circuit that senses changes in leptin and insulin tone, and that the regulation of these neurons is a central mechanism of both leptin and insulin action.

4.1.   Leptin and Insulin Signaling in Diet-induced Obesity

In humans and rodents, obesity induced by a high-fat diet is associated with elevated serum leptin and insulin, and a resistance to the central actions of these hormones [105, 129]. In addition, compelling evidence indicates that obesity-prone rats (selected for sensitivity to a high-energy diet) are less sensitive to centrally administered leptin, even before the development of obesity [130, 131]. These observations indicate that a reduction in central insulin or leptin signaling may promote the development of obesity. This central insulin and leptin resistance is similar to the peripheral insulin resistance that concomitantly develops after exposure to a high-fat diet. Therefore diet-induced decreases in hypothalamic insulin and leptin signaling may predispose the individual to obesity in the same way that peripheral insulin resistance predisposes to diabetes. This hypothesis is supported by recent genetic work demonstrating that mutations that enhance leptin or insulin signaling protect against the development diet-induced obesity [107, 108, 132].

5.   SUMMARY

With the rising prevalence of obesity and insulin resistance syndrome, the need for understanding how humans regulate body weight has grown considerably. The interaction between peripheral signals of energy status from the gut or adipose tissue with neural signals in order to maintain energy homeostasis is enormously complex. Here we have described several, but by no means all, of the molecules involved in this process and how we think they function. Clearly some of these molecules, such as insulin and leptin, are extremely important for normal human health whereas the roles of others may be less critical although still important. For instance, despite the significant role of leptin in physiology, only a handful of obese people have been reported to have defective leptin signaling. So despite its key role as an adipokine leptin, it is unlikely to be the major cause of common human obesity. As insulin resistance syndrome and obesity are likely to be polygenic disorders, it is possible that still more molecules await discovery. The more important task for the future, perhaps, will be to decipher the underlying interactions between all of these signals in order to form a clear picture of the neuroendocrine regulation of food intake.

REFERENCES

[1] Turek FW, Joshu C, Kohsaka A, et al. Obesity and metabolic syndrome in circadian Clock mutant mice. Science 2005;308(5724):1043–1045.
[2] Collins S, Martin TL, Surwit RS, Robidoux J. Genetic vulnerability to diet-induced obesity in the C57BL/6J mouse: Physiological and molecular characteristics. Physiol Behav 2004;81(2):243–248.
[3] Schemmel R, Mickelsen O, Gill JL. Dietary obesity in rats: Body weight and body fat accretion in seven strains of rats. J Nutr 1970;100(9):1041–108.
[4] Reaven GM. Why syndrome X? From Harold Himsworth to the insulin resistance syndrome. Cell Metab 2005;1(1):9–14.
[5] Saper C, Chou T, Elmquist J. The need to feed. Homeostatic and hedonic control of eating. Neuron 2002;36(2):199.
[6] Cone RD. Anatomy and regulation of the central melanocortin system. Nat Neurosci 2005;8(5):571–578.
[7] Grill HJ, Kaplan JM. The neuroanatomical axis for control of energy balance. Front Neuroendocrinol 2002;23(1):2–40.

[8] Cone RD, Low MJ, Elmquist JK, Cameron JL. Neuroendocrinology. In: Larsen PR, Kronenberg HM, Melmed S, Polonsky KS, eds. Williams Textbook of Endocrinology, 10th edn. Philadelphia: Saunders, 2003;81–176.

[9] van den Top M, Lee K, Whyment AD, Blanks AM, Spanswick D. Orexigen-sensitive NPY/AgRP pacemaker neurons in the hypothalamic arcuate nucleus. Nat Neurosci 2004; 7(5):493–494.

[10] Muroya S, Funahashi H, Yamanaka A, et al. Orexins (hypocretins) directly interact with neuropeptide Y, POMC and glucose-responsive neurons to regulate Ca^{2+} signaling in a reciprocal manner to leptin: Orexigenic neuronal pathways in the mediobasal hypothalamus. Eur J Neurosci 2004;19(6):1524–1534.

[11] Mieda M, Yanagisawa M. Sleep, feeding, and neuropeptides: Roles of orexins and orexin receptors. Curr Opin Neurobiol 2002;12(3):339–345.

[12] Yamanaka A, Beuckmann CT, Willie JT, et al. Hypothalamic orexin neurons regulate arousal according to energy balance in mice. Neuron 2003;38(5):701–713.

[13] Mieda M, Williams SC, Sinton CM, Richardson JA, Sakurai T, Yanagisawa M. Orexin neurons function in an efferent pathway of a food-entrainable circadian oscillator in eliciting food-anticipatory activity and wakefulness. J Neurosci 2004;24(46):10493–10501.

[14] Barsh GS, Schwartz MW. Genetic approaches to studying energy balance: Perception and integration. Nat Rev Genet 2002;3(8):589–600.

[15] Jobst EE, Enriori PJ, Cowley MA. The electrophysiology of feeding circuits. Trends Endocrinol Metab 2004;15(10):488–499.

[16] Zigman JM, Elmquist JK. Minireview: From anorexia to obesity—the yin and yang of body weight control. Endocrinology 2003;144(9):3749–3756.

[17] Travagli RA, Hermann GE, Browning KN, Rogers RC. Musings on the wanderer: What's new in our understanding of vago-vagal reflexes? III. Activity-dependent plasticity in vago-vagal reflexes controlling the stomach. Am J Physiol Gastrointest Liver Physiol 2003; 284(2):G180–G187.

[18] Morton GJ, Blevins JE, Williams DL, et al. Leptin action in the forebrain regulates the hindbrain response to satiety signals. J Clin Invest 2005;115(3):703–710.

[19] Small CJ, Bloom SR. Gut hormones and the control of appetite. Trends Endocrinol Metab 2004;15(6):259–263.

[20] Tschop M, Castaneda TR, Joost HG, et al. Physiology: Does gut hormone PYY3-36 decrease food intake in rodents? Nature 2004;430(6996):1 p following 165; discussion 2 p following.

[21] Halatchev IG, Cone RD. Peripheral administration of PYY(3-36) produces conditioned taste aversion in mice. Cell Metab 2005;1(3):159–168.

[22] Kinzig KP, D'Alessio DA, Herman JP, et al. CNS glucagon-like peptide-1 receptors mediate endocrine and anxiety responses to interoceptive and psychogenic stressors. J Neurosci 2003;23(15):6163–6170.

[23] Kinzig KP, D'Alessio DA, Seeley RJ. The diverse roles of specific GLP-1 receptors in the control of food intake and the response to visceral illness. J Neurosci 2002;22(23):10470–10476.

[24] Lachey JL, D'Alessio DA, Rinaman L, Elmquist JK, Drucker DJ, Seeley RJ. The role of central glucagon-like peptide-1 in mediating the effects of visceral illness: Differential effects in rats and mice. Endocrinology 2005;146(1):458–462.

[25] Moran TH. Gut peptides in the control of food intake: 30 years of ideas. Physiol Behav 2004;82(1):175–180.

[26] Moran TH, Kinzig KP. Gastrointestinal satiety signals II. Cholecystokinin. Am J Physiol Gastrointest Liver Physiol 2004;286(2):G183–G188.

[27] Schwartz GJ. Biology of eating behavior in obesity. Obes Res 2004;12(Suppl 2):102S–106S.

[28] Gibbs J, Young RC, Smith GP. Cholecystokinin decreases food intake in rats. J Comp Physiol Psychol 1973;84(3):488–495.

[29] Larsson LI, Rehfeld JF. Distribution of gastrin and CCK cells in the rat gastrointestinal tract. Evidence for the occurrence of three distinct cell types storing COOH-terminal gastrin immunoreactivity. Histochemistry 1978;58(1–2):23–31.

[30] Liddle RA. Regulation of cholecystokinin secretion by intraluminal releasing factors. Am J Physiol 1995;269(3 Pt 1):G319–G327.

[31] Liddle RA, Goldfine ID, Rosen MS, Taplitz RA, Williams JA. Cholecystokinin bioactivity in human plasma. Molecular forms, responses to feeding, and relationship to gallbladder contraction. J Clin Invest 1985;75(4):1144–1152.

[32] Moran TH, McHugh PR. Cholecystokinin suppresses food intake by inhibiting gastric emptying. Am J Physiol 1982;242(5):R491–R497.

[33] West DB, Fey D, Woods SC. Cholecystokinin persistently suppresses meal size but not food intake in free-feeding rats. Am J Physiol 1984;246(5 Pt 2):R776–R787.

[34] Antin J, Gibbs J, Holt J, Young RC, Smith GP. Cholecystokinin elicits the complete behavioral sequence of satiety in rats. J Comp Physiol Psychol 1975;89(7):784–790.

[35] Schwartz GJ, McHugh PR, Moran TH. Integration of vagal afferent responses to gastric loads and cholecystokinin in rats. Am J Physiol 1991;261(1 Pt 2):R64–R69.

[36] Smith GP, Jerome C, Norgren R. Afferent axons in abdominal vagus mediate satiety effect of cholecystokinin in rats. Am J Physiol 1985;249(5 Pt 2):R638–R641.

[37] Chen DY, Deutsch JA, Gonzalez MF, Gu Y. The induction and suppression of c-fos expression in the rat brain by cholecystokinin and its antagonist L364,718. Neurosci Lett 1993;149(1):91–94.

[38] Fraser KA, Davison JS. Cholecystokinin-induced c-fos expression in the rat brain stem is influenced by vagal nerve integrity. Exp Physiol 1992;77(1):225–228.

[39] Fan W, Ellacott KL, Halatchev IG, Takahashi K, Yu P, Cone RD. Cholecystokinin-mediated suppression of feeding involves the brainstem melanocortin system. Nat Neurosci 2004;7(4):335–336.

[40] Tatemoto K, Mutt V. Isolation of two novel candidate hormones using a chemical method for finding naturally occurring polypeptides. Nature 1980;285(5764):417–418.

[41] Medeiros MD, Turner AJ. Processing and metabolism of peptide-YY: Pivotal roles of dipeptidylpeptidase-IV, aminopeptidase-P, and endopeptidase-24.11. Endocrinology 1994;134(5):2088–2094.

[42] Dumont Y, Fournier A, St-Pierre S, Quirion R. Characterization of neuropeptide Y binding sites in rat brain membrane preparations using [125I][Leu31,Pro34]peptide YY and [125I]peptide YY3-36 as selective Y1 and Y2 radioligands. J Pharmacol Exp Ther 1995;272(2):673–680.

[43] Grandt D, Schimiczek M, Rascher W, et al. Neuropeptide Y 3-36 is an endogenous ligand selective for Y2 receptors. Regul Pept 1996;67(1):33–37.

[44] Batterham RL, Bloom SR. The gut hormone peptide YY regulates appetite. Ann NY Acad Sci 2003;994:162–168.

[45] Marsh DJ, Hollopeter G, Huszar D, et al. Response of melanocortin-4 receptor-deficient mice to anorectic and orexigenic peptides. Nat Genet 1999;21(1):119–122.

[46] Batterham RL, Cowley MA, Small CJ, et al. Gut hormone PYY(3-36) physiologically inhibits food intake. Nature 2002;418(6898):650–654.

[47] Cowley MA, Cone RD, Enriori P, Louiselle I, Williams SM, Evans AE. Electrophysiological actions of peripheral hormones on melanocortin neurons. Ann NY Acad Sci 2003;994:175–186.

[48] Halatchev IG, Ellacott KL, Fan W, Cone RD. PYY3-36 inhibits food intake through a melanocortin-4 receptor-independent mechanism. Endocrinology 2004.

[49] Challis BG, Coll AP, Yeo GS, et al. Mice lacking pro-opiomelanocortin are sensitive to high-fat feeding but respond normally to the acute anorectic effects of peptide-YY(3-36). Proc Natl Acad Sci USA 2004;101(13):4695–4700.

[50] Adrian TE, Ferri GL, Bacarese-Hamilton AJ, Fuessl HS, Polak JM, Bloom SR. Human distribution and release of a putative new gut hormone, peptide YY. Gastroenterology 1985;89(5):1070–1077.

[51] Grandt D, Schimiczek M, Beglinger C, et al. Two molecular forms of peptide YY (PYY) are abundant in human blood: Characterization of a radioimmunoassay recognizing PYY 1-36 and PYY 3-36. Regul Pept 1994;51(2):151–159.

[52] Kojima M, Hosoda H, Date Y, Nakazato M, Matsuo H, Kangawa K. Ghrelin is a growth-hormone-releasing acylated peptide from stomach. Nature 1999;402(6762):656–660.

[53] Tomasetto C, Karam SM, Ribieras S, et al. Identification and characterization of a novel gastric peptide hormone: The motilin-related peptide. Gastroenterology 2000;119(2): 395–405.

[54] Wortley KE, Anderson KD, Garcia K, et al. Genetic deletion of ghrelin does not decrease food intake but influences metabolic fuel preference. Proc Natl Acad Sci USA 2004;101(21):8227–8232.

[55] Bailey AR, Von Englehardt N, Leng G, Smith RG, Dickson SL. Growth hormone secretagogue activation of the arcuate nucleus and brainstem occurs via a non-noradrenergic pathway. J Neuroendocrinol 2000;12(3):191–197.

[56] Dickson SL, Luckman SM. Induction of c-fos messenger ribonucleic acid in neuropeptide Y and growth hormone (GH)-releasing factor neurons in the rat arcuate nucleus following systemic injection of the GH secretagogue, GH-releasing peptide-6. Endocrinology 1997;138(2):771–777.

[57] Guan XM, Yu H, Palyha OC, et al. Distribution of mRNA encoding the growth hormone secretagogue receptor in brain and peripheral tissues. Brain Res Mol Brain Res 1997;48(1):23–29.

[58] Tschop M, Smiley DL, Heiman ML. Ghrelin induces adiposity in rodents. Nature 2000; 407(6806):908–913.

[59] Wren AM, Small CJ, Ward HL, et al. The novel hypothalamic peptide ghrelin stimulates food intake and growth hormone secretion. Endocrinology 2000;141(11):4325–4328.

[60] Chen HY, Trumbauer ME, Chen AS, et al. Orexigenic action of peripheral ghrelin is mediated by neuropeptide Y (NPY) and agouti-related protein (AgRP). Endocrinology 2004.

[61] Tschop M, Statnick MA, Suter TM, Heiman ML. GH-releasing peptide-2 increases fat mass in mice lacking NPY: Indication for a crucial mediating role of hypothalamic agouti-related protein. Endocrinology 2002;143(2):558–568.

[62] Druce MR, Wren AM, Park AJ, et al. Ghrelin increases food intake in obese as well as lean subjects. Int J Obes Relat Metab Disord 2005.

[63] Neary NM, Small CJ, Wren AM, et al. Ghrelin increases energy intake in cancer patients with impaired appetite: Acute, randomized, placebo-controlled trial. J Clin Endocrinol Metab 2004;89(6):2832–2836.

[64] Wren AM, Seal LJ, Cohen MA, et al. Ghrelin enhances appetite and increases food intake in humans. J Clin Endocrinol Metab 2001;86(12):5992.

[65] Cummings DE, Purnell JQ, Frayo RS, Schmidova K, Wisse BE, Weigle DS. A prepran-dial rise in plasma ghrelin levels suggests a role in meal initiation in humans. Diabetes 2001;50(8):1714–1719.

[66] le Roux CW, Patterson M, Vincent RP, Hunt C, Ghatei MA, Bloom SR. Postprandial plasma ghrelin is suppressed proportional to meal calorie content in normal-weight but not obese subjects. J Clin Endocrinol Metab 2005;90(2):1068–1071.

[67] Sun Y, Ahmed S, Smith RG. Deletion of ghrelin impairs neither growth nor appetite. Mol Cell Biol 2003;23(22):7973–7981.

[68] Cooper GJ, Willis AC, Clark A, Turner RC, Sim RB, Reid KB. Purification and characterization of a peptide from amyloid-rich pancreases of type 2 diabetic patients. Proc Natl Acad Sci USA 1987;84(23):8628–8632.

[69] Kahn SE, D'Alessio DA, Schwartz MW, et al. Evidence of cosecretion of islet amyloid polypeptide and insulin by beta-cells. Diabetes 1990;39(5):634–638.

[70] Lukinius A, Wilander E, Westermark GT, Engstrom U, Westermark P. Co-localization of islet amyloid polypeptide and insulin in the B cell secretory granules of the human pancreatic islets. Diabetologia 1989;32(4):240–244.

[71] Lutz TA. Pancreatic amylin as a centrally acting satiating hormone. Curr Drug Targets 2005;6(2):181–189.

[72] Reda TK, Geliebter A, Pi-Sunyer FX. Amylin, food intake, and obesity. Obes Res 2002; 10(10):1087–1091.

[73] Rushing PA. Central amylin signaling and the regulation of energy homeostasis. Curr Pharm Des 2003;9(10):819–825.

[74] Chapman I, Parker B, Doran S, et al. Effect of pramlintide on satiety and food intake in obese subjects and subjects with type 2 diabetes. Diabetologia 2005;48(5):838–848.

[75] Poyner DR, Sexton PM, Marshall I, et al. International Union of Pharmacology. XXXII. The mammalian calcitonin gene-related peptides, adrenomedullin, amylin, and calcitonin receptors. Pharmacol Rev 2002;54(2):233–246.

[76] Christopoulos G, Perry KJ, Morfis M, et al. Multiple amylin receptors arise from receptor activity-modifying protein interaction with the calcitonin receptor gene product. Mol Pharmacol 1999;56(1):235–242.

[77] D'Agostino D, Cordle RA, Kullman J, Erlanson-Albertsson C, Muglia LJ, Lowe ME. Decreased postnatal survival and altered body weight regulation in procolipase-deficient mice. J Biol Chem 2002;277(9):7170–7177.

[78] Erlanson-Albertsson C, York D. Enterostatin—a peptide regulating fat intake. Obes Res 1997;5(4):360–372.

[79] Liu M, Shen L, Tso P. The role of enterostatin and apolipoprotein AIV on the control of food intake. Neuropeptides 1999;33(5):425–433.

[80] Mei J, Sorhede-Winzell M, Erlanson-Albertsson C. Plasma enterostatin: Identification and release in rats in response to a meal. Obes Res 2002;10(7):688–694.

[81] Prasad C, Imamura M, Debata C, Svec F, Sumar N, Hermon-Taylor J. Hyperenterostatinemia in premenopausal obese women. J Clin Endocrinol Metab 1999;84(3):937–941.

[82] Rossner S, Barkeling B, Erlanson-Albertsson C, Larsson P, Wahlin-Boll E. Intravenous enterostatin does not affect single meal food intake in man. Appetite 1995;24(1):37–42.

[83] Park M, Lin L, Thomas S, et al. The F1-ATPase beta-subunit is the putative enterostatin receptor. Peptides 2004;25(12):2127–2133.

[84] Nagase H, Nakajima A, Sekihara H, York DA, Bray GA. Regulation of feeding behavior, gastric emptying, and sympathetic nerve activity to interscapular brown adipose tissue by galanin and enterostatin: The involvement of vagal-central nervous system interactions. J Gastroenterol 2002;37(Suppl 14):118–127.

[85] Drucker DJ. Minireview: The glucagon-like peptides. Endocrinology 2001;142(2):521–527.

[86] DeFronzo RA, Ratner RE, Han J, Kim DD, Fineman MS, Baron AD. Effects of exenatide (exendin-4) on glycemic control and weight over 30 weeks in metformin-treated patients with type 2 diabetes. Diabetes Care 2005;28(5):1092–1100.

[87] Anastasi A, Erspamer V, Bucci M. Isolation and structure of bombesin and alytesin, 2 analogous active peptides from the skin of the European amphibians Bombina and Alytes. Experientia 1971;27(2):166–167.

[88] Gibbs J, Smith GP. The actions of bombesin-like peptides on food intake. Ann NY Acad Sci 1988;547:210–216.

[89] Muurahainen NE, Kissileff HR, Pi-Sunyer FX. Intravenous infusion of bombesin reduces food intake in humans. Am J Physiol 1993;264(2 Pt 2):R350–R354.

[90] Wada E, Way J, Lebacq-Verheyden AM, Battey JF. Neuromedin B and gastrin-releasing peptide mRNAs are differentially distributed in the rat nervous system. J Neurosci 1990; 10(9):2917–2930.

[91] Fathi Z, Corjay MH, Shapira H, et al. BRS-3: A novel bombesin receptor subtype selectively expressed in testis and lung carcinoma cells. J Biol Chem 1993;268(8):5979–5984.

[92] Hampton LL, Ladenheim EE, Akeson M, et al. Loss of bombesin-induced feeding suppression in gastrin-releasing peptide receptor-deficient mice. Proc Natl Acad Sci USA 1998;95(6):3188–3192.

[93] Ohki-Hamazaki H, Sakai Y, Kamata K, et al. Functional properties of two bombesin-like peptide receptors revealed by the analysis of mice lacking neuromedin B receptor. J Neurosci 1999;19(3):948–954.

[94] Wada E, Watase K, Yamada K, et al. Generation and characterization of mice lacking gastrin-releasing peptide receptor. Biochem Biophys Res Commun 1997;239(1):28–33.

[95] Ladenheim EE, Hampton LL, Whitney AC, White WO, Battey JF, Moran TH. Disruptions in feeding and body weight control in gastrin-releasing peptide receptor deficient mice. J Endocrinol 2002;174(2):273–281.

[96] Ohki-Hamazaki H, Watase K, Yamamoto K, et al. Mice lacking bombesin receptor subtype-3 develop metabolic defects and obesity. Nature 1997;390(6656):165–169.

[97] Dakin CL, Small CJ, Batterham RL, et al. Peripheral oxyntomodulin reduces food intake and body weight gain in rats. Endocrinology 2004;145(6):2687–2695.

[98] Cohen MA, Ellis SM, Le Roux CW, et al. Oxyntomodulin suppresses appetite and reduces food intake in humans. J Clin Endocrinol Metab 2003;88(10):4696–4701.

[99] Wynne K, Park AJ, Small CJ, et al. Subcutaneous oxyntomodulin reduces body weight in overweight and obese subjects: A double-blind, randomized, controlled trial. Diabetes 2005;54(8):2390–2395.

[100] Bado A, Levasseur S, Attoub S, et al. The stomach is a source of leptin. Nature 1998; 394(6695):790–793.

[101] Peters JH, McKay BM, Simasko SM, Ritter RC. Leptin-induced satiation mediated by abdominal vagal afferents. Am J Physiol Regul Integr Comp Physiol 2005;288(4):R879–R884.

[102] Ladenheim EE, Emond M, Moran TH. Leptin enhances feeding suppression and neural activation produced by systemically administered bombesin. Am J Physiol Regul Integr Comp Physiol 2005;289(2):R473–R477.

[103] Rajala MW, Scherer PE. Minireview: The adipocyte—at the crossroads of energy homeostasis, inflammation, and atherosclerosis. Endocrinology 2003;144(9):3765–3773.

[104] Ravussin E, Smith SR. Increased fat intake, impaired fat oxidation, and failure of fat cell proliferation result in ectopic fat storage, insulin resistance, and type 2 diabetes mellitus. Ann NY Acad Sci 2002;967:363–378.

[105] Munzberg H, Myers MG Jr. Molecular and anatomical determinants of central leptin resistance. Nat Neurosci 2005;8(5):566–570.

[106] Farooqi IS, O'Rahilly S. Monogenic human obesity syndromes. Recent Prog Horm Res 2004;59:409–424.

[107] Howard JK, Cave BJ, Oksanen LJ, Tzameli I, Bjorbaek C, Flier JS. Enhanced leptin sensitivity and attenuation of diet-induced obesity in mice with haploinsufficiency of Socs3. Nat Med 2004;10(7):734–738.

[108] Mori H, Hanada R, Hanada T, et al. Socs3 deficiency in the brain elevates leptin sensitivity and confers resistance to diet-induced obesity. Nat Med 2004;10(7):739–743.

[109] Berthoud HR. Multiple neural systems controlling food intake and body weight. Neurosci Biobehav Rev 2002;26(4):393–428.

[110] Schwartz MW, Woods SC, Porte D Jr, Seeley RJ, Baskin DG. Central nervous system control of food intake. Nature 2000;404(6778):661–671.

[111] Seeley RJ, Woods SC. Monitoring of stored and available fuel by the CNS: Implications for obesity. Nat Rev Neurosci 2003;4(11):901–909.

[112] Kennedy GC. The role of depot fat in the hypothalamic control of food intake in the rat. Proc R Soc Lond B Biol Sci 1953;140(901):578–596.

[113] Coleman DL. Effects of parabiosis of obese with diabetes and normal mice. Diabetologia 1973;9(4):294–298.

[114] Zhang Y, Proenca R, Maffei M, Barone M, Leopold L, Friedman JM. Positional cloning of the mouse obese gene and its human homologue. Nature 1994;372(6505):425–432.

[115] Campfield LA, Smith FJ, Guisez Y, Devos R, Burn P. Recombinant mouse OB protein: Evidence for a peripheral signal linking adiposity and central neural networks. Science 1995;269(5223):546–549.

[116] Halaas JL, Boozer C, Blair-West J, Fidahusein N, Denton DA, Friedman JM. Physiological response to long-term peripheral and central leptin infusion in lean and obese mice. Proc Natl Acad Sci USA 1997;94(16):8878–8883.

[117] Halaas JL, Gajiwala KS, Maffei M, et al. Weight-reducing effects of the plasma protein encoded by the obese gene. Science 1995;269(5223):543–546.

[118] Pelleymounter MA, Cullen MJ, Baker MB, et al. Effects of the obese gene product on body weight regulation in ob/ob mice. Science 1995;269(5223):540–543.

[119] Schwartz MW, Seeley RJ, Campfield LA, Burn P, Baskin DG. Identification of targets of leptin action in rat hypothalamus. J Clin Invest 1996;98(5):1101–1106.

[120] Schwartz MW, Seeley RJ, Woods SC, et al. Leptin increases hypothalamic pro-opiomelanocortin mRNA expression in the rostral arcuate nucleus. Diabetes 1997; 46(12):2119–2123.

[121] Seeley RJ, van Dijk G, Campfield LA, et al. Intraventricular leptin reduces food intake and body weight of lean rats but not obese Zucker rats. Horm Metab Res 1996;28(12): 664–668.

[122] Tartaglia LA, Dembski M, Weng X, et al. Identification and expression cloning of a leptin receptor, OB-R. Cell 1995;83(7):1263–1271.

[123] Woods SC, Chavez M, Park CR, et al. The evaluation of insulin as a metabolic signal influencing behavior via the brain. Neurosci Biobehav Rev 1996;20(1):139–144.

[124] Polonsky KS, Given BD, Hirsch L, et al. Quantitative study of insulin secretion and clearance in normal and obese subjects. J Clin Invest 1988;81(2):435–441.

[125] Woods SC, Lotter EC, McKay LD, Porte D Jr. Chronic intracerebroventricular infusion of insulin reduces food intake and body weight of baboons. Nature 1979;282(5738):503–505.

[126] Bruning JC, Gautam D, Burks DJ, et al. Role of brain insulin receptor in control of body weight and reproduction. Science 2000;289(5487):2122–2125.

[127] Obici S, Feng Z, Karkanias G, Baskin DG, Rossetti L. Decreasing hypothalamic insulin receptors causes hyperphagia and insulin resistance in rats. Nat Neurosci 2002;5(6):566–572.

[128] Cone RD, Lu D, Koppula S, et al. The melanocortin receptors: Agonists, antagonists, and the hormonal control of pigmentation. Recent Prog Horm Res 1996;51:287–317.

[129] De Souza CT, Araujo EP, Bordin S, et al. Consumption of a fat-rich diet activates a pro-inflammatory response and induces insulin resistance in the hypothalamus. Endocrinology 2005.

[130] Levin BE, Dunn-Meynell AA. Reduced central leptin sensitivity in rats with diet-induced obesity. Am J Physiol Regul Integr Comp Physiol 2002;283(4):R941–R948.

[131] Levin BE, Dunn-Meynell AA, Banks WA. Obesity-prone rats have normal blood–brain barrier transport but defective central leptin signaling before obesity onset. Am J Physiol Regul Integr Comp Physiol 2004;286(1):R143–150.

[132] Zabolotny JM, Bence-Hanulec KK, Stricker-Krongrad A, et al. PTP1B regulates leptin signal transduction in vivo. Dev Cell 2002;2(4):489–495.

[133] Cowley MA, Smith RG, Diano S, et al. The distribution and mechanism of action of ghrelin in the CNS demonstrates a novel hypothalamic circuit regulating energy homeostasis. Neuron 2003;37(4):649–661.

[134] Heisler LK, Cowley MA, Tecott LH, et al. Activation of central melanocortin pathways by fenfluramine. Science 2002;297(5581):609–611.

[135] Cowley MA, Smart JL, Rubinstein M, et al. Leptin activates anorexigenic POMC neurons through a neural network in the arcuate nucleus. Nature 2001;411(6836):480–484.

[136] Ibrahim N, Bosch MA, Smart JL, et al. Hypothalamic proopiomelanocortin neurons are glucose responsive and express K(ATP) channels. Endocrinology 2003;144(4):1331–1340.

[137] Yaswen L, Diehl N, Brennan MB, Hochgeschwender U. Obesity in the mouse model of pro-opiomelanocortin deficiency responds to peripheral melanocortin. Nat Med 1999;5(9):1066–1070.

[138] Krude H, Biebermann H, Schnabel D, et al. Obesity due to proopiomelanocortin deficiency: Three new cases and treatment trials with thyroid hormone and ACTH4-10. J Clin Endocrinol Metab 2003;88(10):4633–4640.

[139] Krude H, Biebermann H, Luck W, Horn R, Brabant G, Gruters A. Severe early-onset obesity, adrenal insufficiency and red hair pigmentation caused by POMC mutations in humans. Nat Genet 1998;19(2):155–157.

[140] Fan W, Ellacott KL, Halatchev IG, Takahashi K, Yu P, Cone RD. Cholecystokinin-mediated suppression of feeding involves the brainstem melanocortin system. Nat Neurosci 2004.

[141] Williams DL, Kaplan JM, Grill HJ. The role of the dorsal vagal complex and the vagus nerve in feeding effects of melanocortin-3/4 receptor stimulation. Endocrinology 2000;141(4):1332–1337.

[142] Grill HJ, Ginsberg AB, Seeley RJ, Kaplan JM. Brainstem application of melanocortin receptor ligands produces long-lasting effects on feeding and body weight. J Neurosci 1998;18(23):10128–10135.

[143] Takahashi KA, Cone RD. Fasting induces a large, leptin-dependent increase in the intrinsic action potential frequency of orexigenic arcuate nucleus neuropeptide Y/Agouti-related protein neurons. Endocrinology 2005;146(3):1043–1047.

[144] Segal-Lieberman G, Bradley RL, Kokkotou E, et al. Melanin-concentrating hormone is a critical mediator of the leptin-deficient phenotype. Proc Natl Acad Sci USA 2003; 100(17):10085–10090.

[145] Ludwig DS, Tritos NA, Mastaitis JW, et al. Melanin-concentrating hormone overexpression in transgenic mice leads to obesity and insulin resistance. J Clin Invest 2001;107(3): 379–386.

[146] Ludwig DS, Mountjoy KG, Tatro JB, et al. Melanin-concentrating hormone: A functional melanocortin antagonist in the hypothalamus. Am J Physiol 1998;274(4 Pt 1):E627–E633.

[147] Qu D, Ludwig DS, Gammeltoft S, et al. A role for melanin-concentrating hormone in the central regulation of feeding behaviour. Nature 1996;380(6571):243–247.

[148] Rossi M, Choi SJ, O'Shea D, Miyoshi T, Ghatei MA, Bloom SR. Melanin-concentrating hormone acutely stimulates feeding, but chronic administration has no effect on body weight. Endocrinology 1997;138(1):351–355.

[149] Sakurai T, Amemiya A, Ishii M, et al. Orexins and orexin receptors: A family of hypothalamic neuropeptides and G protein-coupled receptors that regulate feeding behavior. Cell 1998;92(4):573–585.

Chapter 2

Body Composition Assessment of Obesity

Wm. Cameron Chumlea

*Departments of Community Health and Pediatrics, Lifespan Health Research Center,
Wright State University School of Medicine, Dayton, OH 45420, USA*

1.   INTRODUCTION

Obesity is an international health problem for children, adults, and the elderly [1, 2] that can lead to the development of type 2 diabetes, enhance risk factors for cardiovascular and related diseases, and is associated with increased cancer risk and renal failure. Childhood obesity foreshadows its persistence into and through adulthood [3, 4], and obesity is becoming a common problem among the elderly [5–7]. Obesity is generally displayed as excess adipose tissue and a high body weight, but in some elderly persons and others with limited mobility it takes the form of sarcopenic obesity, in which a preferential loss of muscle tissue increases the percentage of body fat [8]. Based on the body mass index (BMI), obesity has a current prevalence of 20% to 30% for non-Hispanic white, non-Hispanic black, and Mexican-American men; 25% to 40% for non-Hispanic white and Mexican-American women; and as high as 46% to 53% for non-Hispanic black women [9]. A similar prevalence exists for portions of the adult and pediatric populations of Europe, and among urban areas of Mexico, the Middle East, India, and China [10–13]. This obesity pandemic is becoming a greater health problem than under-nutrition [14–16].

Current publications indicate that this high prevalence of obesity is a recent phenomenon [9, 17–19]. However, in the 1960s, Cheek and colleagues noted that they were spurred on in their development of new body composition techniques as a result of concern for the high prevalence of obesity among children at that time [20]. Almost 35 years later, there is still a continued need for improved body composition technology applicable to monitoring and treating obese children and adults. Numerous methods and equipment are available to assess fatness and other components of body composition [21, 22]. This chapter discusses the status of those methods applicable for assessing body fatness among obese individuals in clinical and epidemiological settings.

2.   OVERVIEW OF BODY COMPOSITION METHODS

Detailed aspects of body composition methodology, underlying theories and general applications, equipment, and analytical techniques are found in several excellent texts [21–23]. Those interested in specific body composition assessment methods should first consult these references. Body composition methodology is based on assumptions regarding the density of body tissues, concentrations of water and electrolytes, and biological interrelationships between body components and body tissues and their distributions among normal weight individuals. Similar assumptions do not exist for obese persons, whose metabolic and hormonal problems together with accompanying comorbid conditions alter assumptions and interrelationships underlying the validity of body composition methods in normal weight individuals [24]. In addition, the application of body composition technology is limited among most obese adults and many older obese children because their bodies are too large for the available equipment. As a result, epidemiological and national obesity prevalence data are not completely based on actual measures of body fatness because of the difficulty of collecting such data during health surveys from sufficient numbers of obese individuals. It is also difficult to monitor and treat obesity without an easily acceptable assessment method or index and a reference population.

2.1.   Anthropometry

Anthropometric measurements describe body mass, size, shape, and level of fatness. Body size changes with weight gain, which alters the associative power among anthropometric measures and indices. Standardized anthropometric techniques are necessary for comparisons between clinical and research studies, and video and text media describing these techniques are available [25–27]. Those interested in using anthropometric equipment and methods should first consult these several resources.

2.2.   Weight and Stature

Weight is the obvious measure of obesity. Various scales are available for measuring weight, but these must be calibrated regularly. Persons with high body weights tend to have high amounts of body fat although this is not always true among the elderly with sarcopenic obesity, in whom stable or even low body weights occur with increased percent body fatness. Changes in weight reflect corresponding changes in body water, fat, and lean tissue. However, weight is not always the best indicator of obesity because weight is related to stature, i.e., tall people are, on average, heavier than short people. Weight also increases with age in children (because of growth) and in adults (because of fatness). To overcome this lack of specificity, weight is divided by stature squared to create the body mass index or BMI as a descriptive index of body habitus encompassing both the lean and the obese [1].

Stature is also easily measured with a variety of wall-mounted equipment that also needs to be calibrated regularly. In addition, methods are available for predicting stature when it cannot be measured for the handicapped or mobility impaired [28, 29].

2.3.   Body Mass Index

The advantage of BMI as an index of obesity is the availability of extensive national reference data worldwide, its established relationships with levels of body fatness, morbidity, and mortality [1], and it is highly predictive of future risk. High BMI percentile levels based on percentiles on the CDC BMI growth charts and changes in parameters of BMI curves for children are linked to significant levels of risk for adult obesity at corresponding high percentile levels [4, 30]. A boy with a BMI at the 85th percentile at age 12 has a risk of 20% of having a BMI at that same level at 35 years of age (Figure 1). For a girl with

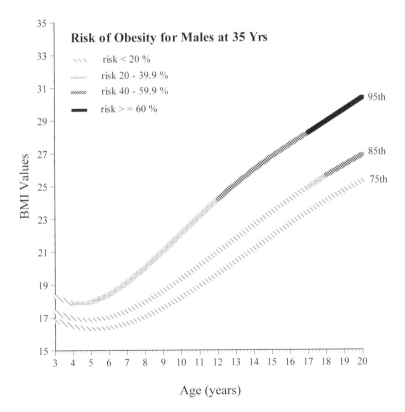

Figure 1. Risk of obesity in boys at age 35 years based on BMI percentiles in childhood [4].

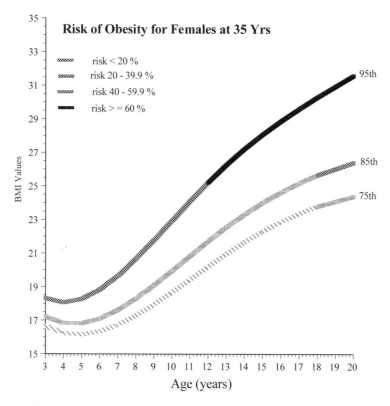

Figure 2. Risk of obesity in girls at age 35 years based on BMI percentiles in childhood [4].

a BMI at the 95th percentile, the corresponding adult risk is greater than 60% (Figure 2). The relationship of obesity as indexed by BMI with mortality has been revised for the US adult population [19]. In the elderly, sarcopenia causes a person of normal weight and BMI to become obese owing to an increased high percentage of body fat. BMI is also useful in monitoring the treatment of obesity, but a weight change of about 3.5 kg is needed to produce a unit change in BMI.

2.4.   Abdominal Circumference

Obesity is frequently associated with increased amounts of intraabdominal fat. A central fat pattern is associated with the deposition of intraabdominal adipose tissue, but subcutaneous abdominal adipose tissue is involved also. The ratio of abdominal circumference (sometime incorrectly referred to as "waist" circumference) to the hip circumference is an early index describing adipose tissue distribution or fat patterning [31, 32]. Ratios greater than 0.85 represent a masculine or central distribution of fat. Most men with a ratio greater than 1.0 and women with a ratio greater than 0.85 are at increased risk

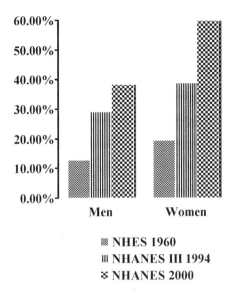

Men **Women**

✺ NHES 1960
Ⅲ NHANES III 1994
✺ NHANES 2000

Figure 3. Change in prevalence of adult from 1960 to 2000. (Data from the National Center for Health Statistics.)

for cardiovascular disease, diabetes, and cancers [33, 34]. However, this ratio is an imperfect indicator of intraabdominal adipose tissue and the use of the abdominal circumference alone provides much the same information [35, 36]. Persons in the upper percentiles for abdominal circumference are considered obese and at increased risk for morbidity, specifically type 2 diabetes and the metabolic syndrome, and mortality [37, 38]. The increased prevalence in abdominal circumference in the general population can be seen in Figure 3 [39]. Circumferences of other body segments such as the arm and leg are possible [25] but there are little available reference data except for arm circumference. The calculation of fat and muscle areas of the arm is not accurate or valid in the obese.

Abdominal thickness is associated with levels of abdominal obesity because a large abdomen should be a thick abdomen [12]. However, there is some inconsistency in standardizing this measurement; should it be taken standing or recumbent, from the small of the back, or from the top of a table when recumbent? There are little available reference data.

2.5. Skinfolds

Skinfolds measure subcutaneous fat thickness, but they are not very useful for the obese. Most skinfold calipers have an upper measurement limit of 45 to 55 mm, which restricts their use to the "moderately" obese or thinner. A few skinfold calipers take larger measurements, but this is not a significant improvement because of the difficulty of grasping and holding a large skinfold, plus the additional problem of reading the caliper dials, all of which create additional errors. The majority of the available national reference data is for triceps and subscapular skinfolds, but the triceps is a sex-specific site and can reflect changes in the underlying triceps muscle rather than an actual change in body fatness. Skinfolds are useful in monitoring changes in fatness in children because of their small body size, and the majority of fat is subcutaneous even in obese children [40, 41]. The statistical relationships of skinfolds with percent and total body fat are often not as strong as that of BMI in both children and adults [42]. Also, we do not know the real upper distribution of subcutaneous fat measurements because most obese children and adults have not had their skinfolds measured.

2.6. Bioelectric Impedance Analysis

Bioelectrical impedance analyzers (BIAs) do not measure any biological quantity or describe any biophysical model related to obesity. The impedance index, stature squared divided by resistance (S^2/R) at a frequency, most often 50 kHz, is an independent variable in regression equations to predict body composition [43–45]. Bioelectrical impedance analyzers use such equations to describe statistical associations based on biological relationships for a specific population, and as such the equations are useful only for subjects that closely match the reference population in body size and shape. BIA has been applied to overweight or obese samples [46, 47] in a few studies; thus the available BIA prediction equations are not applicable to overweight or obese children or adults. The ability of BIA to predict fatness in the obese is difficult because they have a greater proportion of body mass and body water accounted for by the trunk, the hydration of fat-free mass (FFM) is lower in the obese, and the ratio of extracellular water (ECW) to intracellular water (ICW) is increased in the obese.

BIA validity and its estimates of body composition are significant issues for normal weight individuals. BIA is useful in describing mean body composition for groups of individuals, but large errors for an individual limit its clinical application, especially among the obese. The large predictive errors with BIA render it insensitive to small improvements in response to treatment. Commercial BIA analyzers contain all of the problems associated with this methodology.

Recent BIA prediction equations have been published [48] along with body composition mean estimates for non-Hispanic whites, non-Hispanic blacks, and Mexican-American males and females from 12 to 90 years of age [49]. These equations are not recommended for obese individuals or groups.

2.7.   Body Density

Hydrodensitometry estimates body composition using measures of body weight, body volume, and residual lung volume. Historically, body density was converted to the percentage of body weight as fat using the two-compartment models of Siri [50] or Brozek and co-workers [51], but more recently, a multicompartment model is used to calculate body fatness [52]. Body density is plagued with the problem of subject performance because it is difficult if not impossible for an obese adult or child to submerge. Weight belts reduce bouncy, but not all aspects of performance. Air displacement devices [53–55] are limited to adults who are "moderately" obese at best. Regardless, most overweight and obese persons are reluctant to put on a bathing suit and participate in body density measurements.

2.8.   Total Body Water

Total body water (TBW) is easy to measure because it does not require undressing or any real physical participation, but this method is limited in the obese. The major assumption is that FFM is estimated from TBW based on an assumed average proportion of TBW in FFM of 73%, but this proportion ranges from 67% to 80% [49, 50]. In addition, about 15% to 30% of TBW is present in adipose tissue as extracellular fluid, and this proportion increases with the degree of adiposity. These proportions tend to be higher in women than in men, higher in the obese, and produce underestimates of FFM and overestimates of fatness. Variation in the distribution of TBW as a result of disease associated with obesity, such as diabetes and renal failure, affects estimates of FFM and TBF further.

TBW is a potentially useful method applicable to the obese but there are details that need to be considered. The several analytical chemical methods used to quantify the concentration of TBW (and extracellular fluid) have errors of almost a liter. Equilibration times for isotope dilution in relation to levels of body fatness are unknown, because, theoretically, it might (and should) take longer for the dilution dose to equilibrate in an obese person as compared with a normal weight individual. Also, a measure of extracellular space is necessary to correct the amount of FFM in an obese person. Such data could also be very useful in the treatment of end-stage renal disease.

2.9.   Dual-energy x-ray Absorptiometry

Dual energy x-ray absorptiometry (DXA) is the most popular method for quantifying fat, lean, and bone tissues. DXA is fast and user friendly for the subject and the operator, but the machines require regular maintenance and calibration. DXA has inherent assumptions regarding levels of hydration, potassium content, or tissue density in the estimation of fat and lean tissue, and these assumptions vary by manufacturer [56, 57]. DXA estimates of body composition are also affected by differences among manufacturers in the technology, models and software employed, methodological problems, and intra- and intermachine differences [56, 58]. There are physical limitations of body weight, length, thickness and width, and the type of DXA machine, i.e., pencil or fan beam. Most obese adults and many children are often too wide, too thick, and too heavy to receive a whole-body DXA scan although some innovative adaptations have been reported [59]. Pediatric software is available for DXA and should be used according to the manufacturer's recommendations. DXA is a convenient method for measuring body composition in much of the population, and it is currently included in the ongoing National Health and Nutrition Examination Survey (NHANES).

The other imaging systems, such as computed tomography (CT) and magnetic resonance imaging (MRI) are not practical for obese individuals. CT is able to accommodate large body sizes but has high radiation exposures and as such is inappropriate for whole-body assessments, but it has been used to measure intraabdominal fat. MRI is not able to accommodate large body sizes in many instances but can be used for whole body assessments. Both these methods require additional time and software to provide whole-body quantities of fat and lean tissue.

3.   ETHNIC DIFFERENCES IN BODY COMPOSITION

Ethnic differences in body composition and obesity are affected by differences in and associations with socioeconomic status, diet, utilization of health care, and levels of genetic admixture. These associations and effects in some ethnic groups may not be clear because the health status of minority groups is frequently affected by socioeconomic factors. African-American girls are fatter at earlier ages than white girls; they also have an earlier sexual maturation that has been linked to an early onset of obesity [60–64]. At the extremes of body fatness, there are more African-American women than non-Hispanic white women. There are limited body composition data for large samples of African, Hispanic, or Asian Americans and especially for the obese among these groups [34, 65–67]. The exception is that reasonably extensive anthropometric data are available for African, Hispanic and non-Hispanic white Americans from the National Center for Health Statistics in the NHANES.

4.   AVAILABLE REFERENCE DATA

The principal source of national reference data for obesity in the United States comes from the National Center for Health Statistics, Centers for Disease Control and Prevention in the form of the NHANES (http://www.cdc.gov/

nchs/nhanes.htm). The target populations for these surveys consist of all non-institutionalized civilian residents of the continental United States including Alaska, and data from these NCHS surveys presents a picture of the health status of the US population rather than a desired health goal. The current NHANES is the first national survey to include DXA measures of body composition.

The anthropometric data in the NHANES were selected to monitor the health and nutritional status of infants, children, adults, and the elderly. These body measurements follow techniques for corresponding measurements in the *Anthropometric Standardization Reference Manual* [25] and are similar across other NCHS surveys. Mean values and distribution statistics for stature; weight; and selected body circumferences, breadths, and skinfold thicknesses of children and adults are available from all these national health surveys.

5.   RECOMMENDATIONS

A body composition assessment in an obese child or adult depends on several conditions. For most children until they are postpuberty, DXA is the method of choice. This provides an estimate of the amount of fat, lean, and bony tissues, all of which should be monitored along with any change in weight during treatment. For older obese children and adults, the easiest measure to monitor is body weight. This can be combined with a measure of abdominal circumference and BMI to track progress. As fat tissue is reduced and weight is lost, it is important that there is not a greater loss of lean tissue, which can have significant health risks. Other body composition methods that would only be useful in adults as a measure of lean tissue are possibly from DXA or TBW. For overweight and moderately obese individuals, with a managed regimen of diet and exercise, weight will be lost, but some will experience a weight gain as lean tissue is added [68].

Of all the methods available to monitor obesity, BMI is currently the easiest and most informative index. Numerous sets of reference data are available and it is possible to determine, monitor, and track a change in BMI percentiles for children and adults. This, along with changes in weight, will provide a good, clinical estimate of the amount of change that is occurring with treatment for an obese individual.

6.   CONCLUSION

It does not appear that the present epidemic of overweight and obesity will attenuate in the near future. Our ability to diagnosis, monitor, and treat obesity is limited, in part, by our limited ability to assess body fatness easily. There is no universally accepted method of measuring body fatness or for quantifying obesity clearly, and current methods are hampered with problems of nonuniversal assumptions, and limited by application of methodology for obese individuals.

The WHO [10] has made several recommendations concerning obesity. One of these addresses the need for the development and validation of new and existing techniques. In this chapter, we have briefly reviewed many of the existing techniques and their limitations when applied to obese persons. In support of this WHO recommendation, it is clear that existing techniques are not applicable to many obese who are in great need of this technology. This limitation also affects our ability to determine the real prevalence of obesity because the current methods are not applicable to large epidemiological and clinical studies. Obviously much work is yet to be done.

ACKNOWLEDGMENTS

This work was supported by Grants HD-12252 and HL-72838 from the National Institute of Health, Bethesda, MD.

REFERENCES

[1] WHO. Physical Status: The Use and Interpretation of Anthropometry. Geneva: WHO, 1995.

[2] Popkin BM, Doak CM. The obesity epidemic is a worldwide phenomenon. Nutr Rev 1998;56:106–114.

[3] Guo S, Chumlea WC, Roche AF, et al. The predictive value of childhood body mass index values for overweight at age 35 years. Am J Clin Nutr 1994;59:810–819.

[4] Sun SS, Wu W, Chumlea WC, et al. Predicting overweight and obesity in adulthood from body mass index values in childhood and adolescence. Am J Clin Nutr 2002;76:653–658.

[5] Seim HC, Holtmeier KB. Treatment of obesity in the elderly. Am Fam Physician 1993; 47:1183–1189.

[6] Salom IL. Weight control and nutrition: Knowing when to intervene. Geriatrics 1997;33–34.

[7] Arterburn DE, Crane PK, Sullivan SD. The coming epidemic of obesity in elderly Americans. J Am Geriatr Soc 2004;52:1907–1912.

[8] Heber D, Ingles S, Ashley JM, et al. Clinical detection of sarcopenic obesity by bioelectrical impedance analysis. Am J Clin Nutr 1996;64:472S–477S.

[9] Flegal KM, Carroll MD, Ogden CL, et al. Prevalence and trends in obesity among US adults, 1999–2000. JAMA 2002;288:1723–1727.

[10] WHO. Obesity: Preventing and Managing the Global Epidemic. World Health Organization Programme of Nutrition. Geneva: 1998.

[11] Lissau I, Overpeck MD, Ruan WJ, et al. Body mass index and overweight in adolescents in 13 European countries, Israel, and the United States. Arch Pediatr Adolesc Med 2004;158:27–33.

[12] Valsamakis G, Chetty R, Anwar A, et al. Association of simple anthropometric measures of obesity with visceral fat and the metabolic syndrome in male Caucasian and Indo-Asian subjects. Diabet Med 2004;21:1339–1345.

[13] Velazquez-Alva J, Irigoyen M, Zepeda M, et al. Anthropmetric measurements of a sixty-year and older Mexican urban study. J Nutr Health Aging 2004;8:350–354.

[14] Ismail MN. Prevalence of obesity and chronic energy deficiency (CED) in adult Malaysians. Malaysian J Nutr 1995;1:1–10.

[15] Deitel M. Overweight and obesity worldwide now estimated to involve 1.7 billion people. Obes Surg 2003;13:329–330.

[16] James PT. Obesity: The worldwide epidemic. Clin Dermatol 2004;22:276–280.

[17] Kuczmarski R, Flegal K, Campbell S, et al. Increasing prevalence of overweight among US adults. JAMA 1994;272:205–211.

[18] Troiano RP, Flegal KM, Kuczmarski RJ, et al. Overweight prevalence and trends for children and adolescents: The National Health and Nutrition Examination Surveys, 1963 to 1991. Arch Pediatr Adolesc Med 1995;149:1085–1091.

[19] Flegal KM, Graubard BI, Williamson DF, et al. Excess deaths associated with underweight, overweight, and obesity. JAMA 2005;293:1861–1867.

[20] Mellits ED, Cheek DB. The assessment of body water and fatness from infancy to adulthood. Monogr Soc Res Child Dev 1970;35:12–26.

[21] Roche AF, Heymsfield SB, Lohman TG. Human Body Composition. Champaign, IL: Human Kinetics, 1996.

[22] Heymsfield SB, Lohman T, Wang Z, et al. Human Body Composition. Champaign, IL: Human Kinetics, 2005.

[23] Lohman TG. Advances in Body Composition Assessment. Champaign, IL: Human Kinetics, 1992.

[24] Moore FD. The body cell mass and its supporting environment. In: Body Composition in Health and Disease. Philadelphia–London: WB Saunders, 1963.

[25] Lohman T, Martorell R, Roche AF. Anthropometric Standardization Reference Manual. Champaign, IL: Human Kinetics, 1988.

[26] de Onis M, Onyango AW, Van den Broeck J, et al. Measurement and standardization protocols for anthropometry used in the construction of a new international growth reference. Food Nutr Bull 2004;25:S27–S36.

[27] Kuczmarski RJ, Chumlea WC. Third National Health and Nutrition Examination Survey (NHANESIII) Antropometric Procedures Video. J Gerontol 1997;37.

[28] Chumlea WC, Guo SS, Steinbaugh ML. The prediction of stature from knee height for black and white adults and children, with application to the mobility-impaired. J Am Diet Assoc 1994;94:1385–1388, 1391.

[29] Chumlea WC, Guo SS, Wholihan K, et al. Stature prediction equations for elderly non-Hispanic white, non-Hispanic black, and Mexican American persons: From NHANES III (1988-94). J Am Diet Assoc 1998;98:137–142.

[30] Guo SS, Huang C, Maynard LM, et al. BMI during childhood, adolescence, and young adulthood in relation to adult overweight and adiposity: The Fels longitudinal study. Int J Obes Relat Metab Disord 2000;24:1628–1635.

[31] Chumlea WC, Roche AF, Webb P. Body size, subcutaneous fatness and total body fat in older adults. Int J Obes Relat Metab Disord 1984;8:311–317.

[32] Chumlea WC, Baumgartner RN, Garry PJ, et al. Fat distribution and blood lipids in a sample of healthy elderly people. Int J Obes 1992;16:125–133.

[33] Seidell JC, Oosterlee A, Thijssen MAO, et al. Assessment of intra-abdominal and subcutaneous abdominal fat: Relation between anthropometry and computed tomography. Am J Clin Nutr 1987;45:7–13.

[34] Fujimoto WY, Newellmorris LL, Grote M, et al. Visceral fat obesity and morbidity—NIDDM and atherogenic risk in Japanese American men and women. Int J Obes 1991;15:41–44.

[35] Pouliot M, Despres J, Lemieux S, et al. Waist circumference and abdominal sagittal diameter—best simple anthropometric indexes of abdominal visceral adipose tissue accumulation and related cardiovascular risk in men and women. Am J Cardiol 1994;73:460–468.

[36] Despres J, Prudhomme D, Pouliot M, et al. Estimation of deep abdominal adipose-tissue accumulation from simple anthropometric measurements in men. Am J Clin Nutr 1991;54:471–477.

[37] Bray. Obesity. In: Present Knowledge in Nutrition, 7th edn. Washington, DC: International Life Sciences Institute, 1994;19–32.

[38] Nicklas BJ, Penninx BW, Cesari M, et al. Association of visceral adipose tissue with incident myocardial infarction in older men and women: The health, aging and body composition study. Am J Epidemiol 2004;160:741–749.

[39] Okosun IS, Chandra KM, Boev A, et al. Abdominal adiposity in U.S. adults: Prevalence and trends, 1960–2000. Prev Med 2004;39:197–206.

[40] Malina RM, Bouchard C. Subcutaneous fat distribution during growth. In: Fat Distribution During Growth and Later Health Outcomes. New York: Wiley–Liss, 1988;68.

[41] Brambilla P, Manzoni P, Sironi S. Peripheral and abdominal adiposity in childhood obesity. Int J Obes Relat Metab Disord 1994;18:795–800.

[42] Roche AF, Siervogel RM, Chumlea WC, et al. Grading of body fatness from limited anthropometric data. Am J Clin Nutr 1981;34:2831–2838.

[43] Chumlea WC, Guo S. Bioelectrical impedance and body composition: Present status and future direction—reply. Nutr Rev 1994;52:323–325.

[44] Chumlea WC, Sun SS. Bioelectrical impedance analysis. In: Human Body Composition. Champaign, IL: Human Kinetics, 2005.

[45] Sun SS, Chumlea WC. Statistical methods for the development and testing of body composition prediction equations. In: Human Body Composition. Champaign, IL: Human Kinetics, 2005.

[46] Gray DS, Bray GA, Gemayel N, et al. Effect of obesity on bioelectrical impedance. Am J Clin Nutr 1989;2:255–260.

[47] Kushner R, Kunigk A, Alspaugh M, et al. Validation of bioelectrical impedance analysis as a measurement of change in body composition in obesity. Am J Clin Nutr 1990;52:219–223.

[48] Sun SS, Chumlea WC, Heymsfield SB, et al. Development of bioelectrical impedance analysis prediction equations for body composition with the use of a multicomponent model for use in epidemiological surveys. Am J Clin Nutr 2003;77:331–340.

[49] Chumlea WC, Guo SS, Kuczmarski RJ, et al. Body composition estimates from NHANES III bioelectrical impedance data. Int J Obes Relat Metab Disord 2002;1596–1609.

[50] Siri W. Body composition from fluid spaces and density analysis of methods. In: Techniques for Measuring Body Composition. Washington, DC: National Academy Press, 1961;223–244.

[51] Brozek J, Grande F, Anderson J, et al. Densitometric analysis of body composition: Revision of some quantitative assumptions. Ann NY Acad Sci 1963;110:113–140.

[52] Guo SS, Chumlea WC, Roche AF, et al. Age- and maturity-related changes in body composition during adolescence into adulthood: The Fels longitudinal study. Int J Obes Relat Metab Disord 1997;21:1167–1175.

[53] Dempster P, Aitkens S. A new air displacement method for the determination of body composition. Med Sci. Sports Exerc 1995;27:1692–1697.

[54] McCrory MA, Gomez TD, Bernauer EM, et al. Evaluation of a new air displacement plethysmograph for measuring human body composition. Med Sci Sports Exerc 1995;27:1686–1691.

[55] Demerath EW, Guo SS, Chumlea WC, et al. Comparison of percent body fat estimates using air displacement plethysmography and hydrodensitometry in adults and children. Int J Obes Relat Metab Disord 2002;26:389–397.

[56] Roubenoff R, Kehayias J, Dawsonhughes B, et al. Use of dual-energy x-ray absorptiometry in body-composition studies—not yet a gold standard. Am J Clin Nutr 1993;58:589–591.

[57] Kohrt WM. Body composition by DXA: Tried and true? Med Sci Sports Exerc 1995; 27:1349–1353.

[58] Guo SS, Wisemandle W, Tyleshevski FE, et al. Inter-machine and inter-method differences in body composition measures from dual energy x-ray absorptiometry. J Nutr Health Aging 1997;1:29–38.

[59] Tataranni PA, Ravussin E. Use of dual-energy X-ray absorptiometry in obese individuals. Am J Clin Nutr 1995;62:730–734.

[60] Morrison JA, Khoury RR, Chumlea WC, et al. Body composition measures from underwater weighing and dual energy x-ray absorptiometry in black and white girls: A comparative study. Am J Hum Biol 1994;6:481–490.

[61] Herman-Giddens HE, Slora EJ, Hasemeier CM, et al. The prevalence of secondary sexual characteristics in young girls seen in office practice. Am J Dis Child 1993;147:455.

[62] Herman-Giddens ME, Slora EJ, Wasserman RC, et al. Secondary sexual characteristics and menses in young girls seen in office practice. Pediatrics 1997;99:505–512.

[63] Chumlea WC, Schubert CM, Roche AF, et al. Age at menarche and racial comparisons in U.S. girls. Pediatrics 2003;111:110–113.

[64] Sun SS, Schubert CM, Chumlea WC, et al. National estimates of the timing of sexual maturation and racial differences among U.S. children. Pediatrics 2002;110:911–919.

[65] Sparling PB, Millardstafford M, Rosskopf LB, et al. Body composition by bioelectric impedance and densitometry in black women. Am J Hum Biol 1993;5:111–117.

[66] Zillikens MC, Conway JM. Estimation of total body water by bioelectrical impedance analysis in Blacks. Am J Hum Biol 1991;3:25–32.

[67] Fernandez JR, Heo M, Heymsfield SB, et al. Is percentage body fat differentially related to body mass index in Hispanic Americans, African Americans, and European Americans? Am J Clin Nutr 2003;77:71–75.

[68] Friedl KE, Westphal KA, Marchitelli LJ, et al. Evaluation of anthropometric equations to assess body composition changes in young women. Am J Clin Nutr 2001;73:268–275.

Chapter 3

Prevalence of Obesity and the Metabolic Syndrome*

Ali H. Mokdad and Earl S. Ford

Centers for Desease Control and Prevention, 4770 Buford Highway, Atlanta, GA 30341, USA

1. OVERWEIGHT AND OBESITY

Overweight and obesity are terms used to describe excess body fatness, which increases people's risk for morbidity, impaired quality of life, and premature death. They are major clinical and public health problems in the United States [1, 2] and most of the industrialized world [3]. Although precise measurement of a person's amount of body fat requires relatively expensive and sophisticated equipment, practical measures of overweight and obesity exist. One such measure, the body mass index (BMI), is calculated by dividing a person's weight in kilograms by the square of the person's height in meters. Alternatively, BMI can be calculated by multiplying a person's weight in pounds by 703 and dividing by the square of the person's height in inches. Most of the surveillance on overweight and obesity is based on BMI because of the simplicity of the measure.

According to the National Institutes of Health, adults with a BMI of 30 or above are considered obese, and those with a BMI from 25 to 29.9 are considered overweight [4]. Other practical measures of overweight and obesity among adults include abdominal girth and the ratio of waist to hip circumferences. The grid in Figure 1 shows BMI levels for adults of different heights and weights. Although no specific partition values for overweight and obesity have been established for children and adolescents, they are considered overweight if their BMI is at or above the 95th percentile for their sex and age according to the revised Centers for Disease Control and Prevention (CDC) growth charts shown in Figures 2 and 3 [5].

For both youth and adults, the value of BMI in determining public health burden of excess weight is limited in several ways [6]. The BMI by itself does not reflect the distribution of excess fat in the body. Yet another and more serious limitation is that it does not account for differences in body structure;

---

*The findings and conclusions in this report are those of the authors and do not represent the views of the Centers for Disease Control and Prevention.

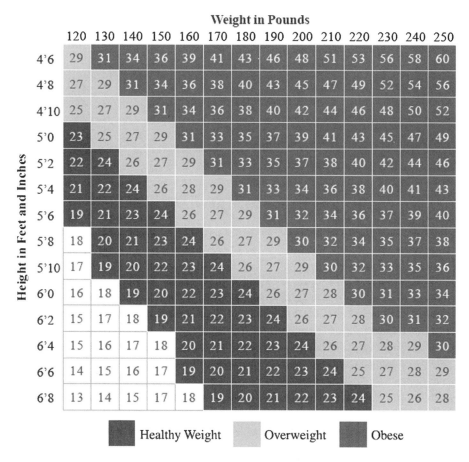

Figure 1. Body mass index in adults: the spectrum of body weights that characterize healthy weight, overweight, and obesity for different levels of body height in adults (from [6].)

a well conditioned athlete might be considered "obese." Moreover, there are ethnic differences for optimal BMI cutoffs. In addition, a BMI as low as 21, which is significantly lower than the current cutoff for overweight, may be associated with the lowest risk for death from coronary heart disease [6].

Figure 4 shows how the prevalence of US residents who are overweight or obese increased from 1960 through 2000. State-based surveillance data from the Behavioral Risk Factors Surveillance System (BRFSS) show a substantial increase in the prevalence of obesity among US adults over the last decade (Figure 5). Overall, the prevalence of obesity among US adults increased from 12% in 1991 to 21.3% in 2002. In 2002, about 2.4% (2.0% of men and 2.8% of women) of the adult population had a BMI of ≥ 40, versus 2.3% in 2001 and 0.9% in 1991. Among races, blacks had the highest rate of obesity (32.4%), primarily because of the high prevalence of obesity among

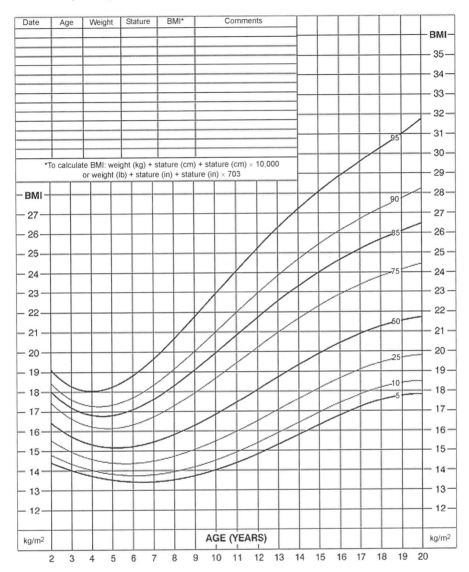

Figure 2. Body mass index-for-age percentiles: girls aged 2 to 20 years (from [6]). Source: developed by the National Center for Health Statistics in collaboration with the National Center for Chronic Disease Prevention and Health Promotion (2000).

black women. West Virginia had the highest rate of obesity (26.6%) and Colorado the lowest (16.1%). In 2002, 58% of adult Americans (66.3% of men and 49.8% of women) who participated in the Behavioral Risk Factor Surveillance Study were overweight. Because these rates are based on self-reported weight and height, they are no doubt substantial underestimates. First, people

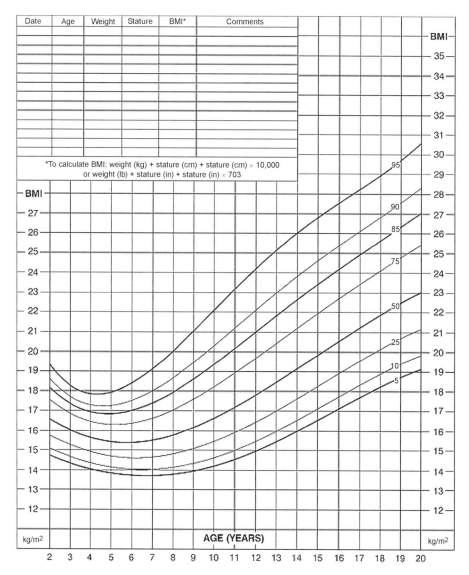

Figure 3. Body mass index-for-age percentiles: boys aged 2 to 20 years (from [6]). Source: developed by the National Center for Health Statistics in collaboration with the National Center for Chronic Disease Prevention and Health Promotion (2000).

without telephones are not included in BRFSS, and such persons are likely to be of low socioeconomic status, a factor associated with both obesity and diabetes [7]. Second, in validation studies of self-reported weight and height, overweight participants tend to underestimate their weight, and all participants tend to overestimate their height [8–10]. Third, those who reported a weight

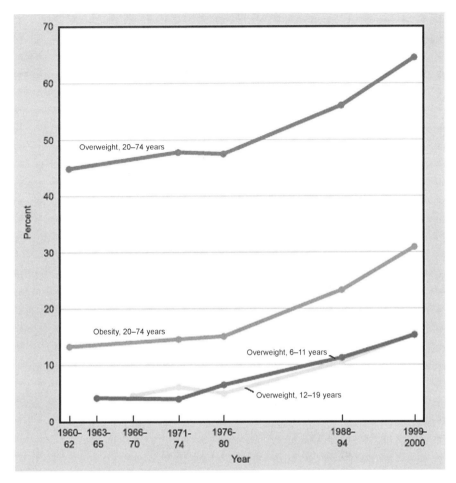

Figure 4. Overweight and obesity by age: United States, 1960–2000. (From Overweight and Obesity by Age, United States, 1960–2000 with Chartbooks on Trends in Health of Americans. Hyattsville, MD: CDC, NCHS, 2003).

greater than 500 pounds or height greater than 7 feet were excluded. The recent estimate of obesity among US adults 20 years of age or older is about 30% based on measured weight and height [11]. In addition to the large state-to-state variation in obesity, Ford et al. showed a wide variation in obesity and its related behaviors between local areas in the United States [12].

Several studies have also shown that a high percentage of US children and young adults are overweight. Rates are especially high in certain subpopulations. For example, Zephier et al. [13] showed that in the Aberdeen Indian Health Service area 39.1% of boys and 38.0% of girls were overweight, and 22.0% of boys and 18.0% of girls were obese. Similar studies suggest widespread increases in the prevalence of overweight and obesity among all US

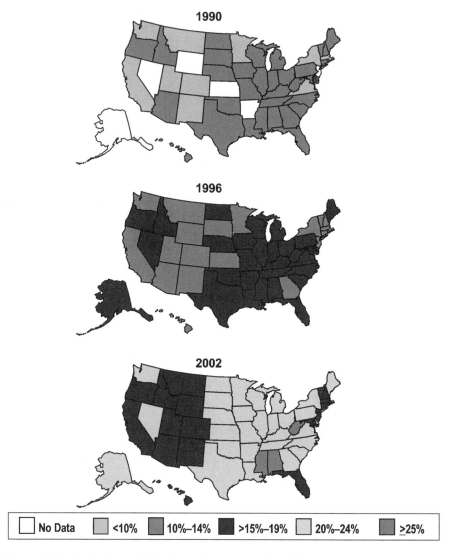

Figure 5. Trends in obesity (defined as a body mass index of 30 or higher) among US adults, BRFSS 1990, 1996, and 2002 (from Behavioral Risk Factor Surveillance System, CDC).

school-age children [14–16]. Other data show that the increasing prevalence of overweight and obesity in schoolchildren, adolescents, and young adults is a worldwide trend [17–20].

Excess weight has multiple causes including environmental, cultural, behavioral, socioeconomic, metabolic, and genetic. While individual behaviors and lifestyle choices are important factors in whether someone will become overweight or obese, environmental factors that influence the choices that individuals make are also crucial. For most people, however, the most proximate determinant of obesity and overweight is the imbalance between energy consumption and energy expenditure.

Excess energy consumption coupled with inadequate physical activity invariably leads to weight gain. The US Surgeon General recommends that adults should engage in at least 30 minutes of moderate physical activity on most days of the week [21]. The US Department of Agriculture recommends that adults should engage in approximately 60 minutes of moderate-to-vigorous-intensity activity on most days of the week while not exceeding the required caloric intake in order to manage body weight and prevent gradual, unhealthy body weight gain [22]. Moderation in calorie intake is also a key to maintaining ideal body weight. Recent data suggest, however, that Americans are eating more, with some performing little or no regular physical activity [23, 24]. Although there is a moderate increase in percentage of Americans engaging in physical activity, the rates are still below what will be needed to attain the healthy weight goals in the United States [1].

Among infants, the risk of being overweight has been associated with caloric intake by the mother during pregnancy as well as maternal smoking and diabetes mellitus [25, 26] and with duration of breastfeeding [27, 28]. For example, at the time they enter school, only 0.8% of children who were breastfed for 12 months or longer were overweight whereas the percentage increased gradually with shorter duration of breastfeeding to reach 4.5% among those who were not breastfed at all [27].

Factors associated with overweight and obesity are listed in Table 1. From a public health perspective, the most important of these factors are lack of physical activity, poor diet, race/ethnicity, and other sociocultural and environmental influences.

The continuing epidemic of overweight and obesity has tremendous implications for future morbidity and mortality rates, health care costs, and quality of life in the United States. Obesity is clearly associated with mortality, although the exact burden is not clear yet [29–31]. Obesity has also been identified as a factor in the increased prevalence of type 2 diabetes mellitus, coronary heart disease, cancers, high blood cholesterol level, high blood pressure, gallbladder disease, and osteoarthritis [32, 33]. Some researchers believe that the epidemic of obesity in the past decade has contributed to a slowing in the decline of blood cholesterol levels and to a decrease in blood pressure levels in the United States [34, 35]. In addition, obesity has a direct cost of $75 billion in the United States (5% to 7% of total annual medical expenditure) and its indirect costs are about $64 billion, which leads to a total cost of about $139 billion (year 2003 dollars) [36]. A recent national survey of health care utilization showed that obese persons had 36% higher inpatient and outpatient expenditures and 77% higher medication costs than normal weight persons [37].

Table 1. Prenatal, early-life, and later-life influences associated with an increased risk of obesity in adulthood

Prenatal and early life influences	*Diet, drugs, and specific disorders*
• High maternal caloric intake during pregnancy	• Excess energy intake and unhealthy eating behaviors
• Maternal smoking	○ Overeating
• Maternal diabetes	○ Frequent eating
• High birth weight	○ High dietary fat intake
• Absence or short duration of breast-feeding	○ Night-eating syndrome
	○ Binge-eating disorder
• Parental obesity	○ Progressive hyperphagic obesity
• Obesity during childhood and adolescence	• Drug and hormone use
	○ Use of antipsychotic drugs
	○ Use of antidepressant drugs
Later-life influences	○ Intense use of insulin
• Pregnancy	• Neuroendocrine disorders
• Postmenopausal factors	• Genetic and congenital disorders
• Sedentary lifestyle	• Disabilities involving physical and sensory impairments
○ No regular physical activity	• Psychological disorders
○ No or little work-related activity	
○ No recreational physical activity	*Other factors*
○ Prolonged television watching	• Smoking cessation
• Absence of policies and environmental factors supporting physical activity and balanced diet	• Ethnicity
	• Socioeconomic factors
	• Poor mental health

Modified from Bray GA. Etiology and Natural History of Obesity.

2.   PREVENTION AND CONTROL PROGRAMS

To be effective, programs to address the obesity epidemic need to be comprehensive and offered through multiple community venues, including schools, faith-based organizations, health care settings, businesses, and work-sites. These programs should focus on increasing physical activity, improving diet, and sustaining these lifestyle changes in order to reduce both body weight and its impact on morbidity and mortality. Programs that address early life influences and programs in schools and after-school settings [38–45] should be as much a priority as programs that target obese adults in community-based settings [46–50]. Programs that specifically target low-income and ethnic minority children are also very important because of the higher rates of obesity in these groups [38, 42–45, 51, 52]. While overweight and obese persons need to reduce their caloric intake and increase their physical activity, many others must play a role to help these individuals and to prevent further increases in obesity and diabetes. Health care providers must counsel their overweight and obese patients. Workplaces must offer healthy food choices in their cafeterias and provide opportunities for employees to be physically active on site. Schools must offer more physical education that encourages lifelong physical activity and provide a balanced diet rich in fruits and vegetables. Urban policymakers must provide more sidewalks, bike paths, and other alternatives to cars. Parents need to reduce the amount of time their children devote to watching television and playing computer games, and encourage active play. In general, restoring physical activity to our daily routines will be crucial to the success of efforts to reduce the percentage of Americans who are overweight or obese.

3.   THE METABOLIC SYNDROME

There is considerable controversy about the metabolic syndrome, including disagreements about its definition and whether it is even a "syndrome" with established outcomes. In general, the term "metabolic syndrome" is used to describe a constellation of risk factors that predispose people to cardiovascular disease (CVD) and its complications. Although there is no universally accepted definition of the metabolic syndrome, abdominal obesity, atherogenic dyslipidemia, high blood pressure, insulin resistance (with or without glucose intolerance), a proinflammatory state, and a prothrombotic state are generally considered to be key components [53]. Commonly used definitions include one proposed by the Third Report of the National Cholesterol Education Program Expert Panel on Detection, Evaluation, and Treatment of High Blood Cholesterol in Adults (Adult Treatment Panel III [ATP III]) [54], one by the World Health Organization (WHO) [55], by the American Association of Clinical Endocrinologists [56], and by the International Diabetes Federation (http://www.idf.org). Criteria for the WHO and NCEP definitions are shown in Tables 2 and 3. Although the WHO and ATP III [54, 55] criteria to diagnose the metabolic syndrome in a population-based sample of noninstitutionalized adults resulted in an overall 86.2% agreement, there were substantial differences in diagnosis for some population subgroups, such as African Americans [57].

Current published data suggest that the metabolic syndrome is highly prevalent in the US adult population [58]. Factors associated with the metabolic syndrome include impaired glucose tolerance and type 2 diabetes [58, 59]. Using the original NCEP definition, Ford et al. showed that about 47 million US residents had the metabolic syndrome and that the overall age-adjusted prevalence of the syndrome was 23.7% and increased substantially with advancing age from 6.7% among Americans 20 through 29 years of age to 43.5% and 42.0% among those 60 through 69 years of age and those 70 years of age or older, respectively [58]. The overall age-adjusted prevalence of the

Table 2. Coexistence of three or more of the following criteria makes a diagnosis
of the metabolic syndrome in accordance with the ATP III criteria

- Abdominal obesity: waist circumference > 102 cm in men and > 88 cm in women
- Hypertriglyceridemia: ≥ 150 mg/dL (1.695 mmol/L)
- Low HDL-cholesterol: < 40 mg/dL (1.036 mmol/L) in men and < 50 mg/dL
  (1.295 mmol/L) in women
- High blood pressure: ≥ 130/85 mm Hg
- High fasting glucose: ≥ 110 mg/dL (6.1 mmol/L)

From [54].

Table 3. The presence of two or more of the following abnormalities in a patient with
diabetes, impaired glucose tolerance, impaired fasting glucose, or insulin resistance
makes a diagnosis of the metabolic syndrome in accordance with the WHO criteria
(1998 definition)

- High blood pressure: > 160/90 mm Hg
- Hyperlipidemia: triglyceride concentration ≥ 150 mg/dL (1.695 mmol/L) and/or HDL
  cholesterol < 35 mg/dL (0.9 mmol/L) in men and < 39 mg/dL (1.0 mmol/L) in women
- Central obesity: waist-to-hip ratio of > 0.90 in men or > 0.85 in women and/or
  BMI ≥ 30 kg/m^2
  Microalbuminuria: urinary albumin excretion rate ≥ 20 mg/min or an albumin-to-creati-
  nine ratio ≥ 20 mg/g.

From [56].

metabolic syndrome was similar for men (24.0%) and women (23.4%), although among African Americans and Mexican Americans women had a 57%
and a 26% higher prevalence than men, respectively and Mexican Americans
had the highest age-adjusted prevalence of the metabolic syndrome among all
ethnic groups (31.9%) [58]. In a recent publication, Ford et al. showed an
increased prevalence of the metabolic syndrome among adults in the United
States [60].

Although many factors may contribute to the pathogenesis of the metabolic
syndrome, insulin resistance is generally considered to be a central mechanism
[61]. Insulin resistance is influenced by other hormonal stimuli and the effects
of free fatty acids [62]. The regulation of the hypothalamic–pituitary adrenal
axis may also be a factor in the pathogenesis of the syndrome [63], given that
this regulation may be disturbed by an environment characterized by abundant
food and few demands for physical activity [64]. Another possible cause of
the metabolic syndrome may be chronic activation of the innate immune system [65], because many people with the metabolic syndrome show evidence
of low-grade inflammation [66–68]. In addition, cytokines and hormones produced by adipocytes may contribute to the physiological perturbations associ-

ated with the metabolic syndrome independent of insulin resistance. However, studies have not shown leptin to be associated with the syndrome [69–71]. Moreover, it is likely that some people may have a genetic predisposition to develop the metabolic syndrome [72]. Finally, sedentary behavior is an important predictor of the metabolic syndrome [73].

People with the syndrome have also been shown to be at increased risk for diabetes and CVD [59, 74, 75]. Hanson et al. [74] showed that during a median follow-up of 4.1 years, 144 of 890 originally nondiabetic participants developed diabetes and that hyperinsulinemia, body size, and lipid levels were significantly associated with participants' diabetes risk whereas their blood pressure was not [74]. Using the NCEP-ATP III criteria for metabolic syndrome, Solymoss et al. showed the prevalence of the syndrome to be 51% in a Canadian population with established coronary artery [75]. Compared with patients without the syndrome, these patients had a worse coronary risk profile, a higher cumulative coronary stenosis score, and a greater likelihood of having had previous myocardial infarction. However, in a detailed review of the prospective studies from 1998 through 2004, Ford [76] concluded that the ability of the metabolic syndrome to predict the future risk of all-cause mortality and cardiovascular mortality may be limited. On the other hand, he showed that the metabolic syndrome is a better predictor of the future risk of diabetes [76].

Even among persons without baseline CVD or diabetes, the presence of the metabolic syndrome was significantly associated with both cardiovascular and all-cause mortality rates. Using the WHO criteria for the metabolic syndrome, Isomaa et al. [59] showed that the risk for coronary heart disease and stroke increased threefold and that the cardiovascular mortality rate was higher among subjects with the metabolic syndrome (12.0 vs. 2.2%, $p < 0.001$).

Similarly, in a population-based, prospective cohort study of 1209 Finnish men 42 to 60 years of age at baseline (1984–1989) who were initially without CVD, cancer, or diabetes Lakka et al. found that both cardiovascular and all-cause mortality rates were significantly higher among men with the metabolic syndrome [77]. Using four definitions based on the NCEP and the WHO criteria and adjusting for conventional cardiovascular risk factors, they showed that men with the metabolic syndrome were 2.9 to 3.3 times more likely to die of coronary heart disease [77].

4.   PREVENTIVE AND CONTROL STRATEGIES

Approaches to the prevention and control of the metabolic syndrome include pharmacologic treatment and behavioral and lifestyle changes such as increasing one's level of physical activity, losing weight, eating a diet rich in fruits and vegetables but low in saturated fat, and eating more foods with a low glycemic index [78–82]. The use of statins, fibrates, angiotensin-converting enzyme inhibitors, and other antihypertensive drugs has been shown to control dyslipidemia and hypertension and thus reduce coronary risk [54, 78, 79]. The thiazolidinediones have also been shown to have beneficial effects on several of the components of the metabolic syndrome, although their long-term safety and effectiveness remain to be proven [83–85].

5.   FUTURE PERSPECTIVES

The rapid increase in obesity in all segments of the population and regions of the country implies that there have been broad sweeping changes in our society that are contributing to weight gain by fostering caloric imbalance [85–92]. Such changes are unlikely to be the result of diminished individual motivation to maintain weight or genetic or other biological changes in the population. Indeed, these changes in behaviors, coupled with an aging US population, will increase the prevalence of obesity and the metabolic syndrome and suggest that the number of people with chronic diseases in general and cardiovascular disease and diabetes in particular is likely to increase dramatically.

The results of scientific research conducted during the last decade provide a sound foundation for efforts to prevent and control chronic diseases. The challenge is in translating these findings into practice. Thus, efforts to identify novel approaches to translate the best science into practice [93] must remain an important research objective. Emphasis must be placed on increasing the acceptance and participation in these preventive programs, particularly among groups who are often seldom reached, such as ethnic minority women and young adults, who are at high risk for the development of obesity, metabolic syndrome, diabetes, and cardiovascular sequelae [94].

Increased resources are also needed to better understand the metabolic syndrome, including its etiology, natural history, genetic and environmental determinants, and clinical outcomes [95] as well as research to identify culturally appropriate interventions to reduce the prevalence of the metabolic syndrome among disproportionately affected groups, particularly Hispanics and African-American women. Therefore, the development and dissemination of community-based interventions that will combat obesity and the metabolic syndrome are also crucial. In all of these research efforts, emphasis must be placed on population-based approaches to developing interventions that address the needs of specific populations in order to reduce and eventually eliminate known health disparities in chronic diseases.

The burden of chronic diseases globally is projected to increase dramatically. The problem is compounded by the aging effects of the population worldwide and the concomitant increased cost of illness at a time when countries struggle to accommodate costs of health care that continue to outstrip growth in their gross domestic product. There is an urgent need to establish a more preventive orientation in health care and public health systems. Indeed, the prevention and control of overweight, obesity, metabolic syndrome, and all related chronic diseases through a balanced diet and increased physical activity must become a priority.

REFERENCES

[1] Mokdad AH, Bowman BA, Ford ES, Vinicor F, Marks JS, Koplan JP. The continuing epidemic of obesity in the United States. JAMA 2001;286:1195–1200.

[2] Ford ES, Mokdad AH, Giles WH. Trends in waist circumference among U.S. adults. Obesity Research 2003;11(10):1223–1231.

[3] World Health Organization. World Health Report 2002: Reducing Risks, Promoting Healthy Life. Geneva, Switzerland: WHO, 2002.

[4] National Institutes of Health, National Heart Lung and Blood Institute. Clinical Guidelines on the Identification, Evaluation, and Treatment of Overweight and Obesity in Adults. Bethesda, MD: United States Department of Health and Human Services, Public Health Service, 1998.

[5] National Center for Health Statistics, Centers for Disease Control and Prevention. CDC growth charts: United States. Available at: http://www.cdc.gov/growthcharts.

[6] Eckel RH, Krauss RM. American Heart Association Call to Action: Obesity as a major risk factor for coronary heart disease. Circulation 1998;97:2099–2100.

[7] Ford ES. Characteristics of survey participants with and without a telephone: Findings from the third National Health and Nutrition Examination Survey. J Clin Epidemiol 1998;1:55–60.

[8] Rowland ML. Self-reported weight and height. Am J Clin Nutr 1990;52:1125–1133.

[9] Palta M, Prineas RJ, Berman R, Hannan P. Comparison of self-reported and measured height and weight. Am J Epidemiol 1982;115:223–230.

[10] Aday LA. Designing and Conducting Health Surveys: A Comprehensive Guide. San Francisco, CA: Jossey-Bass, 1989;79–80.

[11] Hedley AA, Ogden CL, Johnson CL, Carroll MD, Curtin LR, Flegal KM. Prevalence of overweight and obesity among US children, adolescents, and adults, 1999–2002. JAMA 2004;291(23):2847–2850.

[12] Ford ES, Mokdad AH, Giles HW, Galuska DA, Serdula MK. Geographic variation in the prevalence of obesity, diabetes, and obesity-related behaviors. Obes Res 2005;13(1):118–122.

[13] Zephier E, Himes JH, Story M. Prevalence of overweight and obesity in American Indian school children and adolescents in the Aberdeen area: A population study. Int J Obes Relat Metab Disord 1999;23(Suppl 2):S28–30, S28–S30.

[14] Park MK, Menard SW, Schoolfield J. Prevalence of overweight in a triethnic pediatric population of San Antonio, Texas. Int J Obes Relat Metab Disord 2001;25(3):409–416.

[15] Ogden CL, Troiano RP, Briefel RR, Kuczmarski RJ, Flegal KM, Johnson CL. Prevalence of overweight among preschool children in the United States, 1971 through 1994. Pediatrics 1997;99(4):E1.

[16] Melnik TA, Rhoades SJ, Wales KR, Cowell C, Wolfe WS. Overweight school children in New York City: Prevalence estimates and characteristics. Int J Obes Relat Metab Disord 1998;22(1):7–13.

[17] Kitagawa T, Owada M, Urakami T, Yamauchi K. Increased incidence of non-insulin dependent diabetes mellitus among Japanese schoolchildren correlates with an increased intake of animal protein and fat. Clin Pediatr 1998;37(2):111–115.

[18] Likitmaskul S, Kiattisathavee P, Chaichanwatanakul K, Punnakanta L, Angsusingha K, Tuchinda C. Increasing prevalence of type 2 diabetes mellitus in Thai children and adolescents associated with increasing prevalence of obesity. J Pediatr Endocrinol Metab 2003;16(1):71–77.

[19] Wei JN, Sung FC, Lin CC, Lin RS, Chiang CC, Chuang LM. National surveillance for type 2 diabetes mellitus in Taiwanese children. JAMA 2003;290(10):1345–1350.

[20] Ehtisham S, Barrett TG, Shaw NJ. Type 2 diabetes mellitus in UK children—an emerging problem. Diabet Med 2000;17(12):867–871.

[21] United States Department of Health and Human Services, Public Health Service. The Surgeon General's Call to Action to Prevent and Decrease Overweight and Obesity: 2001. Rockville, MD: US Department of Health and Human Services, Public Health Service, Office of the Surgeon General, 2001.

[22] Dietary guidelines for Americans, 2005. U.S. Department of Health and Human Services, U.S. Department of Agriculture. Available at http://www.healthierus.gov/dietaryguidlines.

[23] United States Department of Agriculture (USDA), United States Department of Health and Human Services. Dietary Guidelines for Americans, 5th edn. Washington, DC: USDA, 2000.

[24] United States Department of Health and Human Services. Healthy People 2010. With Understanding and Improving Health, and Objectives for Improving Health, 2nd edn. Washington, DC: Government Printing Office, 2000.

[25] Power C, Jefferis BJ. Fetal environment and subsequent obesity: A study of maternal smoking. Int J Epidemiol 2002;31(2):413–419.

[26] Dabelea D, Hanson RL, Lindsay RS, et al. Intrauterine exposure to diabetes conveys risk for type 2 diabetes and obesity: Study of discordant sibships. Diabetes 2000;49(12):2208–2211.

[27] von Kries R, Koletzko B, Sauerwald T, et al. Breast feeding and obesity: Cross sectional study. BMJ 1999;319(7203):147–150.

[28] Harder T, Bergmann R, Kallischnigg G, Plagemann A. Duration of breastfeeding and risk of overweight: A meta-analysis. Am J Epidemiol 2005;162(5)397–403.

[29] Allison D, Fontaine K, Manson J, Stevens J, Vanltallie K. Annual deaths attributable to obesity in the United States. JAMA 1999;282:1530–1538.

[30] Mokdad AH, Marks JS, Stroup D, Gerberding JL. Actual causes of death in the United States, 2000. JAMA 2004;291:1238–1245.

[31] Flegal KM, Graubard BI, Williamson DF, Gail MH. Excess deaths associated with underweight, overweight, and obesity. JAMA 2005;293(15):1861–1867.

[32] Must A, Spadano J, Coakley EH, Field AE, Colditz G, Dietz WH. The disease burden associated with overweight and obesity. JAMA 1999;282(16):1523–1529.

[33] Ford ES, Moriarty DG, Zack MM, Mokdad AH, Chapman DP. Self-reported body mass index and health-related quality of life: Findings from the Behavioral Risk Factor Surveillance System. Obes Res 2001;9:21–31.

[34] Ford ES, Mokdad AH, Giles WH, Mensah GA. Mean serum total cholesterol concentrations and awareness, treatment, and control of hypercholesterolemia among US adults: Findings from the National Health and Nutrition Examination Survey 1999–2000. Circulation 2003;107:2185–2189.

[35] Hajjar I, Kotchen T. Trends in prevalence, awareness, treatment and control of hypertension in the United States, 1988–2000. JAMA 2003;290:199–206.

[36] Finkelstein EA, Ruhm CJ, Kosa KM. Economic causes and consequences of obesity. Annu Rev Public Health 2005;26:239–257.

[37] Sturm R. The effects of obesity, smoking, and problem drinking on chronic medical problems and health care costs. Health Affairs 2002;21(2):245–253.

[38] Story M, Sherwood NE, Himes JH, et al. An after-school obesity prevention program for African-American girls: The Minnesota GEMS pilot study. Ethn Dis 2003;13(Suppl 1): S54–S64.

[39] Baranowski T, Cullen KW, Nicklas T, Thompson D, Baranowski J. School-based obesity prevention: A blueprint for taming the epidemic. Am J Health Behav 2002;26(6):486–493.

[40] Mo-suwan L, Pongprapai S, Junjana C, Puetpaiboon A. Effects of a controlled trial of a school-based exercise program on the obesity indexes of preschool children. Am J Clin Nutr 1998;68(5):1006–1011.

[41] Neumark-Sztainer D, Story M, Hannan PJ, Rex J. New moves: A school-based obesity prevention program for adolescent girls. Prev Med 2003;37(1):41–51.

[42] Stolley MR, Fitzgibbon ML, Dyer A, Van Horn L, KauferChristoffel K, Schiffer L. Hip-Hop to Health Jr., an obesity prevention program for minority preschool children: Baseline characteristics of participants. Prev Med 2003;36(3):320–329.

[43] Fitzgibbon ML, Stolley MR, Dyer AR, VanHorn L, KauferChristoffel K. A community-based obesity prevention program for minority children: Rationale and study design for Hip-Hop to Health Jr. Prev Med 2002;34(2):289–297.

[44] Davis SM, Going SB, Helitzer DL, et al. Pathways: A culturally appropriate obesity-prevention program for American Indian schoolchildren. Am J Clin Nutr 1999;69 (Suppl 4):796S–802S.

[45] Gittelsohn J, Evans M, Helitzer D, et al. Formative research in a school-based obesity prevention program for native American school children (pathways). Health Educ Res. 1998; 13(2):251–265.

[46] Jeffery RW. Community programs for obesity prevention: The Minnesota Heart Health Program. Obes Res 1995;3(Suppl 2):283s–288s.

[47] Jeffery RW, Gray CW, French SA, et al. Evaluation of weight reduction in a community intervention for cardiovascular disease risk: Changes in body mass index in the Minnesota Heart Health Program. Int J Obes Relat Metab Disord 1995;19(1):30–39.

[48] Wylie-Rosett J, Swencionis C, Peters MH, et al. A weight reduction intervention that optimizes use of practitioner's time, lowers glucose level, and raises HDL cholesterol level in older adults. J Am Diet Assoc 1994;94(1):37–42.

[49] Del Prete L, English C, Caldwell M, Banspach SW, Lefebvre C. Three-year follow-up of Pawtucket Heart Health's community-based weight loss programs. Am J Health Promot 1993;7(3):182–187.

[50] Taylor CB, Fortmann SP, Flora J, et al. Effect of long-term community health education on body mass index. The Stanford Five-City Project. Am J Epidemiol 1991;134(3):235–249.

[51] Kumanyika SK, Obarzanek E, Robinson TN, Beech BM. Phase 1 of the Girls health Enrichment Multi-site Studies (GEMS): Conclusion. Ethn Dis 2003;13(Suppl 1):S88–S91.

[52] Beech BM, Klesges RC, Kumanyika SK, et al. Child- and parent-targeted interventions: The Memphis GEMS pilot study. Ethn Dis 2003;13(Suppl 1):S40–S53.

[53] Grundy SM, Brewer HB Jr, Cleeman JI, et al. Definition of metabolic syndrome: Report of the National Heart, Lung, and Blood Institute/American Heart Association conference on scientific issues related to definition. Arterioscler Thromb Vasc Biol 2004;24:e13–e18.

[54] Third report of the National Cholesterol Education Program (NCEP) Expert Panel on Detection, Evaluation, and Treatment of High Blood Cholesterol in Adults (Adult Treatment Panel III) final report. Circulation 2002;106(25):3143–3421.

[55] Alberti KG, Zimmet PZ. Definition, diagnosis and classification of diabetes mellitus and its complications. Part 1: Diagnosis and classification of diabetes mellitus provisional report of a WHO consultation. Diabet Med 1998;15(7):539–553.

[56] Einhorn D, Reaven GM, Cobin RH, et al. American College of Endocrinology position statement on the insulin resistance syndrome. Endocr Pract 2003;9:237–252.

[57] Ford ES, Giles WH. A comparison of the prevalence of the metabolic syndrome using two proposed definitions. Diabetes Care 2003;26(3):575–581.

[58] Ford ES, Giles WH, Dietz WH. Prevalence of the metabolic syndrome among US adults: Findings from the third National Health and Nutrition Examination Survey. JAMA 2002; 287(3):356–359.

[59] Isomaa B, Almgren P, Tuomi T, et al. Cardiovascular morbidity and mortality associated with the metabolic syndrome. Diabetes Care 2001;24(4):683–689.

[60] Ford ES, Giles WH, Mokdad AH. Increasing prevalence of the metabolic syndrome among US adults. Diabetes Care 2004;27:2444–2449.

[61] Reaven GM. Banting lecture 1988. Role of insulin resistance in human disease. Diabetes 1988;37(12):1595–1607.

[62] Brotman DJ, Girod JP. The metabolic syndrome: A tug-of-war with no winner. Cleve Clin J Med 2002;69(12):990–994.

[63] Bjorntorp P, Rosmond R. The metabolic syndrome—a neuroendocrine disorder? Br J Nutr 2000;83(Suppl 1):S49–S57.

[64] Kreier F, Yilmaz A, Kalsbeek A, Romijn JA, Sauerwein HP, Fliers E, Buijs RM. Hypothesis: Shifting the equilibrium from activity to food leads to autonomic unbalance and the metabolic syndrome. Diabetes 2003;52(11):2652–2656.

[65] Duncan BB, Schmidt MI. Chronic activation of the innate immune system may underlie the metabolic syndrome. Sao Paulo Med J 2001;119(3):122–127.

[66] Frohlich M, Imhof A, Berg G, et al. Association between C-reactive protein and features of the metabolic syndrome: A population-based study. Diabetes Care 2000;23(12):1835–1839.

[67] Festa A, D'Agostino R Jr, Howard G, Mykkanen L, Tracy RP, Haffner SM. Chronic subclinical inflammation as part of the insulin resistance syndrome: The Insulin Resistance Atherosclerosis Study (IRAS). Circulation 2000;102(1):42–47.

[68] Ford ES. The metabolic syndrome and C-reactive protein, fibrinogen, and leukocyte count: Findings from the Third National Health and Nutrition Examination Survey. Atherosclerosis 2003;168(2):351–358.

[69] de Courten M, Zimmet P, Hodge A, et al. Hyperleptinaemia: The missing link in the metabolic syndrome? Diabet Med 1997;14(3):200–208.

[70] Hodge AM, Boyko EJ, de Courten M, et al. Leptin and other components of the metabolic syndrome in Mauritius—a factor analysis. Int J Obes Relat Metab Disord 2001;25(1):126–131.

[71] Ford ES. Factor analysis and defining the metabolic syndrome. Ethn Dis 2003;13(4):429–437.

[72] Groop L. Genetics of the metabolic syndrome. Br J Nutr 2000;83(Suppl 1):S39–S48.

[73] Ford ES, Khol HW 3rd, Mokdad AH, Ajani UA. Sedentary behavior, physical activity, and the metabolic syndrome among U.S. adults. Obes Res 2005;13(3):608–614.

[74] Hanson RL, Imperatore G, Bennett PH, Knowler WC. Components of the metabolic syndrome and incidence of type 2 diabetes. Diabetes 2002;51(10):3120–3127.

[75] Solymoss BC, Bourassa MG, Lesperance J, et al. Incidence and clinical characteristics of the metabolic syndrome in patients with coronary artery disease. Coron Artery Dis 2003;14(3):207–212.

[76] Ford ES. Risk for all-cause mortality, cardiovascular disease, and diabetes associated with the metabolic syndrome. Diabetes Care 2005;28:1769–1778.

[77] Lakka HM, Laaksonen DE, Lakka TA, et al. The metabolic syndrome and total and cardiovascular disease mortality in middle-aged men. JAMA 2002;288(21):2709–2716.

[78] Scott CL. Diagnosis, prevention, and intervention for the metabolic syndrome. Am J Cardiol 2003;92(1A):35i–42i.

[79] Barnard RJ, Wen SJ. Exercise and diet in the prevention and control of the metabolic syndrome. Sports Med 1994;18(4):218–228.

[80] Riccardi G, Rivellese AA. Dietary treatment of the metabolic syndrome—the optimal diet. Br J Nutr 2000;83(Suppl 1):S143–S148.

[81] Marckmann P. Dietary treatment of thrombogenic disorders related to the metabolic syndrome. Br J Nutr 2000;83(Suppl 1):S121–S126.

[82] Steinberger J, Daniels SR. Obesity, insulin resistance, diabetes, and cardiovascular risk in children: An American Heart Association scientific statement from the Atherosclerosis, Hypertension, and Obesity in the Young Committee (Council on Cardiovascular Disease in the Young) and the Diabetes Committee (Council on Nutrition, Physical Activity, and Metabolism). Circulation 2003;107(10):1448–1453.

[83] Greenberg AS. The expanding scope of the metabolic syndrome and implications for the management of cardiovascular risk in type 2 diabetes with particular focus on the emerging role of the thiazolidinediones. J Diabetes Complicat 2003;17(4):218–228.

[84] Komers R, Vrana A. Thiazolidinediones—tools for the research of metabolic syndrome X. Physiol Res 1998;47(4):215–225.

[85] Amos AF, McCarty DJ, Zimmet P. The rising global burden of diabetes and its complications: Estimates and projections to the year 2010. Diabet Med 1997;15(Suppl 5):S1–S5.

[86] Perdue WC, Stone LA, Gostin LO. The built environment and its relationship to the public's health: The legal framework. Am J Public Health 2003;93(9):1390–1394.

[87] Ogden CL, Flegal KM, Carroll MD, Johnson CL. Prevalence and trends in overweight among US children and adolescents, 1999–2000. JAMA 2002;288(14):1728–1732.

[88] Boyle JP, Honeycutt AA, Venkat Narayan KM, et al. Projection of diabetes burden through 2050: Impact of changing demography and disease prevalence in the U.S. Diabetes Care 2001;24(11):1936–1940.

[89] Flegal KM, Troiano RP. Changes in the distribution of body mass index of adults and children in the US population. Int J Obes Relat Metab Disord 2000;24(7):807–818.

[90] Geiss LS. Diabetes Surveillance, 1999. Atlanta, GA: U.S. Department of Health and Human Services, 1999.

[91] Flegal KM, Carroll MD, Kuczmarski RJ, Johnson CL. Overweight and obesity in the United States: Prevalence and trends, 1960–1994. Int J Obes Relat Metab Disord 1998;22(1):39–47.

[92] Troiano RP, Flegal KM. Overweight children and adolescents: Description, epidemiology, and demographics. Pediatrics 1998;101(3 Pt 2):497–504.

[93] California Healthcare Foundation/American Geriatrics Society Panel on Improving Care for Elders with Diabetes. Guidelines for improving the care of the older person with diabetes mellitus. J Am Geriatr Soc 2003;51(Suppl 5):S265–S280.

[94] Sherwood NE, Morton N, Jeffery RW, French SA, Neumark-Sztainer D, Falkner NH. Consumer preferences in format and type of community-based weight control programs. Am J Health Promot 1998;13(1):12–18.

[95] Deedwania PC. Metabolic syndrome and vascular disease: Is nature or nurture leading the new epidemic of cardiovascular disease? Circulation 2004;109:2–4.

Chapter 4

The Genetic Contribution to Obesity

Raul A. Bastarrachea[a,b], Jack W. Kent Jr.[a], Jeff T. Williams[b], Guowen Cai[a], Shelley A. Cole[a] and Anthony G. Comuzzie[a,b]

[a]*Department of Genetics, Southwest Foundation for Biomedical Research, San Antonio, TX 78227, USA*
[b]*Southwest National Primate Research Center, San Antonio, TX 78245, USA*

1.   INTRODUCTION

Common complex diseases can be characterized by quantitative derangements in normal physiological processes (e.g., glucose or lipid levels) that cumulatively act to increase an individual's disease risk. This class of common complex diseases represents a variety of conditions with serious implications for public health including coronary heart disease, hypertension, type 2 diabetes, and obesity. While environmental factors play a significant role in the development of these conditions (e.g., diet), it is the individual's unique genetic background that dictates the response to these environmental pressures. Recent advances in molecular genetics and the biology of adipose tissue have brought to light new genes thought to be involved in the development of obesity. However, most of the genetic variants predisposing to human obesity remain to be identified. Three general approaches have been used to date in the search for genes underlying common, complex diseases, such as obesity. The first approach focuses on *a priori* selected candidate genes believed to have some plausible role in the trait of interest (e.g., obesity) on the basis of their known or presumed biological function. This approach has had limited success in identifying genes involved in the development of disease at the population level. An alternative approach attempts to localize genes and requires no presumptions on the function of the gene, and is based on the detection of unique patterns of segregation among related individuals (chief among this type of approach has been linkage analysis). Recent advances in the ability to evaluate linkage analysis data from large family pedigrees has shown great promise in identifying genomic regions associated with the development of complex phenotypes such as obesity, but the identification of the specific casual genetic variants has remained somewhat elusive. RNA-based technologies have recently begun to prove very useful to identify genes differentially expressed in tissues of healthy and diseased individuals. In this chapter we review the current knowledge of the genetic contribution to the pathogenesis of obesity.

2.   OBESITY AS A COMMON COMPLEX PHENOTYPE

Obesity has now reached epidemic rates in many industrialized nations and has become a significant public health crisis. The World Health Organization has stated that more than 1 billion people are overweight or obese [1]. Almost 61% of the US population is obese or overweight, leading to a dramatic increase in the comorbid diseases of the metabolic syndrome, including type 2 diabetes, and cardiovascular atherosclerotic disease [2, 3]. There is no doubt that this epidemic is on the rise in developing countries as urbanization, increasing reliance on technology, and easy access to large amounts of processed food lead people in those countries toward high-fat, calorie-dense diets, and a more sedentary lifestyle [4]. This broad transition in nutritional status has now reached Asia, Latin America, the Middle East, and Northern Africa, and is causing populations throughout the world to display disease prevalence and trends similar to those seen in the United States. These trends can only be accelerated by economic globalization, which tends to direct job opportunities toward activities demanding less energy expenditure than labor-intensive jobs such as farming, and also promotes sedentary leisure activities such as watching television [5].

Although it is clear that this worldwide marked increase in the prevalence of obesity appears to be attributable to an obesogenic or toxic environment, characterized by the consumption of "super size" portions of energy-dense foods and a lack of appropriate physical activity, research in the past 10 years has shown that genetic factors clearly predispose some individuals to be more susceptible than others to these environmental stressors [6–8].

The search for the cause of this variation has revealed an important heritable contribution to obesity and its related phenotypes [9]. By the end of 2002, more than 300 genes, markers, and chromosomal regions linked with obesity phenotypes had been reported. Genome scans had identified 68 human quantitative trait loci (QTLs), plus 168 QTLs from animal models for obesity. There were 222 studies showing positive associations to 71 candidate genes, with 15 candidate genes supported by at least five positive studies. Causal or strong candidate genes were identified for 23 out of 33 Mendelian syndromes relevant to human obesity [10]. The purpose of this chapter is to present the genetic contribution to the pathogenesis of obesity, in order to evaluate its importance in understanding and treating this serious public health problem.

3. ANCIENT GENES IN A MODERN WORLD: AN EVOLUTIONARY GENETIC PERSPECTIVE ON OBESITY

The vast majority of human evolutionary existence has been spent as hunter-gatherers in environments where access to calories was often restricted. It has only been in recent human history that we find our selves living in what can be termed a readily accessible, energy-rich environment (at least with respect to most of the Westernized world). As a result it has been repeatedly suggested that there is an evolutionary disconnect between the selective pressures of the environment of limited and often unpredictable calories in which our genome evolved and the obesogenic environment (i.e., readily available calories and limited opportunities for energy expenditure) in which those genes now must be expressed [11]. It has been suggested that these environmental pressures favored genetic variants that were more efficient at storing and utilizing available calories (originally referred to as "thrifty" genes [12, 13]), thereby imparting a selective advantage to those who possessed them during periods of famine and deprivation that have often plagued human populations [14, 15]. The human body has a limited capacity to store proteins and carbohydrates, as well as little ability to convert carbohydrate to fat. In this context, the consumption and storage of fat in the adipose tissue as a primary energy reserve constitutes an important evolutionary adaptation [16, 17].

Compared with the conditions that prevailed over evolutionary time, our environment has been drastically altered by 10,000 years of agriculture and especially by 200–300 years of industrialization. Our "thrifty genes" are now exposed to an environment of toxic abundance, which acts as a powerful promoter of chronic diseases such as type 2 diabetes, hypertension, atherosclerosis, and obesity. This environment of excessive calorie intake and a sedentary life style has precipitated an epidemic of obesity [18–20]. However, humans are highly variable in their susceptibility to develop obesity [8, 9, 21–23].

This evolutionary genetic argument has been used to explain phenomena such as the extreme prevalence of obesity and the metabolic syndrome in the Pima Indians of Arizona, where these once evolutionarily favored "thrifty" genes have now become maladaptive in a new environment in which calories are readily available. The relatively small and genetically isolated Pima Indian population has experienced a drastic shift in lifestyle in just over a century, as upstream river diversions eliminated their traditional, physically demanding, irrigated agriculture subsistence [24]. Today, many Pima are employed in sedentary jobs and have shifted to the high-fat, high-caloric-density foods of their non-Indian neighbors. In this environment the Pima have rapidly developed extreme rates of metabolic disease: approximately half of the Arizona Pima have type 2 diabetes, and the rate of obesity exceeds 60% in young adult males and 80% in young adult females [25]. Significantly, a related Mexican population of Pima Indians maintains its traditional diet and active lifestyle and exhibits much lower rates of diabetes and obesity [26].

While some researchers have presented what could be argued to be extreme positions on the role of the environment in the development of the current epidemic of obesity (e.g., [18]), it is generally conceded that it is necessary to assume a synergistic relationship between genes and the environment to explain the development of this complex phenomenon. The result of this interaction of "permissive" genes and "toxic" environments is the expression of a very complex trait. It is this innate complexity that makes the identification of obesity susceptibility genes (as well as those for any common complex disease) such a difficult task. However, the ultimate reward of undertaking such a difficult task is the opportunity to unravel the intimate biological and molecular aspects of the disease, moving us toward a complete understanding of its pathophysiology and ultimately to the design of new medications and more efficacious diagnostic tests [8, 15, 22, 27].

4.   APPROACHES TO OBESITY GENE DISCOVERY

The identification of disease genes through molecular genetic analysis has been very successful for monogenic traits such as cystic fibrosis that exhibit simple patterns of Mendelian inheritance [28]. However, few genes have been identified for the large group of common complex diseases, including obesity, type 2 diabetes, hypertension, cardiovascular disease, asthma, schizophrenia, and cancer. Such diseases are clearly heritable—they exhibit familiality— yet they do not display simple Mendelian (i.e., monogenic) patterns of inheritance. Several factors potentially hamper the study of complex diseases: (a) *genetic (or locus) heterogeneity*, in which different genes influence disease risk in different lineages or populations; (b) *allelic heterogeneity*, in which different variations within the same gene cause similar physiological alterations leading to the development of the disease; (c) *incomplete penetrance*, in which disease-causing mutations are variably expressed, perhaps owing to other compensatory genetic factors, or to random effects; (d) *phenocopy*, in which the sporadic occurrence of the disease is possible even with minimal genetic risk but with a highly permissive environment that increases the risk of disease; and (e) *oligogenic inheritance*, in which depending upon the physiologic structure of the genetic products, mutations must be present in several genes simultaneously for development of the disease [29].

There are currently three fundamental strategies used to identify genes involved in the development of common complex diseases such as obesity.

4.1.   Candidate Gene Association Study

The first and perhaps most traditional approach is the candidate gene association study, which tests the association between a specific genetic variant and a phenotype. Candidate genes for obesity would be those thought to be involved in the development of obesity because of their presumed or known biological effects on mechanisms involved with (a) the regulation of food intake under the control of the central nervous system, (b) the modulation of insulin action and glucose metabolism in target tissues that could contribute to an excess accumulation of adipose tissue or to the development of obesity-induced insulin resistance, or (c) the regulation of energy expenditure and adipose tissue metabolism including lipid oxidation, lipolysis, and lipogenesis. The common procedure to study candidate genes is to identify genetic variants and genotype them in a large sample of unrelated cases and controls. Statistical analyses are performed to detect associations and determine if the disease and a particular allele show significant correlated occurrence [22, 30, 31]. Note that this approach requires that the candidate gene has been identified previously from either biochemical or molecular studies; the question is whether there exist variants in the gene that account for variation observed in the expression of the phenotype or disease state.

4.2.   Genome Scan

The second approach, the genome scan, detects chromosomal regions known as quantitative trait loci or QTLs, and potential genes or gene clusters within such regions, where linkage with the target phenotype can be shown. Linkage analysis, utilizing polymorphic markers evenly spaced throughout the complete genome, identifies chromosomal regions with statistically significant cosegregation with the quantitative phenotype. The genome scan strategy does not require assuming the function of the genes in the susceptible loci, but relies on the detection of the unique pattern of segregation of markers and phenotypes across generations of related individuals. The genomic region found in a linkage study is usually large (10 to 30 cM—a region that can encompass many genes); consequently, fine mapping is necessary to pinpoint a QTL to a narrower genomic region to eventually be able to identify the causative genes [27, 32, 33].

At present most genome-wide linkage studies make use of approximately 400 to 600 polymorphic markers (e.g., microsatellites) per person distributed fairly evenly throughout the human genome. Once each member of a pedigree is genotyped for these markers, one can estimate the probability that two individuals share any given chromosomal region identically by descent. One then estimates the correlation of the disease phenotype between related pairs, to estimate what proportion of variance in the phenotype is "explained" by these shared regions. Regions that show significant linkage to the trait are the QTLs, interpreted as rough locations of causative genes for the disease. The next step is to refine the genetic location, aided by the availability of high-resolution human genetic maps [34–36]. The localized genes found within the implicated region can be sequenced to try to identify the genetic alteration present in affected individuals but absent in unaffected pedigreed members. Such genetic alterations are considered as causes of the disease.

The technique of positional cloning is enhanced by the availability of the human genome sequence, which identifies both known and probable genes [37, 38]. The main difference between a positional candidate gene and a traditional candidate gene is that each positional candidate gene is considered based solely on its proximity to a QTL previously identified through a linkage analysis in a genome scan. Therefore, the genome-wide scan approach offers the potential of identifying novel or previously unsuspected genes affecting a given phenotype. This does not, of course, exclude the possibility that a previously suspected candidate gene could be responsible for the QTL [39], in which case the linkage analysis strengthens that gene's "candidacy."

4.3.   mRNA

The third approach to identifying genes is based on variations in the profile of tissue gene expression, whether in lean versus obese individuals or in different tissues within individuals. This specific approach uses messenger RNA (mRNA), unlike the two previously described approaches which are based on the use of DNA. The collection of mRNA from tissue samples can be somewhat problematic in human studies when compared to the DNA approach. RNA is less stable chemically than DNA, and requires special care to avoid the degradation of the sample. More importantly, while DNA can be collected from blood, collection of samples of other tissues typically requires surgical biopsy [31].

5.   EVIDENCE FROM ANIMAL MODELS FOR THE GENETIC CONTRIBUTION TO OBESITY

5.1.   Monogenic Obesity

There are several spontaneous forms of monogenic obesity in rodents, some of which have been known for decades. The genes responsible for many of these have been cloned, revealing interesting candidate genes to be considered in studies of human obesity [40, 41]. Six single genes that have been shown to cause obesity have been identified from several strains of rodents, and have been termed *ob*, *db*, *agouti*, *fat*, *tubby*, and *mahogany*. They all express protein molecules that seem to interact with physiological pathways involved in energy homeostasis, body weight regulation, and adipose tissue storage [42].

The two best described animal models of monogenic obesity are the mutant rodents *ob* (*obese*) and *db* (*diabetes*). These rodents present a complete deficiency in the expression of the circulating adipostatic hormone leptin, or its receptor respectively, owing to gene defects in the structural genes for these proteins. Both mutations were identified positionally; characterization of leptin, the *ob* gene product, was a breakthrough in our understanding of adipostatic regulation. The lack of leptin or a functional signaling receptor leads to an increased food intake and the development of obesity and type 2 diabetes. It seems that the genes coding for leptin and its receptor play a key role in the development of fat tissue accumulation at early stages of life [43–45].

The *agouti* yellow mouse presents a dominant mutation, conferring to the mutant mice an obese phenotype with increased linear growth and a yellow coat color. The mutation expresses an ectopic protein whose action is to antagonize melanocortin receptors. While peripheral agouti causes abnormal pigmentation via the melanocortin receptor 1 (MC1R), ectopic expression of agouti in brain affects the central melanocortin receptor 4 (MC4R), directly altering the hypothalamic neuroendocrine system and leading to the melanocortin-obesity syndrome. In humans there is a similar phenotype due to mutations in the gene for MC4R (see later) [46–48]. A natural suppression of the mutation induced by *agouti* has been observed during the study of two natural autosomal recessive mutations called *mahogany* (*mg*) and *mahoganoid* (*md*). These appear to be caused by the gene *Atrn* (attractin). Both mutations are capable of deviating melanogenesis from synthesis of pheomelanin to that of eumelanin. They also strongly prevent the development of obesity induced by ectopic agouti [49–51].

Other recessive mutations in rodents resulting in phenotypes associated with obesity are also accompanied by endocrine and metabolic disturbances. This is seen with homozygotic mutation of the carboxipeptidase E enzyme (Cpe) in the strain of *fat* rodents which is biochemically manifested by elevated plasma pancreatic proinsulin concentrations. The Cpe gene is similar to the proconvertase-1 gene in humans [52, 53]. Mutations in the *tubby* gene lead to multiple sensory deficits with a moderate obesity phenotype which starts in the adult life of the mutant, differing from *fat* strains in that *tubby* mutants present insulin resistance [54, 55]. Although the differences between animal species and humans cannot allow a complete comparative analogy in their biological functions, we cannot deny that the existence of a variety of animal models has been an important tool to understand many aspects of the genetics and physiology of human obesity [54, 56, 57]. These models, particularly rodents, have been the subjects of extensive research to pursue the identification of genes in humans. Manufacture of genetically modified mutant strains has enabled researchers to elucidate several metabolic pathways influencing the regulation of body weight [58].

5.2.   Oligogenic Obesity

A quantitative genetic approach to the study of body weight in rodents gives us an opportunity to investigate important aspects regarding its genetic architecture. This kind of approach can be addressed using an animal model system in which both environmental and genetic effects can be maintained [59]. Another important advantage when using rodents or other laboratory animals as model systems in quantitative genetics is the capability to select specific phenotypes such as energy expenditure [60] that would be more difficult to measure in humans. The spectrum of the existing genetic variants, combined with a short generation time and the low cost of maintenance, allows animal systems to be considered as appropriate models for this kind of approach. Identification of QTLs can proceed efficiently from mating of inbred strains that differ in obesity-related traits. A thorough analysis of the various QTLs gives us the opportunity to determine if some genes exert control on energy expenditure independently of adiposity or food intake, or if another group of genes may act in a coordinated fashion on all the components of the regulation of energy balance [56, 61]. The relative ease of identifying QTLs for obesity in rodents compared to humans has led to integrated genetic maps for polygenic obesity in different mouse strains; these maps are highly reliable but bewilderingly dense [29, 47].

Perhaps the most striking variable for the development of obesity in humans is the accessibility and composition of the diet. Animal models are readily maintained on controlled dietary regimens. Several studies have shown that barely noticeable differences in body composition and fat tissue accumulation between rodent strains bred on normocaloric diets become magnified when calorie-dense saturated fat diets are offered. Intentionally manipulating environmental variables teaches us that in the presence of gene × environment interactions, the effects of genetic susceptibility become fully apparent when amplified by environmental risk factors [62–65].

Several of the QTLs related to adiposity, body weight and related phenotypes have been detected near the positions for single-gene mutations involved in the development of obesity. Loci on chromosomes 6 and 7 have been identified in strains of BSB mice. Linkage in the former was found near the leptin gene while the latter exhibited linkage with body fat, total cholesterol, and hepatic lipase activity [66]. Similarly, a locus in chromosome 4 identified in the strain SWR/J × AKR/J includes the gene for the leptin receptor [45]. Because long stretches of mouse and human genomes contain genes that code for the same proteins, in roughly the same order, rodent QTLs can implicate homologous regions in humans. Examples of this are the two mouse obesity QTLs, obesity-1 (mob-1) and obesity qt-1 (obq1), which are homologous with the human uncoupling proteins 2 and 3 (UCP 2 and 3) genes [67].

In the past years, transgenic technology has created several rodent models of obesity that have helped in clarifying the functions of several specific proteins and genes regarding their influence in the peripheral and central pathways that control energy homeostasis [43, 68, 69]. With the advent of DNA recombinant technology, researchers have been able to modulate transgene (Tg) expression; the ability to introduce and overexpress genes makes this technique one of the most useful approaches in molecular genetics of obesity. A related procedure using a knockout (KO) gene or homologous recombination permits the interruption of specific endogenous gene expression by replacing the native gene with a nonfunctional allele [70, 71]. Both techniques have allowed physiologists to understand the relative importance of the genetic components that control body weight regulation, through observation of abnormalities resulting from interrupted or overexpressed genes. As with rodent QTL studies, results in animal models implicate homologous genes in humans. Thirty-nine KO and Tg genes have been introduced into the last update of the human genetic map [10, 42, 43].

6.   EVIDENCE FOR THE GENETIC CONTRIBUTION TO OBESITY IN HUMANS

6.1.   The Genetic Contribution to Rare Forms of Human Obesity

6.1.1.   Syndromic forms of human obesity. An abnormal and excessive distribution of adipose tissue is characteristic of some syndromic forms of obesity, where the excess of body fat is one of the many manifestations of the disorder but not the dominant feature. Prader–Willi syndrome is a dominant autosomal illness; it is the best characterized and is the most common syndromic obesity in humans. Its estimated prevalence and clinical characteristics have been described in many studies [72, 73]. Approximately 70% of patients present an abnormality in several genes located on their paternally inherited chromosome 15. Most of the remaining cases present a maternal disomy of the same chromosome. Recent studies have shown that translocations or mutations in the small C/D box of nucleolar RNAs within the nucleoriboprotein gene *SNRPN* cause an important loss of function, triggering the development of this syndrome [74].

The prevalence of the Bardet–Biedl (BBS) syndrome ranges from 1:160,000 in England to 1:13,500 in the Middle East where consanguineous marriages are more common. Causative genes have been identified in three different loci of BBS, named *BBS2*, *BBS4*, and *BBS6* [75]. The mutation of the *BBS2* gene [76] was identified on chromosome 16q21 and the function of this gene has not yet been determined. *BBS4* has been identified on chromosome 15q22.3–q23 and the protein product shows a strong similarity to the *O*-linked *N*-acetylglucosamine transferase that in humans has been related to insulin resistance [77]. *BBS6* is caused by mutations in the gene *MKKS* (McKussick–Kaufman syndrome) that presents a high similarity with a chaperone bacterial protein believed to play a key role in the regulation of protein integrity [78]. A mutation in a second locus identified on chromosome 11q34 has also been described; it has been designated *BBS1*. The identification of another protein named BBS7, sharing properties with BBS1 and BBS2, has recently been reported [79, 80].

Other syndromic forms of obesity include Cohen, Borjeson, Albright Hereditary Osteodystrophy, Wilson–Turner, and Alstrom syndromes. Most of these syndromic forms have been genetically mapped at different chromosomal regions but the causative genes have been very hard to isolate because of the extreme rarity of these mutations. Moreover, polymorphic markers in these regions do not cosegregate with obesity in families that do not express these syndromes, perhaps suggesting heterogeneity in the causes of syndromic and nonsyndromic obesity [81].

6.1.2.   Monogenic forms of human obesity.   Several rare obesogenic mutations found in humans are homologous to those identified in rodents; they characteristically belong to the same metabolic pathway controlling hunger, satiety, and energy homeostasis, with obesity as the dominant feature and independent of environmental factors. From an historical perspective [82, 83], the spontaneous mutations found in extremely obese mice generated innovative experiments of parabiosis, in which surgical cross-anastomosis of the circulatory systems of obese mutants and their wild-type littermates resulted in a dramatic body weight reduction in the obese mice. These results led to the prediction of a regulatory loop system between the adipose tissue and the brain, and culminated many years later with the positional cloning in mouse of the obese (*ob*) gene, its receptor, LepR, and characterization of the *ob* protein product leptin [43–45, 84, 85]. One of the main functions of leptin is the communication to the brain of the magnitude of the long-term fat storage. When this hormone reaches the hypothalamus, it triggers a series of neuroendocrine responses on the anabolic NPY and AgRP and catabolic prohormone proopiomelanocortin (POMC)-containing neurons, regions already known to be involved in the regulation of fat metabolism [86, 87].

The genes responsible for monogenic forms of human obesity include the genes coding for leptin, the leptin receptor, and POMC. Mutations in these genes lead to very rare recessive forms of obesity associated with multiple en-docrine aberrations [88]. Two related children (cousins) and an unrelated male child of Pakistani origin were homozygous for a mutation in the leptin gene involving the loss of a single guanine nucleotide in codon 133 [89–91]. This mutation results in the complete loss of function of the gene product, produc-ing a phenotype characterized by extreme obesity from the first week of life, substantial increase of appetite, hyperphagia, central hypothyroidism, and hy-pogonadotropic hypogonadism [92, 93]. The heterozygous relatives of these children presented subnormal levels of leptin, a higher prevalence of obesity and a higher body fat percentage when compared with controls matched for age and ethnicity. Another mutation located in the codon 105 was found in the homozygous state in three adults and a child in a consanguineous fam-ily, resulting in the same phenotype as the affected children with the mutation in codon 133. Subcutaneous leptin administration has been shown to reverse most of the phenotypic abnormalities associated with human congenital leptin deficiency [94, 95]. Only three individuals within a family have been identi-fied as homozygous for a mutation in the leptin receptor, resulting in a G–T substitution in exon 16. The mutant receptor is truncated in the anterior part of its transmembrane domain, entirely blocking leptin signaling inside the hy-pothalamus. The homozygous subjects have a phenotype of extreme obesity and pituitary dysfunction similar to that observed in congenital leptin defi-ciency. However, obese individuals carrying the leptin receptor mutation have marked elevation of serum leptin levels. A striking difference between patients with the leptin gene mutation and with the ones carrying a mutation in the re-ceptor is that the latter have significant growth retardation and hypothalamic hypopituitarism [96].

The significant role of the melanocortin system in the regulation of body weight in humans has been well documented by the discovery of mutations in the POMC gene [97] that result in extreme obesity. This gene is expressed in the brain, intestines, placenta, and pancreas in humans. POMC is the precursor for several hormones of the hypothalamic–pituitary–adrenal axis, mainly the α-melanocyte-stimulating hormone (α-MSH), adrenocorticotropic hormone and β-endorphin. α-MSH is a physiological ligand for the central nervous sys-tem receptor MC4R. The production of α-MSH is under the control of leptin and the signal generated by this neurotransmitter upon binding to the MC4R receptor promotes catabolism and appetite inhibition [98–100]. Homozygous or compound heterozygous individuals for mutations in the POMC gene re-sulting in loss of function have been detected in children with early-onset ex-treme obesity, adrenal insufficiency, and red hair pigmentation, which reflects the lack of pituitary neuropeptides acting as ligands for MC4R, MC1R, and MC2R, respectively [101–103].

Several nonsyndromic monogenic forms of obesity are related to mutations in the melanocortin MC4R receptor gene [104]. More than 30 different mutations of the MC4R receptor have been described in French [105], English [106], Italian [107], Japanese [108], and Spanish [109] populations. The general endocrine and metabolic phenotype presents as moderate to severe obesity; slight and nonsignificant alteration of the hypothalamic–pituitary–adrenal axis; and normal neuroendocrine functions regarding growth, reproduction, and thyroid function. When analyzed, these mutations present haploinsufficiency instead of a negative dominant mechanism. In contrast to the very rare mutations of the leptin gene, the leptin receptor, or POMC, the frequency of mutations in the MC4R gene ranges from 1% to 5% in different populations and in subjects with a BMI > 40 [43, 47, 104], although other groups have reported frequencies as low as 0.5% [110]. In a recent study that included 500 extremely obese children, 29 had mutations for the MC4R gene [111]. Children homozygous for such mutations had a BMI higher than heterozygous controls. The heterozygous carriers of a total loss-of-function mutation had a BMI higher than heterozygotes carrying a partial signaling mutation of the receptor. The signaling properties of the mutant receptor assayed in cell culture were correlated with the severity of obesity. These findings show that obesity secondary to mutations in the MC4R gene is associated with a codominant inheritance and highly resembles common complex obesity rather than the other monogenic disorders; however, its appearance begins at a very early age and the patients have hyperphagia that tends to disappear toward adulthood. It has also been suggested that the altered signaling of the mutant MC4R could be related to the development of hyperinsulinemia. Such a relationship leads one to consider the MC4R as a "real" thrifty gene through its action in promoting energy expenditure, making the receptor an excellent target for the development of drugs for treatment of the metabolic syndrome [111–114].

6.2.   Genetic Contribution to Common Human Obesity

6.2.1.   Candidate gene studies.   The candidate genes that have been studied extensively include the ones involved in the regulation of energy balance such as uncoupling proteins (UCPs), the nuclear receptor PPARγ, and the β-adrenergic receptor β3-AR, as well as the genes for leptin and the leptin receptor, discussed above. Positive associations with phenotypes for obesity have currently been reported in more than 70 genes [10]. Two examples of variants in candidate genes are (a) a mutation Trp64Arg in β3-AR [115, 116] and (b) another common variant, Pro12Ala, of the isoform γ2 in the gene of the PPARγ receptor [117]. It has been suggested that the variant Trp64Arg of β3-AR acts as a modifier of other candidate genes. Such gene × gene interaction is proposed to increase the probability that a given subject will accumulate more adipose tissue if the adrenergic receptor variant coexists with other variants already identified, such as a variant of the α_{2b}-adrenoceptor gene [118], the isoform PPARγ2, or the coactivator of PPARγ, PPARGC1 [23, 119].

In mature adipocytes of the brown adipose tissue, stimulation of the β-adrenergic receptor by norepinephrine activates UCP-1 via cyclic adenosine monophosphate (cAMP). The UCP are transporters of the inner mitochondrial membrane that dissipate the proton gradient, releasing stored energy as heat [120]. An A-3826G variant in UCP-1 has been associated with an increase in fat mass in a Quebec family study [121]. Additional effects between the allele A-3826G and the mutation Trp64Arg of the β3-AR receptor were found in a morbidly obese French population [122]. Synergistic effects between the same allele of UCP-1 and the mutation of the adrenergic receptor have been shown to diminish sympathetic nervous activity and affect serum lipid concentration in Japanese populations [123, 124]. Similarly, associations have been found between uncoupling protein polymorphisms (UCP2-UCP3) and energy metabolism/obesity in Pima Indians [125]. The Trp64Arg mutation has been correlated with weight gain, obesity, and insulin resistance in Pima Indians, French, and Finnish populations [126–128]. On the other hand, discordant studies have also been published regarding this particular topic, including family studies in Quebec and Sweden [129]. Thus the status of Trp64Arg remains controversial, illustrating the difficulties facing the candidate gene approach.

The conflicting results from some candidate gene studies require deeper investigation. Possible reasons for not being able to reproduce results include the admixture and stratification of the populations being studied, small sample sizes yielding low statistical power, different genes operating in different populations, variation in linkage disequilibrium among populations [130], or low likelihood that the genes would be involved in the general risk for the development of the disease [131].

To obtain reliable results it has been suggested that the size of the studied sample should be large, that the experimental design include case-control studies based in families, and that the findings should be replicated in other populations of similar ethnic origin. It is also important to choose a plausible candidate gene based on some criteria, which may include that its chromosomal location be very near to a locus linked to obesity in humans or animal models (positional candidate); that its expression profile be able to respond to environmental modifications in, for example, adipocyte, muscle, or hypothalamus; that its expression be shown to be regulated by food intake or physical activity; or that its overexpression or knockout be feasible and shown to manipulate the body weight in animal models. Ideally, a candidate gene should fulfill at least two of these recommendations prior to the screening of a large number of individuals [132–135].

6.2.2.   Genome scan studies.   All research designs using genome scans involve the use of genetic polymorphisms frequently and [ideally] uniformly distributed throughout the genome. The kind of polymorphism most commonly used is the microsatellite marker, owing to its abundance and high heterozygosity. Analysis is usually performed on either sibling pairs or extended pedigrees; the latter provide much more information but may present additional difficulties in recruitment. The latter design includes families extended to several generations, including second- and third-degree relatives, and makes it easier to correlate the given phenotype to markers inherited identical by descent (IBD) [10, 136, 137]. Computer simulations show that with the appropriate study design and a pedigreed sample of adequate size, individual genes that contribute as little as 10% of the variance in a trait can be localized to specific chromosomal regions (QTLs) using the variance component approach [138].

Since the publication of the first human genome scans for phenotypes related to obesity nearly a decade ago, a fair number of studies have reported highly significant linkages, with several findings being replicated.

Among the first, and still perhaps one of the strongest, QTL effects in humans for a phenotype related to obesity comes from the San Antonio Family Heart Study (SAFHS) [139]. A locus influencing serum leptin levels was found on chromosome 2p22 using the variance components approach, with highly significant linkage measured as a log odds ratio (LOD) score of 7.5 [139, 140]. (The LOD score compares the probability of linkage at a given locus to the null probability of no linkage; a LOD of at least 3 is taken as significant evidence of linkage [34].) This QTL has been replicated in both French (LOD = 2.4–2.7) and African-American [141, 142] family studies. Significant linkage has also been detected in the SAFHS on chromosome 8 for both leptin (LOD = 3.1) and BMI (LOD = 3.2), as well as on chromosome 17 for BMI (LOD = 3.2) [143–145]. The QTL on chromosome 2 is very close to the locus for the POMC gene, making this a very strong candidate. In Caucasians, this region of chromosome 2 has shown promising linkage with adiponectin, an adipocyte-derived protein that is inversely expressed with body fat content, and it is believed that it plays a key role in the risk of developing diabetes or coronary artery disease [33, 146, 147]. There has also been evidence of linkage with this chromosomal region and type 2 diabetes in French families (LOD = 2.3).

This last piece of evidence could indicate that the same genes contribute pleiotropically to obesity and diabetes [148]. To date, QTLs have been published for chromosomes 1q21–q24, 2q24, 2q37, 3p21–p24, 3q27, 5q13, 5q31–q33, 6q22–q23, 7p15, 8p21–p22, 9p13–q21, 10q22–q26, 11q21–q24, 12q24, 15q13–q21, 17p11–p12, 18p11, and 20q11–q13 [10, 31, 137]. The identification of these regions in the genome is beginning to show a consistent evidence for linkage with type 2 diabetes [149] and obesity. It is noteworthy that three of these genomic regions (3p, 15p, 20q) show particularly solid linkage for both diabetes and obesity, suggesting an underlying common causative genetic architecture consistent with the epidemiological observations of the cluster of metabolic abnormalities that are simultaneously present in individuals with these pathologies [31, 137]. Several potential candidate genes have been identified in these three regions, notably on chromosome 3, the *APM1* gene, which encodes the adipose cytokine adiponectin; the glucose transporter gene *GLUT2*; and the *ApoD* gene, which encodes an integral part of the structure of the high-density lipoprotein HDL; on chromosome 15, the gene for the insulin-like growth factor 1 receptor (IGF-1R); and on chromosome 20, the gene encoding the agouti-signaling protein (ASIP), a potent inhibitor of MC3R and MC4R; *GNAS1*, whose variants have been associated to Albright hereditary osteodystrophy; and the gene *CEBPB* (CAAT/enhancer-binding-protein β), which plays a significant role in adipocyte differentiation [31].

A recent significant finding from a genome-wide scan for obesity was obtained from more than 10,000 individuals. The authors found a locus in chromosome 4p15–p14 with a non-parametric linkage score of 11.3, showing a significant linkage with severe obesity in women. The genetic variants within the linkage region have not yet been described [150].

6.2.3.   LD mapping and expression studies.   *SNPs.* The use of single nucleotide polymorphisms (SNPs) has recently become of great interest within the genetic community. A SNP can be a functional mutation or can be in linkage disequilibrium with a functional variant. SNPs are the most abundant variants in the human genome: they can be found on an average of once each 1.3 kb within the genome, and they are usually biallelic. As they are very common, by targeting them it is possible to narrow the region in the genome that must be searched for genes [151]. Traditional microsatellite-based linkage studies generally identify relatively large genomic regions of 10 to 30 centiMorgans (cM), so that extensive efforts of fine mapping are necessary to accurately pinpoint a QTL toward a narrower genomic region of less than 1 cM [152].

The use of linkage disequilibrium mapping has recently been proposed as more efficient than the traditional linkage analysis to detect more precise genomic regions involved in the biology of complex diseases such as obesity, through the development of several genome scans combined with linkage disequilibrium to map pertinent genes [153]. Theoretically, it is assumed that a useful level of linkage disequilibrium is confined to an average distance of less than 3 kb in the general population, which implies that approximately 50,000 SNPs are required for a whole-genome linkage disequilibrium study [154]. However, other investigators have suggested that this number could be reduced to 30,000 SNPs, which would make SNP-based genome scanning adaptable to chip-based technology [155].

Linkage disequilibrium. A very strong aspect directing the interest in this approach is evidence that the SNPs assemble themselves in linkage disequilibrium blocks or allelic associations, such that genotyping a single SNP would predict the genotype of other nearby SNPs. This fact indicates that it is feasible to identify haplotype blocks in extensive parts of the genome, by genotyping several "key" informative SNPs, making this approach highly attractive once haplotype blocks have been identified within the human genome [156]. This approach seems to represent a more accessible way to identify causative genetic variations by genotyping a selection of evenly spaced SNPs, relying on linkage disequilibrium between the disease variant and a nearby typed marker. Therefore, once gene candidates have been identified in the genome scan, the screening of SNPs in these genes may eventually lead us to identify those variants contributing to complex disease generation [157, 158].

Attempts to define these blocks of linkage disequilibrium to generate a haplotype map have already started. If this map is obtained, only a few key SNPs would be required to identify the haplotypes. There is no doubt that this approach would greatly accelerate the search for disease-susceptibility genes when combined with population-based association studies [159, 160]. The completion of the human genome sequence, the construction of the SNP map (also known as the "HapMap" [156]), and the characterization of the linkage disequilibrium patterns in human populations has resulted in the successful identification of a susceptibility gene for type 2 diabetes, *NIDDM1*, on chromosome 2 in Mexican-Americans and a Northern European Finnish population. *NIDDM1* encodes a member of the family of calpain-like cysteine proteases, calpain-10 (CAPN10) [160].

Nevertheless, it has been noted that the degree and the extent of linkage disequilibrium vary enormously throughout the genome and are highly unpredictable, implying that a causative variation of the disease could be juxtaposed to a genotyped marker yet produce no noticeable disequilibrium [161, 162]. This fact has led to a hot debate between genetic experts and remains an important question to be resolved [163].

6.2.4.   Expression studies.   Application of association methods would benefit from more efficient identification of candidate genes. A recent approach uses mRNA expression in tissue samples to identify genes that may be important in the development of complex diseases, especially when expression differs in normal and disease states. A wide variety of RNA-based technologies can be used to identify changes in the genetic expression of several tissues in obesity and type 2 diabetes [164]. The most solid techniques comprise differential display polymerase chain reaction (ddPCR), representational difference analysis (RDA), selective subtraction hybridization (SSH), and cDNA microarrays. All of these techniques could be applied to human tissues in expression studies, but for reasons related to feasibility, or to the inherent risk of biopsy of the pertinent tissues, such approaches are more commonly applied to animal models that reflect the pathologic human condition under investigation [165].

An outstanding animal model for the study of obesity and type 2 diabetes is the Israeli sand rat *Psammomys obesus* (*P. obesus*). These animals are native to North Africa and the Middle East and when in the wild state are slim and normoglycemic. When in captivity and fed conventional rat chow diets, 50% of adults at 16 weeks of age develop obesity, and among these, 30% eventually develop type 2 diabetes [166]. Using RNA ddPCR techniques in this animal model, a new gene has been encountered with properties appearing to play a key role in the pathophysiology of type 2 diabetes. It was named tanis, which means "fasting" in Hebrew. Its primary expression is in the liver and is markedly increased in diabetic sand rats in the fasting state. The complete sequence of the tanis mRNA in *P. obesus* has been obtained. It consists of 1,155 base pairs, and the encoded protein product has 189 amino acids. The corresponding human gene has been located in the chromosome 15q26.3 and the expected human tanis protein is estimated to be 187 amino acids long with a molecular mass of 21 kDa. Hepatic expression of tanis secondary to a 24-hour fasting in *P. obesus* with type 2 diabetes showed a threefold greater increase than in the nondiabetic control group of sand rats. Multiple linear regression analysis showed that only blood glucose concentrations were independently associated with the genetic expression of tanis. Taking these data together, the results show strong evidence indicating that the glucose levels are the key regulators of hepatic tanis expression, and that this gene is differentially expressed in type 2 diabetes. A very interesting observation is the strong interaction between tanis protein and the hepatic acute-phase reactant serum amyloid A (SAA). It appears that tanis possesses receptor properties that allow it to bind the inflammatory protein SAA. This and other acute-phase proteins have been the center of recent attention as risk markers for cardiovascular disease. The authors suspect that tanis and the acute-phase protein SAA may be a strong mechanistic link between obesity, type 2 diabetes, inflammation, and cardiovascular disease [167, 168].

In isolation, either DNA-based or RNA-based methods have limitations in their ability to identify candidate genes for complex diseases. As noted, genome-wide scans identify large DNA regions containing hundreds or perhaps thousands of genes, and fine-mapping is often costly and time-consuming. On the other hand, RNA-based methodologies can identify hundreds of differentially expressed genes, requiring detailed functional assays to determine which genes are actually important in the development of a given disease. For these reasons, recent attempts have been made to combine information from differential expression studies with data obtained from genome scans. With this approach, researchers have been able to achieve a substantial synergy in the identification of candidate genes [139].

An example of this combined approach is the recent discovery of beacon, a novel protein that appears to play a key role in the regulation of energy balance. This protein is differentially expressed in the hypothalamus of lean and obese *Psammomys obesus*. Its sequencing has revealed a mRNA of 413 bp encoding a 73-amino-acid protein with a predicted size of 8.6 kDa. High levels of expression of this protein in the hypothalamus of *P. obesus* have already been confirmed. A linear relationship has been established between the expression of the beacon gene and either body weight or percentage of body fat [169]. Beacon is predominantly expressed in the retrochiasmatic nucleus of the hypothalamus, a region already known for its involvement in the control of appetite, through neurons that express orexigenic and anorexigenic neuropeptides such as neuropeptide Y (NPY), agouti-related protein (AgRP), cocaine-amphetamine regulated transcriptor, proopiomelanocortine (POMC), α-melanocyte stimulating hormone (α-MSH), among others. This pattern of expression suggests the strong possibility that beacon could interact with these anabolic and catabolic intrahypothalamic systems that centrally control food intake and energy balance [170]. The beacon human homolog was identified as the ubiquitin-like 5 gene, localized to chromosome 19p13. Several studies have previously shown linkage and/or association between this genomic region and traits related to obesity, such as plasma leptin concentrations and body fat content. Genomic regions linked to obesity in rat and mouse and syntenic with human chromosome 19p13 have also been identified [171, 172]. Therefore it seems evident that one or several genes located in chromosome 19q13 may definitively be involved in the control of adipose tissue metabolism. Beacon is an excellent candidate gene for obesity based both on its genomic location and its pattern of expression in the sand rat. Recent studies indicate that beacon genetic expression increases in the hypothalamus of *P. obesus* before their increase in body weight in those animals with a genetic predisposition for the development of obesity and type 2 diabetes. This fact might indicate that this elevation could be an early marker for the metabolic abnormalities seen in both pathologies [173].

7.   CONCLUSION

Obesity is a complex disease involving multiple genes and strong interactions between gene–environment interaction. Underlying variation that went unnoticed (and may have been beneficial) when food was scarce and humans led more physically active lifestyles, has contributed to an epidemic of metabolic disease in an increasingly Westernized, technological world. Because of its complex causation, obesity, like many other common disorders, does not yield to simple Mendelian analysis. The development of tools adequate for analysis of complex disease is relatively new.

Despite its complexity, much progress has been made in understanding the causes of obesity and its related disorders. Insights have come from animal models and from rare monogenic disorders that reveal individual components of the complex pathways regulating energy homeostasis. For common complex human obesity, a range of techniques has become available. Candidate genes identified from known biochemical pathways can be evaluated by association analysis and expression studies to learn if natural variation in these genes is responsible for variation in the disease. Genome linkage analyses of related individuals offer the chance to identify novel genes and pathways as well as to confirm and prioritize candidate genes.

All these techniques continue to offer surprises. While research continues into variation in energy expenditure, we have also discovered the unexpected importance of the neuroendocrine control of appetite. For example, identification of leptin from linkage studies, first in mice and subsequently in humans, has revealed an intricate pathway of feedback control and has changed our view of adipose tissue from passive storage to active endocrine organ. As discoveries multiply, we gain new opportunities for therapeutic intervention in a potentially devastating disease. We also gain new appreciation for the exquisite systems that regulate energy acquisition, storage, and use.

ACKNOWLEDGMENTS

This work was supported by Grants HL28972, MH59490, and RR013986 from the National Institutes of Health.

REFERENCES

[1] World Health Organization. Obesity: Preventing and Managing the Global Epidemic. Geneva: World Health Organization, 1998.

[2] Froguel P, Boutin P. Genetics of pathways regulating body weight in the development of obesity in humans. Exp Biol Med 2001;226:991–996.

[3] Wyatt HR. The prevalence of obesity. Prim Care 2003;30:267–279.

[4] Friedrich MJ. Epidemic of obesity expands its spread to developing countries. JAMA 2002;287:1382–1386.

[5] Popkin BM, Lu B, Zhai F. Understanding the nutrition transition: Measuring rapid dietary changes in transitional countries. Public Health Nutr 2002;5:947–953.

[6] Comuzzie AG, Williams JT, Martin LJ, Blangero J. Searching for genes underlying normal variation in human adiposity. J Mol Med 2001;79:57–70.

[7] Wadden TA, Brownell KD, Foster GD. Obesity: Responding to the global epidemic. J Consult Clin Psychol 2002;70:510–525.

[8] Loos RJ, Bouchard C. Obesity—is it a genetic disorder? J Intern Med 2003;254:401–425.

[9] Comuzzie AG, Allison DB. The search for human obesity genes. Science 1998;280: 1374–1377.

[10] Chagnon YC, Rankinen T, Snyder EE, et al. The human obesity gene map: The 2002 update. Obes Res 2003;11:313–367.

[11] Eaton SB, Konner M, Shostak M. Stone agers in the fast lane: Chronic degenerative diseases in evolutionary perspective. Am J Med 1988;84:739–749.

[12] Neel JV, Weder A, Julius S. Type II diabetes, essential hypertension and obesity as "syndromes of impaired genetic homeostasis": The "thrifty genotype" hypothesis enters the 21st century. Perspect Biol Med 1998;42:44–74.

[13] Neel JV. Diabetes mellitus: A "thrifty" genotype rendered detrimental by "progress"? 1962. Bull World Health Organ 1999;77:694–703.

[14] Bjorntorp P. Thrifty genes and human obesity. Are we chasing ghosts? Lancet 2001;358: 1006–1008.

[15] Kagawa Y, Yanagisawa Y, Hasegawa K, et al. Single nucleotide polymorphisms of thrifty genes for energy metabolism: Evolutionary origins and prospects for intervention to prevent obesity-related diseases. Biochem Biophys Res Commun 2002;295:207–222.

[16] Flatt JP. The difference in the storage capacities for carbohydrate and for fat, and its implications in the regulation of body weight. Ann NY Acad Sci 1987;499:104–123.

[17] Stubbs RJ, Mazlan N, Whybrow S. Carbohydrates, appetite and feeding behavior in humans. J Nutr 2001;131:2775S–2781S.

[18] Poston WS II, Foreyt JP. Obesity is an environmental issue. Atherosclerosis 1999;146: 201–209.

[19] Jequier E. Pathways to obesity. Int J Obes Relat Metab Disord 2002;26(Suppl 2):S12–S17.

[20] Zimmet P, Thomas CR. Genotype, obesity and cardiovascular disease—has technical and social advancement outstripped evolution? J Intern Med 2003;254:114–125.

[21] Arner P. Obesity—a genetic disease of adipose tissue? Br J Nutr 2000;83(1):S9–S16.

[22] Clement K, Boutin P, Froguel P. Genetics of obesity. Am J Pharmacog 2002;2:177–187.

[23] Shuldiner AR, Munir KM. Genetics of obesity: More complicated than initially thought. Lipids 2003;38:97–101.

[24] National Institute of Diabetes and Digestive and Kidney Diseases (NIDDK). The Pima Indians: Pathfinders for health. 2002;http://diabetes.niddk.nih.gov/dm/pubs/pima/index. htm

[25] Knowler WC, Pettit DJ, Saad MF, et al. Obesity in the Pima Indians: its magnitude and relationship with diabetes. Am J Clin Nutr 1991;53(Suppl 6):1543S–1551S.

[26] Ravussin E, Valencia ME, Esparza J, et al. Effects of a traditional lifestyle on obesity in Pima Indians. Diabetes Care 1994;17:1067–1074.

[27] Liu YJ, Araujo S, Recker RR, Deng HW. Molecular and genetic mechanisms of obesity: Implications for future management. Curr Mol Med 2003;3:325–340.

[28] Zielenski J, Tsui LC. Cystic fibrosis: Genotypic and phenotypic variations. Annu Rev Genet 1995;29:777–807.

[29] Broeckel U, Schork NJ. Identifying genes and genetic variation underlying human diseases and complex phenotypes via recombination mapping. J Physiol 2004;554(1):40–45.

[30] Rankinen T, Perusse L, Weisnagel SJ, et al. The human obesity gene map: The 2001 update. Obes Res 2002;10:196–243.

[31] Walder K, Segal D, Jowett J, Blangero J, Collier GR. Obesity and diabetes gene discovery approaches. Curr Pharm Des 2003;9:1357–1372.

[32] Rogers J, Mahaney MC, Almasy L, Comuzzie AG, Blangero J. Quantitative trait linkage mapping in anthropology. Am J Phys Anthropol Suppl 1999;29:127–151.

[33] Comuzzie AG, Funahashi T, Sonnenberg G, et al. The genetic basis of plasma variation in adiponectin, a global endophenotype for obesity and the metabolic syndrome. J Clin Endocrinol Metab 2001;86:4321–4325.

[34] Lander E, Kruglyak L. Genetic dissection of complex traits: Guidelines for interpreting and reporting linkage results. Nat Genet 1995;11:241–247.

[35] McPherson JD, Marra M, Hillier L, et al. A physical map of the human genome. Nature 2001;409:934–941.

[36] Wille A, Leal SM. Novel selection criteria for genome scans of complex traits. Genet Epidemiol 2001;21(Suppl 1):S800–S804.

[37] Blangero J, Williams JT, Almasy L. Variance component methods for detecting complex trait loci. Adv Genet 2001;42:151–181.

[38] Venter JC, Adams MD, Myers EW, et al. The sequence of the human genome. Science 2001;291:1304–1351.

[39] Comuzzie AG. The emerging pattern of the genetic contribution to human obesity. Best Pract Res Clin Endocrinol Metab 2002;16:611–621.

[40] Echwald SM. Genetics of human obesity: Lessons from mouse models and candidate genes. J Intern Med 1999; 245:653–666.

[41] Sorensen TI, Echwald SM. Obesity genes. BMJ 2001;322:630–631.

[42] Brockmann GA, Bevova MR. Using mouse models to dissect the genetics of obesity. Trends. Genet 2002;18:367–376.

[43] Zhang Y, Proenca R, Maffei M, Barone M, Leopold L, Friedman JM. Positional cloning of the mouse obese gene and its human homologue. Nature 1994;372:425–432.

[44] Tartaglia LA, Dembski M, Weng X, et al. Identification and expression cloning of a leptin receptor, OB-R. Cell 1995;83:1263–1271.

[45] Chen H, Charlat O, Tartaglia LA, et al. Evidence that the diabetes gene encodes the leptin receptor: Identification of a mutation in the leptin receptor gene in db/db mice. Cell 1996;84:491–495.

[46] Miller MW, Duhl DM, Vrieling H, et al. Cloning of the mouse agouti gene predicts a secreted protein ubiquitously expressed in mice carrying the lethal yellow mutation. Genes Dev 1993;7:454–467.

[47] Barsh GS, Farooqi IS, O'Rahilly S. Genetics of body-weight regulation. Nature 2000; 404:644–651.

[48] Robinson SW, Dinulescu DM, Cone RD. Genetic models of obesity and energy balance in the mouse. Annu Rev Genet 2000;34:687–745.

[49] Miller KA, Gunn TM, Carrasquillo MM, Lamoreux ML, Galbraith DB, Barsh GS. Genetic studies of the mouse mutations mahogany and mahoganoid. Genetics 1997;146:1407–1415.

[50] Gunn TM, Miller KA, He L, et al. The mouse mahogany locus encodes a transmembrane form of human attractin. Nature 1999;398:152–156.

[51] Nagle DL, McGrail SH, Vitale J, et al. The mahogany protein is a receptor involved in suppression of obesity. Nature 1999;398:148–152.

[52] Jackson RS, Creemers JW, Ohagi S, et al. Obesity and impaired prohormone processing associated with mutations in the human prohormone convertase 1 gene. Nat Genet 1997;16:303–306.

[53] Cawley NX, Rodríguez YM, Maldonado A, Loh YP. Trafficking of mutant carboxypeptidase E to secretory granules in a beta-cell line derived from Cpe(fat)/Cpe(fat) mice. Endocrinology 2003;144:292–298.

[54] Augustine KA, Rossi RM. Rodent mutant models of obesity and their correlations to human obesity. Anat Rec 1999;257:64–72.

[55] Santagata S, Boggon TJ, Baird CL, et al. G-protein signaling through tubby proteins. Science 2001;292:2041–2050.

[56] Fisler JS, Warden CH. Mapping of mouse obesity genes: A generic approach to a complex trait. J Nutr 1997;127:1909S–1916S.

[57] Pomp D. Animal models of obesity. Mol Med Today 1999;5:459–460.

[58] Inui A. Obesity—a chronic health problem in cloned mice? Trends Pharmacol Sci 2003; 24:77–80.

[59] Pomp D. Genetic dissection of obesity in polygenic animal models. Behav Genet 1997; 27:285–306.

[60] Moody DE, Pomp D, Nielsen NK, Van Vleck LD. Identification of quantitative trait loci influencing traits related to energy balance in selection and inbred lines of mice. Genetics 1999;152:699–711.

[61] Smith BK, Andrews PK, West DB. Macronutrient diet selection in thirteen mouse strains. Am J Physiol Regul Integr Comp Physiol 2000; 278:R797–R805.

[62] Paigen B. Genetics of responsiveness to high-fat and high-cholesterol diets in the mouse. Am J Clin Nutr 1995;62:458S–462S.

[63] West DB, Waguespack J, McColister S. Dietary obesity in the mouse: Interaction of strain with diet composition. Am J Physiol 1995;268:R658–R665.

[64] Maeda N, Shimomura I, Kishida K, et al. Diet-induced insulin resistance in mice lacking adiponectin/ACRP30. Nat Med 2002;8:731–737.

[65] Smith Richards BK, Belton BN, Poole AC, et al. QTL analysis of self-selected macro-nutrient diet intake: Fat, carbohydrate, and total kilocalories. Physiol Genomics 2002;11: 205–217.

[66] Warden CH, Fisler JS, Shoemaker SM. Identification of four chromosomal loci determining obesity in a multifactorial mouse model. J Clin Invest 1995;95:1545–1552.

[67] York B, Truett AA, Monteiro MP, et al. Gene-environment interaction: A significant diet-dependent obesity locus demonstrated in a congenic segment on mouse chromosome 7. Mamm Genome 1999;10:457–462.

[68] Livingston JN. Genetically engineered mice in drug development. J Intern Med 1999;245: 627–635.

[69] Lee K, Villena JA, Moon YS, et al. Inhibition of adipogenesis and development of glucose intolerance by soluble preadipocyte factor-1 (Pref-1). J Clin Invest 2003;111:453–461.

[70] Stubdal H, Lynch CA, Moriarty A, et al. Targeted deletion of the tub mouse obesity gene reveals that tubby is a loss-of-function mutation. Mol Cell Biol 2000;20:878–882.

[71] Majdic G, Young M, Gomez-Sanchez E, et al. Knockout mice lacking steroidogenic factor 1 are a novel genetic model of hypothalamic obesity. Endocrinology 2002;143:607–614.

[72] Gunay-Aygun M, Cassidy SB, Nicholls RD. Prader–Willi and other syndromes associated with obesity and mental retardation. Behav Genet 1997;27:307–324.

[73] Wigren M, Hansen S. Prader–Willi syndrome: Clinical picture, psychosocial support and current management. Child Care Health Dev 2003;29: 449–456.

[74] Gallagher RC, Pils B, Albalwi M, Francke U. Evidence for the role of PWCR1/HBII-85 C/D box small nucleolar RNAs in Prader–Willi syndrome. Am J Hum Genet 2002;71: 669–678.

[75] Sheffield VC, Nishimura D, Stone EM. The molecular genetics of Bardet–Biedl syndrome. Curr Opin Genet Dev 2001;11:317–321.

[76] Nishimura DY, Searby CC, Carmi R, et al. Positional cloning of a novel gene on chromosome 16q causing Bardet–Biedl syndrome (BBS2). Hum Mol Genet 2001;10:865–874.

[77] Mykytyn K, Braun T, Carmi R, et al. Identification of the gene that, when mutated, causes the human obesity syndrome BBS4. Nat Genet 2001;28:188–191.

[78] Slavotinek AM, Searby C, Al-Gazali L, et al. Mutation analysis of the MKKS gene in McKusick–Kaufman syndrome and selected Bardet–Biedl syndrome patients. Hum Genet 2002;110:561–567.

[79] Badano JL, Ansley SJ, Leitch CC, Lewis RA, Lupski JR, Katsanis N. Identification of a novel Bardet–Biedl syndrome protein, BBS7, that shares structural features with BBS1 and BBS2. Am J Hum Genet 2003;72:650–658.

[80] Mykytyn K, Nishimura DY, Searby CC, et al. Evaluation of complex inheritance involving the most common Bardet–Biedl syndrome locus (BBS1). Am J Hum Genet 2003;72:429–437.

[81] Reed DR, Ding Y, Xu W, Cather C, Price RA. Human obesity does not segregate with the chromosomal regions of Prader–Willi, Bardet–Biedl, Cohen, Borjeson or Wilson–Turner syndromes. Int J Obes Relat Metab Disord 1995;19:599–603.

[82] Coleman DL. Effects of parabiosis of obese with diabetes and normal mice. Diabetologia 1973;9:294–298.

[83] Coleman DL. Inherited obesity–diabetes syndromes in the mouse. Prog Clin Biol Res 1981;45:145–158.

[84] Jeanrenaud B, Rohner-Jeanrenaud F. Effects of neuropeptides and leptin on nutrient partitioning: Dysregulations in obesity. Annu Rev Med 2001; 52:339–351.

[85] Margetic S, Gazzola C, Pegg GG, Hill RA. Leptin: A review of its peripheral actions and interactions. Int J Obes Relat Metab Disord 2002;26:1407–1433.

[86] Cummings DE, Schwartz MW. Genetics and pathophysiology of human obesity. Annu Rev Med 2003;54:453–471.

[87] Schwartz MW, Woods SC, Seeley RJ, Barsh GS, Baskin DG, Leibel RL. Is the energy homeostasis system inherently biased toward weight gain? Diabetes 2003;52:232–238.

[88] Montague CT, Farooqi IS, Whitehead JP, et al. Congenital leptin deficiency is associated with severe early-onset obesity in humans. Nature 1997;387:903–908.

[89] Strobel A, Issad T, Camoin L, Ozata M, Strosberg AD. 1998. A leptin missense mutation associated with hypogonadism and morbid obesity. Nat Genet 1998;18:213–215.

[90] Rau H, Reaves BJ, O'Rahilly S, Whitehead JP. Truncated human leptin (delta133) associated with extreme obesity undergoes proteasomal degradation after defective intracellular transport. Endocrinology 1999;140:1718–1723.

[91] Farooqi IS, Keogh JM, Kamath S, et al. Partial leptin deficiency and human adiposity. Nature 2001;414:34–35.

[92] Farooqi S, Rau H, Whitehead J, O'Rahilly S. ob gene mutations and human obesity. Proc Nutr Soc 1998;57:471–475.

[93] Ozata M, Ozdemir IC, Licinio J. Human leptin deficiency caused by a missense mutation: Multiple endocrine defects, decreased sympathetic tone, and immune system dysfunction indicate new targets for leptin action, greater central than peripheral resistance to the effects of leptin, and spontaneous correction of leptin-mediated defects. J Clin Endocrinol Metab 1999;84:3686–3695.

[94] Farooqi IS, Jebb SA, Langmack G, et al. Effects of recombinant leptin therapy in a child with congenital leptin deficiency. N Engl J Med 1999;341:879–884.

[95] Farooqi IS, Matarese G, Lord GM, et al. Beneficial effects of leptin on obesity, T cell hyporesponsiveness, and neuroendocrine/metabolic dysfunction of human congenital leptin deficiency. J Clin Invest 2002;110:1093–1103.

[96] Clement K, Vaisse C, Lahlou N, et al. A mutation in the human leptin receptor gene causes obesity and pituitary dysfunction. Nature 1998;392:398–401.

[97] Challis BG, Pritchard LE, Creemers JW, et al. A missense mutation disrupting a dibasic prohormone processing site in pro-opiomelanocortin (POMC) increases susceptibility to early-onset obesity through a novel molecular mechanism. Hum Mol Genet 2002;11:1997–2004.

[98] MacNeil DJ, Howard AD, Guan X, et al. The role of melanocortins in body weight regulation: Opportunities for the treatment of obesity. Eur J Pharmacol 2002;450:93–109.

[99] Pritchard LE, Turnbull AV, White A. Pro-opiomelanocortin processing in the hypothalamus: Impact on melanocortin signalling and obesity. J Endocrinol 2002;172:411–421.

[100] Voisey J, Carroll L, van Daal A. Melanocortins and their receptors and antagonists. Curr Drug Targets 2003;4:586–597.

[101] Wardlaw SL. Clinical review 127: Obesity as a neuroendocrine disease: Lessons to be learned from proopiomelanocortin and melanocortin receptor mutations in mice and men. J Clin Endocrinol Metab 2001;86:1442–1446.

[102] Krude H, Biebermann H, Gruters A. Mutations in the human proopiomelanocortin gene. Ann NY Acad Sci 2003a;994:233–239.

[103] Krude H, Biebermann H, Schnabel D, et al. Obesity due to proopiomelanocortin deficiency: Three new cases and treatment trials with thyroid hormone and ACTH4-10. J Clin Endocrinol Metab 2003b;88:4633–4640.

[104] Hinney A, Schmidt A, Nottebom K, et al. Several mutations in the melanocortin-4 receptor gene including a nonsense and a frameshift mutation associated with dominantly inherited obesity in humans. Clin Endocrinol Metab 1999;84:1483–1486.

[105] Vaisse C, Clement K, Durand E, Hercberg S, Guy-Grand B, Froguel P. Melanocortin-4 receptor mutations are a frequent and heterogeneous cause of morbid obesity. Clin Invest 2000;106:253–262.

[106] Farooqi IS, Yeo GS, Keogh JM, et al. Dominant and recessive inheritance of morbid obesity associated with melanocortin 4 receptor deficiency. Clin Invest 2000;106:271–279.

[107] Miraglia Del Giudice E, Cirillo G, Nigro V, et al. Low frequency of melanocortin-4 receptor (MC4R) mutations in a Mediterranean population with early-onset obesity. Int J Obes Relat Metab Disord 2002;26:647–651.

[108] Kobayashi H, Ogawa Y, Shintani M, et al. A novel homozygous missense mutation of melanocortin-4 receptor (MC4R) in a Japanese woman with severe obesity. Diabetes 2002;51:243–246.

[109] Marti A, Corbalan MS, Forga L, Martinez JA, Hinney A, Hebebrand J. A novel nonsense mutation in the melanocortin-4 receptor associated with obesity in a Spanish population. Int J Obes Relat Metab Disord 2003;27:385–388.

[110] Jacobson P, Ukkola O, Rankinen T, et al. Melanocortin 4 receptor sequence variations are seldom a cause of human obesity: The Swedish Obese Subjects, the HERITAGE Family Study, and a Memphis cohort. J Clin Endocrinol Metab 2002;87: 4442–4446.

[111] Farooqi IS, Keogh JM, Yeo GS, Lank EJ, Cheetham T, O'Rahilly S. Clinical spectrum of obesity and mutations in the melanocortin-4 receptor gene. N Engl J Med 2003;348: 1085–1095.

[112] Cone RD. Haploinsufficiency of the melanocortin-4 receptor: Part of a thrifty genotype? J Clin Invest 2000;106:185–187.

[113] Branson R, Potoczna N, Kral JG, Lentes KU, Hoehe MR, Horber FF. Binge eating as a major phenotype of melanocortin 4 receptor gene mutations. N Engl J Med 2003; 348:1096–1103.

[114] Lubrano-Berthelier C, Cavazos M, Le Stunff C, et al. The human MC4R promoter: Characterization and role in obesity. Diabetes 2003;52:2996–3000.

[115] Lonnqvist F, Krief S, Strosberg AD, Nyberg S, Emorine LJ, Arner P. Evidence for a functional beta 3-adrenoceptor in man. Br J Pharmacol 1993;110:929–936.

[116] Clement K, Vaisse C, Manning BS, et al. Genetic variation in the beta 3-adrenergic receptor and an increased capacity to gain weight in patients with morbid obesity. N Engl J Med 1995;333:352–354.

[117] Stumvoll M, Haring H. The peroxisome proliferator-activated receptor-gamma2 Pro12Ala polymorphism. Diabetes 2002;51:2341–2347.

[118] Dionne IJ, Turner AN, Tchernof A, et al. Identification of an interactive effect of beta3- and alpha2b-adrenoceptor gene polymorphisms on fat mass in Caucasian women. Diabetes 2001;50:91–95.

[119] Hsueh WC, Cole SA, Shuldiner AR, et al. Interactions between variants in the beta3-adrenergic receptor and peroxisome proliferator-activated receptor-gamma2 genes and obesity. Diabetes Care 2001a;24:672–677.

[120] Argyropoulos G, Harper ME. Uncoupling proteins and thermoregulation. J Appl Physiol 2002;92:2187–2198.

[121] Cassard-Doulcier AM, Bouillaud F, Chagnon M, et al. The Bcl I polymorphism of the human uncoupling protein (ucp) gene is due to a point mutation in the 5′-flanking region. Int J Obes Relat Metab Disord 1996;20:278–279.

[122] Clement K, Ruiz J, Cassard-Doulcier AM, et al. Additive effect of A → G (-3826) variant of the uncoupling protein gene and the Trp64Arg mutation of the beta 3-adrenergic receptor gene on weight gain in morbid obesity. Int J Obes Relat Metab Disord 1996;20:1062–1066.

[123] Shihara N, Yasuda K, Moritani T, et al. Synergistic effect of polymorphisms of uncoupling protein 1 and beta3-adrenergic receptor genes on autonomic nervous system activity. Int J Obes Relat Metab Disord 2001;25:761–766.

[124] Matsushita H, Kurabayashi T, Tomita M, Kato N, Tanaka K. Effects of uncoupling protein 1 and beta3-adrenergic receptor gene polymorphisms on body size and serum lipid concentrations in Japanese women. Maturitas 2003;45:39–45.

[125] Walder K, Norman RA, Hanson RL, et al. Association between uncoupling protein polymorphisms (UCP2-UCP3) and energy metabolism/obesity in Pima Indians. Hum Mol Genet 1998;7:1431–1435.

[126] Widen E, Lehto M, Kanninen T, Walston J, Shuldiner AR, Groop LC. Association of a polymorphism in the beta 3-adrenergic-receptor gene with features of the insulin resistance syndrome in Finns. N Engl J Med 1995;333:348–351.

[127] Clement K, Manning BS, Basdevant A, Strosberg AD, Guy-Grand B, Froguel P. Gender effect of the Trp64Arg mutation in the beta 3 adrenergic receptor gene on weight gain in morbid obesity. Diabetes Metab 1997;23:424–427.

[128] Oizumi T, Daimon M, Saitoh T, et al. Funagata Diabetes Study. Genotype Arg/Arg, but not Trp/Arg, of the Trp64Arg polymorphism of the beta(3)-adrenergic receptor is associated with type 2 diabetes and obesity in a large Japanese sample. Diabetes Care 2001;24:1579–1583.

[129] Gagnon J, Mauriege P, Roy S, et al. The Trp64Arg mutation of the beta3 adrenergic receptor gene has no effect on obesity phenotypes in the Quebec Family Study and Swedish Obese Subjects cohorts. J Clin Invest 1996;98:2086–2093.

[130] Hirschhorn JN, Lohmueller K, Byrne E, Hirschhorn K. A comprehensive review of genetic association studies. Genet Med 2002;4:45–61.

[131] Risch NJ. Searching for genetic determinants in the new millennium. Nature 2000;405:847–856.

[132] Cardon LR, Bell JI. Association study designs for complex diseases. Nat Rev Genet 2001;2:91–99.

[133] Deng HW, Lai DB, Conway T, et al. Characterization of genetic and lifestyle factors for determining variation in body mass index, fat mass, percentage of fat mass, and lean mass. J Clin Densitom 2001a;4:353–361.

[134] Deng HW, Li J, Recker RR. LOD score exclusion analyses for candidate genes using random population samples. Ann Hum Genet 2001b;65(Pt 3):313–329.

[135] Cooper DN, Nussbaum RL, Krawczak M. Proposed guidelines for papers describing DNA polymorphism-disease associations. Hum Genet 2002;110: 207–208.

[136] Blangero J, Almasy L. Multipoint oligogenic linkage analysis of quantitative traits. Genet Epidemiol 1997;14:959–964.

[137] Elbein SC. Perspective: The search for genes for type 2 diabetes in the post-genome era. Endocrinology 2002;143:2012–2018.

[138] Dyer TD, Blangero J, Williams JT, Goring HH, Mahaney MC. The effect of pedigree complexity on quantitative trait linkage analysis. Genet Epidemiol 2001;21(Suppl 1): S236–S243.

[139] Comuzzie AG, Hixson JE, Almasy L, et al. A major quantitative trait locus determining serum leptin levels and fat mass is located on human chromosome 2. Nat Genet 1997; 15:273–276.

[140] Almasy L, Blangero J. Multipoint quantitative-trait linkage analysis in general pedigrees. Am J Hum Genet 1998;62:1198–1211.

[141] Hager J, Dina C, Francke S, et al. A genome-wide scan for human obesity genes reveals a major susceptibility locus on chromosome 10. Nat Genet 1998;20:304–308.

[142] Rotimi CN, Comuzzie AG, Lowe WL, Luke A, Blangero J, Cooper RS. The quantitative trait locus on chromosome 2 for serum leptin levels is confirmed in African-Americans. Diabetes 1999;48:643–644.

[143] Mitchell BD, Cole SA, Comuzzie AG. A major quantitative trait locus on chromosome 17 is linked to body mass index in Mexican Americans. Circulation 1989;98(Suppl):459.

[144] Mitchell BD, Cole SA, Comuzzie AG, et al. A quantitative trait locus influencing BMI maps to the region of the beta-3 adrenergic receptor. Diabetes 1999;48:1863–1867.

[145] Martin LJ, Cole SA, Hixson JE, et al. Genotype by smoking interaction for leptin levels in the San Antonio Family Heart Study. Genet Epidemiol 2002;22:105–115.

[146] Ouchi N, Kihara S, Funahashi T, Matsuzawa Y, Walsh K. 2003. Obesity, adiponectin and vascular inflammatory disease. Curr Opin Lipidol 2003;14:561–566.

[147] Stefan N, Stumvoll M, Vozarova B, et al. Plasma adiponectin and endogenous glucose production in humans. Diabetes Care 2003;26:3315–3319.

[148] Vionnet N, Hani El-H, Dupont S, et al. Genomewide search for type 2 diabetes-susceptibility genes in French whites: Evidence for a novel susceptibility locus for early-onset diabetes on chromosome 3q27-qter and independent replication of a type 2-diabetes locus on chromosome 1q21-q24. Am J Hum Genet 2000;67:1470–1480.

[149] Duggirala R, Almasy L, Blangero J, et al. and American Diabetes Association GENNID Study Group. Further evidence for a type 2 diabetes susceptibility locus on chromosome 11q. Genet Epidemiol 2003;24:240–242.

[150] Stone S, Abkevich V, Hunt SC, et al. A major predisposition locus for severe obesity at 4p15-p14. Am J Hum Genet 2002;70(6):1459–1468.

[151] Syvanen AC. Accessing genetic variation: Genotyping single nucleotide polymorphisms. Nat Rev Genet 2001; 2:930–942.

[152] Deng HW, Chen WM, Recker RR. QTL fine mapping by measuring and testing for Hardy–Weinberg and linkage disequilibrium at a series of linked marker loci in extreme samples of populations. Am J Hum Genet 2000;66:1027–1045.

[153] Bahring S, Aydin A, Luft FC. The study of gene polymorphisms. How complex is complex genetic disease? Methods Mol Med 2003;86:221–235.

[154] Kruglyak L. Prospects for whole-genome linkage disequilibrium mapping of common disease genes. Nat Genet 1999;22:139–144.

[155] Jorde LB. Linkage disequilibrium and the search for complex disease genes. Genome Res 2000;10:1435–1444.

[156] Gibbs RA, Belmont JW, Hardenbol P, et al. The International HapMap Project. Nature 2003;426:789–796.

[157] Daly MJ, Rioux JD, Schaffner SF, Hudson TJ, Lander ES. High-resolution haplotype structure in the human genome. Nat Genet 2001;29:229–232.

[158] Gabriel SB, Schaffner SF, Nguyen H, et al. The structure of haplotype blocks in the human genome. Science 2002;296:2225–2229.

[159] Cardon LR, Abecasis GR. Using haplotype blocks to map human complex trait loci. Trends Genet 2003;19:135–140.

[160] Horikawa Y, Oda N, Cox NJ, et al. Genetic variation in the gene encoding calpain-10 is associated with type 2 diabetes mellitus. Nat Genet 2000;26:163–175.

[161] Abecasis GR, Noguchi E, Heinzmann A, et al. Extent and distribution of linkage disequilibrium in three genomic regions. Am J Hum Genet 2001;68:191–197.

[162] Reich DE, Cargill M, Bolk S, et al. Linkage disequilibrium in the human genome. Nature 2001;411:199–204.

[163] Couzin J. Genomics. New mapping project splits the community. Science 2002;296:1391–1393.

[164] Cox LA, Birnbaum S, VandeBerg JL. Identification of candidate genes regulating HDL cholesterol using a chromosomal region expression array. Genome Res 2002;12:1693–1702.

[165] Burgess JK. Gene expression studies using microarrays. Clin Exp Pharmacol Physiol 2001;28:321–328.

[166] Walder KR, Fahey RP, Morton GJ, Zimmet PZ, Collier GR. Characterization of obesity phenotypes in *Psammomys obesus* (Israeli sand rats). Int J Exp Diabetes Res 2000b;1:177–184.

[167] Walder K, Kantham L, McMillan JS, et al. Tanis: A link between type 2 diabetes and inflammation? Diabetes 2002a;51:1859–1866.

[168] Gao Y, Walder K, Sunderland T, et al. Elevation in Tanis expression alters glucose metabolism and insulin sensitivity in H4IIE cells. Diabetes 2003;52:929–934.

[169] Collier GR, McMillan JS, Windmill K, et al. Beacon: A novel gene involved in the regulation of energy balance. Diabetes 2000;49:1766–1771.

[170] Sainsbury A, Cooney GJ, Herzog H. Hypothalamic regulation of energy homeostasis. Best Pract Res Clin Endocrinol Metab 2002;16:623–637.

[171] Morwessel NJ.The genetic basis of diabetes mellitus. AACN Clin Issues 1998;9:539–554.

[172] Cheverud JM, Vaughn TT, Pletscher LS, et al. Genetic architecture of adiposity in the cross of LG/J and SM/J inbred mice. Mamm Genome 2001;12:3–12.

[173] Walder K, Ziv E, Kalman R, et al. Elevated hypothalamic beacon gene expression in *Psammomys obesus* prone to develop obesity and type 2 diabetes. Int J Obes Relat Metab Disord 2002b;26:605–609.

Chapter 5

Etiology of Obesity: The Problem of Maintaining Energy Balance

Barry E. Levin[a,b] and Deborah J. Clegg[c]

[a]*Department of Neurology and Neurosciences, New Jersey Medical School, University of Medicine and Dentistry of New Jersey, Newark, NJ 07103, USA*
[b]*Neurology Service, VA Medical Center, 385 Tremont Ave., E. Orange, NJ 07018-1095, USA*
[c]*Department of Psychiatry, Genome Research Institute, 2170 East Galbraith Rd., Cincinnati, OH 45237, USA*

1. INTRODUCTION: OBESITY AND THE CONCEPT OF DEFENDED BODY WEIGHT

The proposition that body weight is defended assumes that there is a homeostatic process by which energy intake, expenditure, and storage are monitored and then actively maintained within specified limits. Our ideas about such homeostatic controls of bodily functions originated with Cannon [1]. Blood pressure, temperature, fluid and electrolyte balance, and glucose metabolism are examples of such regulated systems in which small deviations from a given set-point are rapidly detected and corrected by the brain using inputs from the internal and external environments. Richter called the sensors for such inputs "interoceptors" and "exteroceptors," respectively [2] (Figure 1). Both Cannon and Richter recognized that control of regulated systems required a constant dialogue between the brain and the internal and external environments. However, regulation of body weight differs from that of other systems in that the regulated elements, carbohydrate, protein and fat, are stored in depots [3]. Fat is more energy dense and more readily stored in large depots than are carbohydrate and protein and is the major form of stored energy in the body. Storage of fat in depots allows wide swings in energy intake, storage, and expenditure to occur while still providing a rapidly mobilizable pool of nutrients to fuel the immediate metabolic needs of the body. Thus, fat depots act as the buffer between energy intake and expenditure.

Food supplies have not been readily available throughout most of human history. Thus, survival depended on the presence of a strong internal drive to seek, ingest, and store as much energy as possible as fat in times of plenty and a mechanism for reducing energy expenditure to preserve adipose stores during times of scarcity [4–9]. In other words, anabolic processes must take precedence over catabolic ones in the hierarchy of systems controlling body weight.

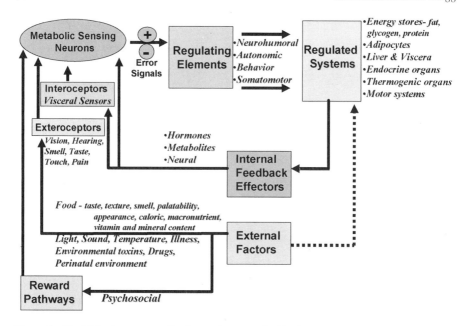

Figure 1. Model for factors contributing to the control of body weight. There are many internal and external signals that converge upon and are integrated by a distributed network of metabolic sensing neurons. The sensitivities of these sensing neurons are genetically and environmentally determined and provide the "set-point" at which body weight is regulated. These signals alter the intake, storage, and expenditure of energy through regulation of neuroendocrine and metabolic pathways. Inherent plasticity in the system allows for either homeostasis at a given level or upward resetting of the defended body weight.

This regulatory strategy would be particularly useful in both hunter-gatherer and agricultural societies where periods of famine occurred at regular intervals [9]. While such a "thrifty gene" [10] would confer a competitive survival advantage, it would also predispose such individuals to become obese when highly palatable, energy-dense foods were plentiful and obtainable at low energetic cost. This would not be a problem if obesity had no health consequences and if weight gain were reversible. Unfortunately, for reasons unknown, each incremental gain in adiposity in obesity-prone individuals is avidly defended against all attempts to lower it [5, 11–16]. This progressive, upward resetting of the defended body weight is very different from the way in which other regulated systems function and probably accounts for the high rate of recidivism in the treatment of obesity [17, 18].

Some have argued that body weight and fat stores are regulated simply by "settling" about a given homeostatic level without active controls or an actual set-point [3, 19]. However, the basic premise of this review is that body weight is actively regulated about a set-point which resides within a distributed network of specialized "metabolic sensing" neurons in the brain. We further speculate that the level at which this set-point operates is determined initially by an individual's genetic background and then modified by a host of environmental factors that promote and perpetuate the obese state by permanently altering metabolic sensing neurons and the central systems regulating body weight.

2.   NEURAL CONTROL OF THE DEFENDED BODY WEIGHT

Hetherington and Ranson [20] first demonstrated the importance of the brain in the regulation of body weight by showing that lesions of the ventromedial area of the hypothalamus (VMH) led to a striking hyperphagia and obesity. Since that time, a number of sites within the brain have been identified in which lesions can alter energy homeostasis, i.e., the balance among energy intake, expenditure, and storage [21–26]. Originally, this was taken as evidence that such sites represent "centers" for the control of hunger and satiety [27, 28]. However, it is more likely that the control of most neural functions, including energy homeostasis, resides within distributed, integrated networks of neurons throughout the brain [29]. Nevertheless, sites at which lesions alter body weight regulation do represent important nodes within such networks. These nodes contain neurons that produce neuropeptides and transmitters involved in the regulation of energy homeostasis. Many of these neurons are specialized metabolic sensors [30, 31]. They have evolved receptors, transporters, and metabolic pathways that allow them to utilize metabolic and hormonal signals from the periphery to control their membrane potential and firing rate. Whereas most neurons use substrates to fuel their activity-based energy needs, metabolic sensing neurons also utilize these substrates as signaling molecules to control their firing rate [30, 31]. First called "glucosensing neurons" because of their ability to use glucose as a signaling molecule [28, 32], it is now clear that many of these same neurons also utilize fatty acids, ketone bodies, lactate, and other substrates as signaling molecules to control their activity [33–37]. Many also have receptors for leptin and insulin [38–40] that provide direct [41–43] and indirect [44, 45] signals to the brain related to the amount of fat stored in adipose depots. Both of these hormones, as well as most substrates, cross the blood–brain barrier by a saturable facilitated transport processes [46–49]. In addition, many metabolic sensing neurons are located next to circumventricular organs such as the median eminence in the hypothalamus and area postrema in the brain stem. Because these structures have no blood–brain barrier, hormones and metabolites can diffuse from the circulation directly into the surrounding brain [50, 51]. Many metabolic sensing neurons also lie close to the cerebral ventricles into which hormones and metabolites are transported and then diffuse into the surrounding brain [49, 52–54]. Finally, metabolic sensing neurons are "hard-wired" into ascending neural pathways from peripheral metabolic sensors in the liver, gut, and other organs [55, 56], as well as sensors that monitor the external environment [57] (Figure 1). Metabolic sensing neurons are also integrated into pathways mediating reward, motivation, memory, and learning [58–60]. Signals from all of these sources arrive with differing temporal patterns and are integrated to alter membrane potential, firing rate, transmitter and peptide release, and gene transcription. The output of metabolic sensing neurons goes to effector systems that regulate energy homeostasis and body weight (Figure 1).

Metabolic sensing neurons are highly localized in brain areas in which lesions either raise [20, 25, 26, 61] or lower [62–64] body weight. Among these, only lesions of the VMH actually disrupt the defense of body weight [65, 66]. For example, rats with lesions of the lateral hypothalamus (LH) reduce their body weight and then defend it avidly against all attempts to drive them above or below their new lesion-induced set-point [62, 67–69]. However, if VMH-lesioned rats are fed unpalatable or low-calorie diets, their weights decline to that of unlesioned rats and obesity will not develop if those diets are present from lesioning [65, 70]. Their resting metabolic rate is substantially lower than expected from their metabolic mass and they fail to display the expected downward adjustment in metabolic rate associated with weight reduction [66].

The fact that VMH lesions disrupt the physiological defense of body weight while lesions in other areas do not supports a unique role for the VMH in the regulation of energy homeostasis. The VMH is composed of the ventromedial and arcuate (ARC) nuclei. Of these two nuclei, the ARC appears to be the more important in the control of body weight. Only VMH lesions that include the ARC produce the full VMH syndrome [20, 71, 72] and isolated lesions of the ARC or its connections produce hyperphagia and obesity [73]. The ARC contains neuropeptide Y (NPY) and proopiomelanocortin (POMC) neurons the primary purpose of which appears to be the regulation of energy homeostasis [74–80]. They are also prototypic metabolic sensing neurons that alter their firing rate when ambient glucose levels change [81, 82] and have receptors for and are responsive to a variety of peripheral hormones involved in energy homeostasis such as leptin [39, 83–85], insulin [40, 85], ghrelin [86], and PYY [87]. They lie adjacent to the median eminence, which has no blood–brain barrier [88] and next to the third cerebral ventricle, from which various hormones and substrates can diffuse. ARC POMC neurons produce α-melanocyte stimulating hormone (α-MSH), a catabolic peptide that acts at melanocortin-3 and -4 receptors (MC3/4-R) in the LH and paraventricular nucleus to produce anorexia and increased thermogenesis [76, 80, 89, 90]. ARC NPY neurons project to the same target areas as do POMC neurons and NPY release in these areas produces marked hyperphagia and reduced thermogenesis and fat oxidation [74, 75, 89, 91]. ARC NPY neurons are unique because they also produce agouti-related peptide (AgRP), a selective inverse agonist (effectively an antagonist) for MC3/4-R [92, 93]. This provides a mechanism for interaction between NPY and POMC neurons at their overlapping target areas. In addition, NPY and POMC cell bodies lie in close anatomical proximity in the ARC. This facilitates cross-talk between them and incoming peptide and hormone signals from the periphery [83, 87]. Finally, leptin and insulin both inhibit NPY [94, 95] and stimulate POMC expression [96, 97]. These multiple interactions between the metabolic sensing ARC NPY and POMC neurons provide a critical anabolic/catabolic balance for the hypothalamic control of energy homeostasis.

The LH also contains metabolic sensing neurons that use glucose [98, 99] and fatty acids [100] as signaling molecules. Although it is not completely certain that they are metabolic sensing neurons [101–107], both LH orexin (hypocretin) [108–111] and melanin concentrating hormone (MCH) [112] increase food intake when injected into the brain. However, unlike ARC NPY and POMC neurons which project to a limited number of overlapping targets and whose primary function is the regulation of energy expenditure, orexin and MCH neurons project widely throughout the neuraxis and participate in a number of other functions such as arousal, motivation, and motor activity [113–119]. In fact, it is likely that the effects of orexin and MCH on energy homeostasis are mediated through their connections with ARC neurons as part of more generalized processes such as arousal and changes in motor activity [110, 111, 114, 120].

While the hypothalamus is historically recognized for its role in the regulation of body weight, the brain stem also plays a prominent role that is less appreciated. Areas such as the nucleus tractus solitarius (NTS) contain metabolic sensing neurons [56, 121] that are integrated within the distributed network of neurons involved in energy homeostasis. The NTS lies under the floor of the fourth cerebral ventricle and is adjacent to the area postrema, a circumventricular organ [51]. Unlike the hypothalamus, which receives only relayed neural inputs from the periphery and visceral sensors, NTS neurons receive direct afferents [122, 123]. Neurons in the rostral NTS also receive gustatory and sensory afferents from the tongue, pharynx, and mouth [124]. The NTS and other brain stem nuclei contain metabolic sensing neurons (including populations of POMC and NPY neurons) that project upward to various forebrain areas involved in energy homeostasis and reward [125, 126]. They also project caudally through vagal parasympathetic and spinal sympathetic outflow areas for visceromotor, metabolic, and endocrine control [127, 128]. Thus, areas within both the hypothalamus and brain stem represent important nodes of metabolic sensing neurons within a distributed network capable of integrating multiple metabolic, hormonal, and neural signals from the periphery for the regulation of body weight.

3. OBESITY AND THE PROBLEM OF MAINTAINING BODY WEIGHT

Obesity becomes a problem in humans because of its associations with diseases such as diabetes, hypertension, and cardiovascular disease [129]. In our distant past, it is unlikely that many humans ever became obese enough or lived long enough to develop these comorbidities because famine and intermittent availability of food were common [9]. These selection pressures appear to have biased the defense of body weight heavily toward filling and resisting the depletion of energy stores rather than preventing their overload. Of the three macronutrients, fat is the most energy dense (9 kcal/g vs. 4 kcal/g for carbohydrate and protein) and the most readily stored in large excess. Protein is stored primarily as structural components of organs and is used as an energy source mainly when all other depots are depleted. Hepatic and muscle glycogen stores are adequate for only single day's reserve [130]. On the other hand, fatty acids stored in adipose tissue comprise a large, energy-dense, and mobile reserve. However, because the amount of fat ingested in a single day represents only a small fraction of total body stores, small incremental changes in fat ingestion may slip below the detection threshold of the system and produce obesity in genetically predisposed individuals [3, 131].

The discovery of leptin [132] provided the long sought after signal from adipose tissue to the brain [133]. Leptin is produced by adipocytes in direct proportion to adipose mass [134] and is secreted into the blood where it enters the brain parenchyma by facilitated transport across the blood–brain barrier [46], as well as diffusion from cerebrospinal fluid [52] and circumventricular organs [46]. Leptin interacts with its receptor on metabolic sensing neurons where it regulates membrane potential, firing rate, and neuropeptide transcription [83, 97, 135, 136]. Activation of central receptors leads to reduced food intake and increased thermogenesis [137, 138]. Insulin acts on many of these same neurons through intracellular pathways that converge with the leptin signaling cascade [85, 139]. Insulin, like leptin, reflects the size of the body's adipose stores [44, 45]. The typical model posits a negative feedback system whereby increases in adipose mass lead to increases in leptin and insulin levels which then feed back to central sites to reduce intake and increase expenditure [140]. However, the system is really more heavily biased toward preventing a downward than an upward level of adipose stores [141]. Overeating produces little change in short-term leptin levels in obesity-resistant subjects [142, 143], while caloric restriction leads to a rapid fall in plasma leptin and insulin levels so that they no longer accurately reflect the size of adipose stores [41]. Because both leptin and insulin stimulate catabolic POMC and inhibit anabolic NPY neurons [95–97, 136], their withdrawal leads to a net anabolic state with a strong drive to seek food and conserve energy stores by decreasing metabolic rate [95, 144–146].

Because the typical intake of fat represents such a small percentage of total body stores, even moderate amounts of fat ingestion may not activate systems that inhibit further intake [143, 147, 148], particularly in obesity-prone individuals [131]. Even in obesity-resistant individuals, it takes up to a week to make the appropriate downward corrections for overconsumption when the fat and caloric densities of the diet are increased [143, 147]. Neither do such individuals appropriately increase their metabolic rate under these circumstances. Also, some obesity-prone individuals oxidize less fat than carbohydrate, leading to increased fat storage [149–152]. On the other hand, when energy intake is restricted, both obesity-prone and -resistant individuals readily decrease their metabolic rate to conserve energy [4, 5, 11, 12, 14, 41, 153]. On refeeding, they become hyperphagic and maintain a reduced metabolic rate until the lost adipose stores are regained [15, 41, 148, 154]. Thus, humans [131, 141, 147, 155] and rodents [143, 148] compensate more readily for decreases than increases in caloric intake. As obesity develops, leptin and insulin levels rise and saturate blood–brain barrier transporters [46, 47]. Ingestion of high-fat diets reduces both leptin transport [156, 157] and central leptin and insulin signaling [158, 159], effects that can occur in the absence of either obesity or elevated leptin and insulin levels [156, 159]. Thus, intake of high-fat diets reduces the physiological salience of negative feedback signals from adipose stores by altering the lipid composition and biomechanical properties of membranes of metabolic sensing neurons in which receptors, transporters, and ion channels reside [160–162].

In rats, this unique property of high-fat diets produces obesity in predisposed individuals who are born with an already raised detection threshold for catabolic signals from the periphery. Lean, obesity-prone rats on low-fat diets have reduced sensitivities to the anorectic effects of leptin [157, 163] and insulin [157] and to the signaling properties of glucose [164–170]. Despite early elevations of leptin and insulin levels produced by intake of high-fat diets, these animals fail to reduce their intake until they have become irreversibly obese [143, 148, 171, 172]. At any given point along their upward body weight gain trajectory, obesity-prone rats avidly defend that specific body weight and adipose mass when calorically restricted [4, 14, 15, 148, 154]. Plastic change within neural pathways (or even peripheral organs [173, 174] involved in energy homeostasis) might underlie this progressive and irreversible increase in the level of defended body weight in obesity-prone individuals. For example, manipulations of the maternal environment, the development of obesity itself and repeated changes in dietary composition in neonatal and adult rats all produce progressive and permanent alterations in such neuronal systems in association with a permanent upward resetting of the defended body weight [161, 175–180].

4.   HOW IS BODY WEIGHT REALLY REGULATED?

While leptin and insulin are clearly important in the regulation of body weight, rodents with defective leptin signaling can still regulate their body weight fairly normally. They just do so at an elevated level [3, 13, 181]. Also, obesity-resistant rats do not become obese even after they lose their central sensitivity to the anorectic effects of insulin [159]. Thus, it is clear that there must be other factors besides leptin and insulin which are monitored in regulation of body weight. A partial list of such candidates includes fatty acids [182], glucose [183–187], amino acids [188], nutrient oxidation [183, 189–194], thermogenesis [195, 196], core temperature [197], gastric distention [198], energy density [147, 185], and hepatic ATP production [199]. It is likely that one or more of these factors plays a role in body weight regulation under a variety of conditions and some may become even more important regulators in the absence of leptin and insulin signaling.

Diet palatability and psychosocial factors related to food intake are also major contributors to the development of obesity in humans. Intake of palatable diets can override all of the normal homeostatic controls of intake and produce hyperphagia and massive obesity indexobesity [200–203] even in LH-lesioned [69, 204] and obesity-resistant rats [41, 200]. Such "nonhomeostatic" intake persists in the face of very high levels of leptin and insulin [41, 200] and is independent of defects in leptin signaling [181]. Intake of highly palatable diets is driven by the rewarding orosensory and postingestive properties of food [205] and psychosocial factors attendant to meal taking [206, 207]. However, weight gained because of hyperphagia produced by such highly palatable diets may not be sustained; when palatability is reduced, rats rapidly reduce their intakes and body weights [41, 200, 203]. Nevertheless, when the highly palatable diet is reintroduced, rats rapidly regain lost weight to the level of others kept on the palatable diet throughout [200]. Thus, there are different "set-points" for body weight, each of which may depend on the caloric density, fat content, or palatability of the diet. It is likely that each is mediated by different sets of distributed neuronal circuits [29, 208]. The homeostatic pathways generally involve the hypothalamic and brain stem areas described above while a separate set of reward pathways mediates intake of palatable diets [209–212]. While these two networks are largely anatomically and neurochemically distinct, they are also highly interconnected and interdependent [29, 208] (Figure 1).

5. FACTORS THAT LOWER THE DEFENDED BODY WEIGHT

Other than brain lesions, illness, toxins, and surgical interventions, very few manipulations can permanently lower the defended body weight in obese individuals. While chronic administration of drugs that target central pathways involved in energy homeostasis offer some hope for lowering the defended body weight, none that meet minimal criteria of being safe, effective, inexpensive, and acceptable to a broad range of patients are currently available. Chronic intake of drugs such as fenfluramine (now off the market) and sibutramine alter monoamine metabolism and lower the defended body weight [213–216]. Sibutramine appears to do this by preventing the upregulation of anabolic ARC NPY and downregulation of catabolic POMC expression that normally occur with loss of adipose stores [213]. Because the main effect of sibutramine is on NPY and POMC neurons, it will probably require the use of a drug that targets a different set of central or peripheral systems involved in body weight regulation if additional weight loss is required.

Exercise also lowers the defended body weight in male (but not female) [217] rats without producing a compensatory increase in food intake [218, 219]. Exercise has a similar short-term effect on appetite in humans [220, 221]. As with sibutramine, this effect may be the result of an exercise-induced normalization of central peptides involved in energy homeostasis [218, 219]. But this effect lasts only as long as the individual continues to exercise [219]. However, when exercise is begun early in life, it prevents the development of obesity in obesity-prone rats fed a moderate fat diet and this effect persists long after cessation of exercise [222]. This suggests that exercise begun while the brain is still developing might have a beneficial effect on neural pathways involved in energy homeostasis. A case for exercise as an adjunct to obesity treatment also comes from studies showing that high levels of exercise are a common characteristic of some of the few formerly obese humans who are successful at long-term weight loss [223, 224]. This may be due to an exercise-induced normalization of resting metabolic rate [224] as opposed to the chronically reduced metabolic rate seen in sedentary formerly obese subjects [11]. Unfortunately, it is unlikely that the majority of obese individuals will be able to maintain the high levels of exercise necessary to correct the reduced metabolic rate associated with chronic weight loss.

6. IMPLICATIONS FOR FUTURE RESEARCH

We have come a long way in our understanding of the way in which body weight is regulated. The extremely high recidivism rate in the treatment of obesity [17, 18] reinforces the fact that there is a near-permanent upward resetting of the defended body weight that occurs when genetically predisposed individuals become obese. Thus, prevention would be the best method of stemming the increasing obesity epidemic. To do this, we will need a better understanding of the factors that promote and perpetuate that upward resetting of body weight during both the perinatal and adult periods of life. We believe that a focus on the factors that regulate the detection thresholds of metabolic sensing neurons for various signals will be particularly profitable. We already have identified many central and peripheral signals that affect such neurons and these may provide potential pharmacological targets for the development of safe, effective drugs for the chronic treatment of already obese individuals. However, the redundancy and plasticity of the anabolic systems designed to prevent weight loss makes it likely that effective long-term treatment will require more than one drug that targets more than one system. Some surgical interventions have been successful in producing chronic weight loss in some individuals [225]. Yet we know almost nothing about the way in which such interventions alter central and peripheral pathways involved in body weight regulation. Further studies in this area may uncover previously unknown mechanisms for weight control. Finally, we need a better understanding of the mechanisms that underlie the considerable gender-specific differences in the way in which males and females defend their body weights [226].

In conclusion, we have presented evidence that obesity results from the synergy between genetic and environmental factors. Our genetic background provides a hard-wired neural template that promotes storage and minimizes depletion of energy stores. Our environment plays on that genetic predilection by providing us with an almost limitless supply of highly palatable, energy-dense foods that can be obtained at little energetic cost. We postulate that the set-point for the defended body weight is encoded within distributed networks of metabolic sensing neurons that integrate incoming signals from the internal and external environment in order to regulate somatosensory, visceral, and hormonal outputs that control energy homeostasis. It may be that permanent changes within this distributed network are responsible for the observation that the set-point for the defended body weight can move upward but rarely moves downward in genetically predisposed individuals.

REFERENCES

[1] Cannon WB. The Wisdom of the Body. New York: Norton, 1939.
[2] Richter CP. Total self regulatory functions of animals and human beings. Harvey Lecture Series 1942–1943;38:63.
[3] Flatt JP. Physiological and metabolic control of macronutrient balance. In: Berthoud H-R, Seeley RJ, eds. Neural and Metabolic Control of Macronutrient Intake. Boca Raton: CRC Press, 2000;143–164.

[4]   Corbett SW, Stern JS, Keesey RE. Energy expenditure in rats with diet-induced obesity. Am J Clin Nutr 1986;44:173–180.

[5]   Leibel RL, Rosenbaum M, Hirsch J. Changes in energy expenditure resulting from altered body weight. N Engl J Med 1995;332:621–628.

[6]   Elliot DL, Goldberg L, Kuehl KS, Bennett WM. Sustained depression of the resting metabolic rate after massive weight loss. Am J Clin Nutr 1989;49(1):93–96.

[7]   Herberg LJ, Winn P. Body-weight regulatory mechanisms and food hoarding in hereditarily obese (fa/fa) and lean (Fa/Fa) Zucker rats. Physiol Behav 1982;29(4):631–635.

[8]   Fantino M, Cabanac M. Body weight regulation with a proportional hoarding response in the rat. Physiol Behav 1980;24(5):939–942.

[9]   Diamond J. Guns, Germs and Steel. NY, London: W.W. Norton, 1997.

[10] Neel V. Diabetes mellitus: A "thrifty" genotype rendered detrimental by progress. Am J Hum Genet 1962;14:353–362.

[11] Leibel RL, Hirsch J. Diminished energy requirements in reduced-obese patients. Metabolism 1984;33:164–170.

[12] Boyle PC, Storlien LH, Keesey RE. Increased efficiency of food utilization following weight loss. Physiol Behav 1978;21(2):261–264.

[13] Keesey RE, Corbett SW. Adjustments in daily energy expenditure to caloric restriction and weight loss by adult obese and lean Zucker rats. Int J Obes 1990;14:1079–1084.

[14] MacLean PS, Higgins JA, Johnson GC, Fleming-Elder BK, Peters JC, Hill JO. Metabolic adjustments with the development, treatment, and recurrence of obesity in obesity-prone rats. Am J Physiol Regul Integr Comp Physiol 2004.

[15] MacLean PS, Higgins JA, Johnson GC, et al. Enhanced metabolic efficiency contributes to weight regain after weight loss in obesity-prone rats. Am J Physiol 2004; 287(6):R1306–R1315.

[16] Levin BE. Metabolic imprinting and the obesity epidemic. Curr Opin Endocrinol Diabet 2002;9:375–380.

[17] Kramer FM, Jeffery RW, Forster JL, Snell MK. Long-term follow-up of behavioral treatment for obesity: Patterns of weight regain among men and women. Int J Obes 1989;13(2):123–136.

[18] Klem ML, Wing RR, Lang W, McGuire MT, Hill JO. Does weight loss maintenance become easier over time? Obes Res 2000;8(6):438–444.

[19] Wirtshafter D, Davis JD. Set points, settling points, and the control of body weight. Physiol Behav 1977;19:75–78.

[20] Hetherington AW, Ranson SW. Hypothalamic lesions and adiposity in the rat. Anat Rec 1940;78:149–172.

[21] Bernardis LL, Bellinger LL. Somatic, endocrine and metabolic changes in controls pairfed for six weeks to rats with dorsomedial hypothalamic nucleus lesions (DMNL rats). Physiol Behav 1990;48:789–794.

[22] Rollins BL, King BM. Amygdala-lesion obesity: What is the role of the various amygdaloid nuclei? Am J Physiol Regul Integr Comp Physiol 2000;279(4):R1348–R1356.

[23] Edwards GL, White BD, Zhao W, He B, Dean RG, Martin RJ. Lesions of the area postrema/adjacent nucleus of the solitary tract result in enhanced hypothalamic neuropeptide Y levels. Ann NY Acad Sci 1994;739:337–338.

[24] Edwards GL, White BD, He B, Dean RG, Martin RJ. Elevated hypothalamic neuropeptide Y levels in rats with dorsomedial hindbrain lesions. Brain Res 1997;755(1):84–90.

[25] Ahlskog JE, Hoebel BG. Overeating and obesity from damage to a noradrenergic system in the brain. Science 1973;182:166–169.

[26] Tokunaga K, Fukushima M, Kemnitz JW, Bray GA. Comparison of ventromedial and paraventricular lesions in rats that become obese. Am J Physiol 1986;251:R1221–R1227.

[27] Stellar E. The physiology of motivation. Psychol Rev 1954;5:5–22.

[28] Anand BK, Chhina GS, Sharma KN, Dua S, Singh B. Activity of single neurons in the hypothalamus feeding centers: Effect of glucose. Am J Physiol 1964;207:1146–1154.

[29] Berthoud HR. Multiple neural systems controlling food intake and body weight. Neurosci Biobehav Rev 2002;26(4):393–428.

[30] Levin BE. Metabolic sensors: Viewing glucosensing neurons from a broader perspective. Physiol Behav 2002;76:397–401.

[31] Levin BE, Routh VH, Kang L, Sanders NM, Dunn-Meynell AA. Neuronal glucosensing: What do we know after 50 years? Diabetes 2004;53(10):2521–2528.

[32] Oomura Y, Kimura K, Ooyama H, Maeo T, Iki M, Kuniyoshi N. Reciprocal activities of the ventromedial and lateral hypothalamic area of cats. Science 1964;143:484–485.

[33] Puthuraya KP, Oomura Y, Shimizu N. Effects of endogenous sugar acids on the ventromedial hypothalamic nucleus of the rat. Brain Res 1985;332(1):165–168.

[34] Minami T, Shimizu N, Duan S, Oomura Y. Hypothalamic neuronal activity responses to 3-hydroxybutyric acid, an endogenous organic acid. Brain Res 1990;509:351–354.

[35] Song Z, Routh VH. Differential effects of glucose and lactate on glucosensing neurons in the ventromedial hypothalamic nucleus. Diabetes 2005;54(1):15–22.

[36] Yang X, Kow L-M, Funabashi T, Mobbs CV. Hypothalamic glucose sensor. Similarities to and differences from pancreatic β-cell mechanisms. Diabetes 1999;48:1763–1772.

[37] Yang XJ, Kow LM, Pfaff DW, Mobbs CV. Metabolic pathways that mediate inhibition of hypothalamic neurons by glucose. Diabetes 2004;53(1):67–73.

[38] Kang L, Routh VH, Kuzhikandathil EV, Gaspers L, Levin BE. Physiological and molecular characteristics of rat hypothalamic ventromedial nucleus glucosensing neurons. Diabetes 2004;53:549–559.

[39] Baskin DG, Breininger JF, Schwartz MW. Leptin receptor mRNA identifies a subpopulation of neuropeptide Y neurons activated by fasting in rat hypothalamus. Diabetes 1999;48:828–833.

[40] Benoit SC, Air EL, Coolen LM, et al. The catabolic action of insulin in the brain is mediated by melanocortins. J Neurosci 2002;22:9048–9052.

[41] Levin BE, Keesey RE. Defense of differing body weight set-points in diet-induced obese and resistant rats. Am J Physiol 1998;274:R412–R419.

[42] Rosenbaum M, Nicolson M, Hirsch J, Murphy E, Chu F, Leibel RL. Effects of weight change on plasma leptin concentrations and energy expenditure. J Clin Endocrinol Metab 1997;82(11):3647–3654.

[43] Weigle DS, Duell PB, Connor WE, Steiner RA, Soules MR, Kuijper JL. Effect of fasting, refeeding, and dietary fat restriction on plasma leptin levels. J Clin Endocrinol Metab 1997;82:561–565.

[44] Bagdade JD, Bierman EL, Porte D Jr. The significance of basal insulin levels in the evaluation of the insulin response to glucose in diabetic and nondiabetic subjects. J Clin Invest 1967;46(10):1549–557.

[45] Polonsky KS, Given BD, Van Cauter E. Twenty-four-hour profiles and pulsatile patterns of insulin secretion in normal and obese subjects. J Clin Invest 1988;81(2):442–448.

[46] Banks WA, Kastin AJ, Huang W, Jaspan JB, Maness LM. Leptin enters the brain by a saturable system independent of insulin. Peptides 1996;17:305–311.

[47] Banks WA, Jaspan JB, Huang W, Kastin AJ. Transport of insulin across the blood–brain barrier: Saturability at euglycemic doses of insulin. Peptides 1997;18(9):1423–1429.

[48] Banks WA, Clever CM, Farrell CL. Partial saturation and regional variation in the blood-to-brain transport of leptin in normal weight mice. Am J Physiol 2000;278:E1158–E1171.

[49] Schwartz MW, Sipols A, Kahn SE, et al. Kinetics and specificity of insulin uptake from plasma into cerebrospinal fluid. Am J Physiol 1990;259:E278–E283.

[50] Krisch B, Leonhardt H, Buchheim W. The functional and structural border between the CSF- and blood-milieu in the circumventricular organs (organum vasculosum laminae terminalis, subfornical organ, area postrema) of the rat. Cell Tissue Res 1978;195(3):485–497.

[51] Ganong WF. Circumventricular organs: Definition and role in the regulation of endocrine and autonomic function. Clin Exp Pharm Physiol 2000;27(5–6):422–427.

[52] Schwartz MW, Peskind E, Raskind M, Boyko EJ, Porte D Jr. Cerebrospinal fluid leptin levels: Relationship to plasma levels and to adiposity in humans. Nat Med 1996;2:589–593.

[53] Baura GD, Foster DM, Porte D Jr, et al. Saturable transport of insulin from plasma into the central nervous system of dogs in vivo: A mechanism for regulated insulin delivery to the brain. J Clin Invest 1993;92(4):1824–1830.

[54] Ono T, Steffens AB, Sasaki K. Influence of peripheral and intracerebroventricular glucose and insulin infusions on peripheral and cerebrospinal fluid glucose and insulin levels. Physiol Behav 1983;30(2):301–306.

[55] Shimizu N, Oomura Y, Novin D, Grijava CV, Cooper PH. Functional correlations between lateral hypothalamic glucose-sensitive neurons and hepatic portal glucose-sensitive units in rat. Brain Res 1983;265:49–54.

[56] Adachi A, Shimizu N, Oomura Y, Kobashi M. Convergence of heptoportal glucose-sensitive afferent signals to glucose-sensitive units within the nucleus of the solitary tract. Neurosci Lett 1984;46:215–218.

[57] Hamilton RB, Norgren R. Central projections of gustatory nerves in the rat. J Comp Neurol 1984;222:560–577.

[58] Aou S, Oomura Y, Lenard L, et al. Behavioral significance of monkey hypothalamic glucose-sensitive neurons. Brain Res 1984;302:69–74.

[59] Sikdar SK, Oomura Y. Selective inhibition of glucose-sensitive neurons in rat lateral hypothalamus by noxious stimuli and morphine. J Neurophysiol 1985;53(1):17–31.

[60] Aou S, Takaki A, Karadi Z, Hori T, Nishino H, Oomura Y. Functional heterogeneity of the monkey lateral hypothalamus in the control of feeding. Brain Res Bull 1991;27(3–4):451–455.

[61] Bovetto S, Richard D. Lesion of central nucleus of amygdala promotes fat gain without preventing effect of exercise on energy balance. Am J Physiol 1995;269:2–6.

[62] Boyle PC, Keesey RE. Chronically reduced body weight in rats sustaining lesions of the lateral hypothalamus and maintained on palatable diets and drinking solutions. J Comp Physiol Psychol 1975;88(1):218–223.

[63] Bernardis LL, Bellinger LL. Production of weanling rat ventromedial and dorsomedial hypothalamic syndromes by electrolytic lesions with platinum–iridium electrodes. Neuroendocrinology 1976;22(2):97–106.

[64] Ungerstedt U. Adipsia and aphagia after 6-hydroxydopamine induced degeneration of the nigro-striatal dopamine system. Acta Physiol Scand (Suppl) 1971;367:95–122.

[65] Weingarten HP, Chang P, Jarvie KR. Reactivity of normal and VMH-lesioned rats to quinine-adulterated foods: Negative evidence for negative finickiness. Behav Neurol 1983;97:221–233.

[66] Vilberg TR, Keesey RE. Ventromedial hypothalamic lesions abolish compensatory reduction in energy expenditure to weight loss. Am J Physiol 1990;258:R476–R480.

[67] Mitchel JS, Keesey RE. Defense of a lowered weight maintenance level by lateral hypothalamically lesioned rats: Evidence from a restriction-refeeding regimen. Physiol Behav 1977;18:1121–1125.

[68] Milam KM, Stern JS, Storlien LH, Keesey RE. Effect of lateral hypothalamic lesions on regulation of body weight and adiposity in rats. Am J Physiol 1980;239(3):R337–R343.

[69] Corbett SW, Wilterdink EJ, Keesey RE. Resting oxygen consumption in over- and under-fed rats with lateral hypothalamic lesions. Physiol Behav 1985;35:971–977.

[70] Sclafani A, Springer D, Kluge L. Effect of quinine-adulterated diet upon body weight maintenance in male rats with ventromedial hypothalamic lesions. J Comp Physiol Psychol 1975;89:478–488.

[71] Shimizu N, Oomura Y, Plata-Salaman CR, Morimoto M. Hyperphagia and obesity in rats with bilateral ibotenic acid-induced lesions of the ventromedial hypothalamic nucleus. Brain Res 1987;416:153–156.

[72] Scallet AC, Olney JW. Components of hypothalamic obesity: Biperidyl-mustard lesions add hyperphagia to monosodium glutamate-induced hyperinsulinemia. Brain Res 1986;374:380–384.

[73] Bell ME, Bhatnagar S, Akana SF, Choi S, Dallman MF. Disruption of arcuate/paraventricular nucleus connections changes body energy balance and response to acute stress. J Neurosci 2000;20(17):6707–6713.

[74] Billington CJ, Briggs JE, Grace M, Levine AS. Effects of intracerebroventricular injection of neuropeptide Y on energy metabolism. Am J Physiol 1991;260:R321–R327.

[75] Stanley BG, Leibowitz SF. Neuropeptide Y injected in the paraventricular hypothalamus: A powerful stimulant of feeding behavior. Proc Natl Acad Sci USA 1985;82:3940–3943.

[76] Tsujii S, Bray GA. Acetylation alters the feeding response to MSH and beta-endorphin. Brain Res Bull 1989;23(3):165–169.

[77] Fan W, Boston BA, Kesterson RA, Hruby VJ, Cone RD. Role of melanocortinergic neurons in feeding and the agouti obesity syndrome. Nature 1997;385:165–168.

[78] Marsh DJ, Hollopeter G, Kafer KE, Palmiter RD. Role of the Y5 neuropeptide Y receptor in feeding and obesity. Nat Med 1998;4:718–721.

[79] Giraudo SQ, Billington CJ, Levine AS. Feeding effects of hypothalamic injection of melanocortin 4 receptor ligands. Brain Res 1998;302–306.

[80] Haynes WG, Morgan DA, Djalali A, Mark AL. Activation of melanocortin-4 receptors enhances thermogenic sympathetic nerve activity to brown adipose tissue. Hypertension 1998;32:620A.

[81] Muroya S, Yada T, Shioda S, Takigawa M. Glucose-sensitive neurons in the rat arcuate nucleus contain neuropeptide Y. Neurosci Lett 1999;264:113–116.

[82] Ibrahim N, Bosch MA, Smart JL, et al. Hypothalamic proopiomelanocortin neurons are glucose responsive and express K(ATP) channels. Endocrinology 2003;144(4):1331–1340.

[83] Cowley MA, Smart JL, Rubinstein M, et al. Leptin activates anorexigenic POMC neurons through a neural network in the arcuate nucleus. Nature 2001;411(6836):480–484.

[84] Pinto S, Roseberry AG, Liu H, et al. Rapid rewiring of arcuate nucleus feeding circuits by leptin. Science 2004;304(5667):110–115.

[85] Xu AW, Kaelin CB, Takeda K, Akira S, Schwartz MW, Barsh GS. PI3K integrates the action of insulin and leptin on hypothalamic neurons. J Clin Invest 2005;115:951–958.

[86] Cowley MA, Smith RG, Diano S, et al. The distribution and mechanism of action of ghrelin in the CNS demonstrates a novel hypothalamic circuit regulating energy homeostasis. Neuron 2003;37(4):649–661.

[87] Batterham RL, Cowley MA, Small CJ, et al. Gut hormone PYY(3-36) physiologically inhibits food intake. Nature 2002;418(6898):650–654.

[88] Broadwell RD, Brightman MW. Entry of peroxidase into neurons of the central and peripheral nervous systems from extracerebral and cerebral blood. J Comp Neurol 1976; 166(3):257–283.

[89] Elias CF, Aschkenasi C, Lee C, et al. Leptin differentially regulates NPY and POMC neurons projecting to the lateral hypothalamic area. Neuron 1999;23(4):775–786.

[90] Mountjoy KG, Mortrud MT, Low MJ, Simerly RB, Cone RD. Localization of the melanocortin-4 receptor (mc4-r) in neuroendocrine and autonomic control circuits in the brain. Mol Endocrinol 1994;8(10):1298–1308.

[91] Billington CJ, Briggs JE, Harker S, Grace M, Levine AS. Neuropeptide Y in hypothalamic paraventricular nucleus: A center coordinating energy metabolism. Am J Physiol 1994;266:R1765–R1770.

[92] Ollmann MM, Wilson BD, Yang YK, et al. Antagonism of central melanocortin receptors in vitro and in vivo by agouti-related protein. Science 1997;278(5335):135–138.

[93] Hahn TM, Breininger JF, Baskin DG, Schwartz MW. Colocalization of Agouti-related protein and neuropeptide Y in arcuate nucleus neurons activated by fasting ***NB to be changed? Nat Neurosci 1998;1:271–272.

[94] Stephens TW, Basinski M, Bristow PK, et al. The role of neuropeptide Y in antiobesity action of the obese gene product. Nature 1995;377:530–532.

[95] White JD, Olchovsky D, Kershaw M, Berelowitz M. Increased hypothalamic content of preproneuropeptide-Y messenger ribonucleic acid in streptozotocin-diabetic rats. Endocrinology 1990;126:765–772.

[96] Kim E-M, Grace MK, Welch CC, Billington CJ, Levine AS. STZ-induced diabetes decreases and insulin normalizes POMC mRNA in arcuate nucleus and pituitary in rats. Am J Phsyiol 1999;276:R1320–R1326.

[97] Schwartz MW, Seeley RJ, Woods SC, et al. Leptin increases hypothalamic pro-opiomelanocortin mRNA expression in the rostral arcuate nucleus. Diabetes 1997; 46:2119–2123.

[98] Oomura Y, Ono T, Ooyama H, Wayner MJ. Glucose and osmosensitive neurons of the rat hypothalamus. Nature 1969;222:282–284.

[99] Shibata S, Oomura Y, Kita H. Ontogenesis of glucose sensitivity in the rat lateral hypothalamus: A brain slice study. Brain Res 1982;281(1):114–117.

[100] Oomura Y, Nakamura T, Sugimori M, Yamada Y. Effect of free fatty acid on the rat lateral hypothalamic neurons. Physiol Behav 1975;14(04):483–486.

[101] Moriguchi T, Sakurai T, Nambu T, Yanagisawa M, Goto K. Neurons containing orexin in the lateral hypothalamic area of the adult rat brain are activated by insulin-induced acute hypoglycemia. Neurosci Lett 1999;264(1–3):101–104.

[102] Griffond B, Risold PY, Jacquemard C, Colard C, Fellmann D. Insulin-induced hypoglycemia increases preprohypocretin (orexin) mRNA in the rat lateral hypothalamic area. Neurosci Lett 1999;262(2):77–80.

[103] Muroya S, Uramura K, Sakurai T, Takigawa M, Yada T. Lowering glucose concentrations increases cytosolic Ca^{2+} in orexin neurons of the rat lateral hypothalamus. Neurosci Lett 2001;309:165–168.

[104] Dunn-Meynell AA, Routh VH, Kang L, Gaspers L, Levin BE. Glucokinase is the likely mediator of glucosensing in both glucose excited and glucose inhibited central neurons. Diabetes 2002;51:2056–2065.

[105] Bayer L, Poncet F, Fellmann D, Griffond B. Melanin-concentrating hormone expression in slice cultures of rat hypothalamus is not affected by 2-deoxyglucose. Neurosci Lett 1999;267(2):77–80.

[106] Sergeyev V, Broberger C, Gorbatyuk O, Hökfelt T. Effect of 2-mercaptoacetate and 2-deoxy-D-glucose administration on the expression of NPY, AGRP, POMC, MCH and hypocretin/orexin in the rat hypothalamus. Neuroreport 2000;11(1):117–121.

[107] Burdakov D, Gerasimenko O, Verkhratsky A. Physiological changes in glucose differentially modulate the excitability of hypothalamic melanin-concentrating hormone and orexin neurons in situ. J Neurosci 2005;25(9):2429–2433.

[108] Lin L, Faraco J, Li R, et al. The sleep disorder canine narcolepsy is caused by a mutation in the hypocretin (orexin) receptor 2 gene. Cell 1999;98(3):365–376.

[109] Date Y, Ueta Y, Yamashita H, et al. Orexins, orexigenic hypothalamic peptides, interact with autonomic, neuroendocrine and neuroregulatory systems. Proc Natl Acad Sci USA 1999;96(2):748–753.

[110] Trivedi P, Yu H, MacNeil DJ, Van der Ploeg LH, Guan XM. Distribution of orexin receptor mRNA in the rat brain. FEBS Lett 1998;438(1–2):71–75.

[111] Elias CF, Saper CB, Maratos-Flier E, et al. Chemically defined projections linking the mediobasal hypothalamus and the lateral hypothalamic area. J Comp Neurol 1998;402(4):442–459.

[112] Marsh DJ, Weingarth DT, Novi DE, et al. Melanin-concentrating hormone 1 receptor-deficient mice are lean, hyperactive, and hyperphagic and have altered metabolism. Proc Natl Acad Sci 2002;99(5):3240–3245.

[113] Yamanaka A, Kunii K, Nambu T, et al. Orexin-induced food intake involves neuropeptide Y pathway. Brain Res 2000;859(2):404–409.

[114] Peyron C, Tighe DK, van den Pol AN, et al. Neurons containing hypocretin (orexin) project to multiple neuronal systems. J Neurosci 1998;18:9996–10015.

[115] Chemelli RM, Willie JT, Sinton CM, et al. Narcolepsy in orexin knockout mice: Molecular genetics of sleep regulation. Cell 1999;98(4):437–451.

[116] Hara J, Beuckmann CT, Nambu T, et al. Genetic ablation of orexin neurons in mice results in narcolepsy, hypophagia, and obesity. Neuron 2001;30(2):345–354.

[117] Wang J, Osaka T, Inoue S. Orexin-A-sensitive site for energy expenditure localized in the arcuate nucleus of the hypothalamus. Brain Res 2003;971(1):128–134.

[118] Kiwaki K, Kotz CM, Wang C, Lanningham-Foster L, Levine JA. Orexin A (hypocretin 1) injected into hypothalamic paraventricular nucleus and spontaneous physical activity in rats. Am J Physiol Endocrinol Metab 2004;286(4):E551–E559.

[119] Shimada M, Tritos NA, Lowell BB, Flier JS, Maratos-Flier E. Mice lacking melanin-concentrating hormone are hypophagic and lean. Nature 1998;396(6712):670–674.

[120] Broberger C, De Lecea L, Sutcliffe JG, Hökfelt T. Hypocretin/orexin- and melanin-concentrating hormone-expressing cells form distinct populations in the rodent lateral hypothalamus: Relationship to the neuropeptide Y and agouti gene-related protein systems. J Comp Neurol 1998;402(4):460–474.

[121] Mizuno Y, Oomura Y. Glucose responding neurons in the nucleus tractus solitarius of the rat, in vitro study. Brain Res 1984;307:109–116.

[122] Niijima A. Glucose-sensitive afferent nerve fibres in the hepatic branch of the vagus nerve in the guinea-pig. J Physiol 1982;332:315–323.

[123] Niijima A. Glucose-sensitive afferent nerve fibers in the liver and their role in food intake and blood glucose regulation. J Auton Nerv Syst 1983;9(1):207–220.

[124] Travers SP, Pfaffmann C, Norgren R. Convergence of lingual and palatal gustatory neural activity in the nucleus of the solitary tract. Brain Res 1986;365:305–320.

[125] Ricardo JA, Koh ET. Anatomical evidence of direct projections from the nucleus of the solitary tract to the hypothalamus, amygdala, and other forebrain structures in the rat. Brain Res 1978;153(1):1–26.

[126] Ritter S, Bugarith K, Dinh TT. Immunotoxic destruction of distinct catecholamine subgroups produces selective impairment of glucoregulatory responses and neuronal activation. J Comp Neurol 2001;432:197–216.

[127] Norgren R. Projections from the nucleus of the solitary tract in the rat. Neuroscience 1978;3:207–218.

[128] Loewy AD, Burton H. Nuclei of the solitary tract: Efferent projections to the lower brain stem and spinal cord of the cat. J Comp Neurol 1978;181(2):421–449.

[129] Must A, Spadano J, Coakley EH, Field AE, Colditz G, Dietz WH. The disease burden associated with overweight and obesity. JAMA 1999;282(16):1523–1529.

[130] Flatt JP. Use and storage of carbohydrate and fat. Am J Clin Nutr 1995;61(Suppl 4):959S.

[131] McDevitt RM, Poppitt SD, Murgatroyd PR, Prentice AM. Macronutrient disposal during controlled overfeeding with glucose, fructose, sucrose, or fat in lean and obese women. Am J Clin Nutr 2000;72(2):369–377.

[132] Zhang Y, Proenca R, Maffei M, Barone M, Leopold L, Friedman JM. Positional cloning of the mouse obese gene and its human homologue. Nature 1994;372:425–432.

[133] Kennedy GC. The role of depot fat in the hypothalamic control of food intake in the rat. Proc R Soc Lond B Biol Sci 1953;611:221–235.

[134] Frederich RC, Hamann A, Anderson S, Lollmann B, Lowell BB, Flier JS. Leptin levels reflect body lipid content in mice: Evidence for diet-induced resistance to leptin action. Nat Med 1995;1(12):1311–1314.

[135] Spanswick D, Smith MA, Groppi VE, Logan SD, Ashford ML. Leptin inhibits hypothalamic neurons by activation of ATP-sensitive potassium channels. Nature 1997; 390(6659):521–525.

[136] Schwartz MW, Baskin DG, Bukowski TR, et al. Specificity of leptin action on elevated blood glucose levels and hypothalamic neuropeptide Y gene expression in ob/ob mice. Diabetes 1996;45:531–535.

[137] Campfield LA, Smith FJ, Guisez Y, Devos R, Burn P. Recombinant mouse OB protein: Evidence for a peripheral signal linking adiposity and central neural networks. Science 1995;269:546–549.

[138] Mistry AM, Swick AG, Romsos DR. Leptin rapidly lowers food intake and elevates metabolic rates in lean and ob/ob mice. J Nutr 1997;127:2065–2072.

[139] Niswender KD, Schwartz MW. Insulin and leptin revisited: Adiposity signals with overlapping physiological and intracellular signaling capabilities. Front Neuroendocrinol 2003;24:1–10.

[140] Schwartz MW, Woods SC, Porte D Jr, Seeley RJ, Baskin DG. Central nervous system control of food intake. Nature 2000;404(6778):661–671.

[141] Prentice A, Jebb S. Energy intake/physical activity interactions in the homeostasis of body weight regulation. Nutr Rev 2004;62(7 Pt 2):S98–S104.

[142] Murgatroyd PR, Fruhbeck G, Goldberg GR, et al. Leptin does not respond to 48 h fat deposition or mobilization in women. Int J Obes Relat Metab Disord 2003;27(4):457–462.

[143] Levin BE, Dunn-Meynell AA, Ricci MR, Cummings DE. Abnormalities of leptin and ghrelin regulation in obesity-prone juvenile rats. Am J Physiol 2003;285(5):E949–E957.

[144] Hardie LJ, Rayner DV, Holmes S, Trayhurn P. Circulating leptin levels are modulated by fasting, cold exposure and insulin administration in lean but not Zucker (*fa/fa*) rats as measured by ELISA. Biochem Biophys Res Commun 1996;223:660–665.

[145] Larue-Achagiotis C, Le Magnen J. Fast-induced changes in plasma glucose, insulin and free fatty acid concentration compared in rats during the night and day. Physiol Behav 1983;30(1):93–96.

[146] Friedman MI. Hyperphagia in rats with experimental diabetes mellitus: A response to a decreased supply of utilizable fuels. J Comp Physiol Psychol 1978;92(1):109–117.

[147] Bell EA, Castellanos VH, Pelkman CL, Thorwart ML, Rolls BJ. Energy density of foods affects energy intake in normal-weight women. Am J Clin Nutr 1998;67(3):412–420.

[148] Rolls BJ, Rowe EA, Turner RC. Persistent obesity in rats following a period of consumption of a mixed, high energy diet. J Physiol 1980;298:415–427.

[149] Chang S, Graham B, Yakubu F, Lin D, Peters JC, Hill JO. Metabolic differences between obesity-prone and obesity-resistant rats. Am J Physiol Regul Integr Comp Physiol 1990;259:R1103–R1110.

[150] Astrup A, Buemann B, Toubro S, Raben A. Defects in substrate oxidation involved in predisposition to obesity. Proc Nutr Soc 1996;55:817.

[151] Verboeket-van de Venne WP, Westerterp KR, ten Hoor F. Substrate utilization in man: Effects of dietary fat and carbohydrate. Metabolism 1994;43(2):152–156.

[152] Zurlo F, Lillioja S, Esposito-Del Puente A, et al. Low ratio of fat to carbohydrate oxidation as predictor of weight gain: Study of 24-h RQ. Am J Physiol 1990;259:E650–E657.

[153] Boyle PC, Storlien LH, Harper AE, Keesey RE. Oxygen consumption and locomotor activity during restricted feeding and realimentation. Am J Physiol 1981;241(5):R392–R397.

[154] Levin BE, Dunn-Meynell AA. Defense of body weight against chronic caloric restriction in obesity-prone and -resistant rats. Am J Physiol 2000;278:R231–R237.

[155] Mattes RD, Pierce CB, Friedman MI. Daily caloric intake of normal-weight adults: Response to changes in dietary energy density of a luncheon meal. Am J Clin Nutr 1988; 48(2):214–219.

[156] Banks WA, Coon AB, Robinson SM, et al. Triglycerides induce leptin resistance at the blood–brain barrier. Diabetes 2004;53(5):1253–1260.

[157] Levin BE, Dunn-Meynell AA, Banks WA. Obesity-prone rats have normal blood–brain barrier transport but defective central leptin signaling prior to obesity onset. Am J Physiol 2003;286:R143–R150.

[158] El-Haschimi K, Pierroz DD, Hileman SM, Bjorbaek C, Flier JS. Two defects contribute to hypothalamic leptin resistance in mice with diet-induced obesity. J Clin Invest 2000;105:1827–1832.

[159] Clegg DJ, Benoit SC, Reed JA, Woods SC, Levin BE. Reduced anorexic effects of insulin in obesity-prone rats and rats fed a moderate fat diet. Am J Physiol 2005;288:R981–R986.

[160] Taghibiglou C, Bradley CA, Wang Y, Wang Y. High cholesterol levels in neuronal cells impair the insulin signaling pathway and interfere with insulin's neuromodulatory action. Soc Neurosci Abstr 2004;34:Abst 633.13.

[161] Levin BE, Hamm MW. Plasticity of brain α-adrenoceptors during the development of diet-induced obesity in the rat. Obes Res 1994;2:230–238.

[162] Field CJ, Ryan EA, Thomson AB, Clandinin MT. Diet fat composition alters membrane phospholipid composition, insulin binding, and glucose metabolism in adipocytes from control and diabetic animals. J Biol Chem 1990;265(19):11143–11150.

[163] Levin BE, Dunn-Meynell AA. Reduced central leptin sensitivity in rats with diet-induced obesity. Am J Physiol 2002;283:R941–R948.

[164] Levin BE, Dunn-Meynell AA, Routh VH. Brain glucose sensing and body energy homeostasis: Role in obesity and diabetes. Am J Physiol 1999;276:R1223–R1231.

[165] Levin BE. Intracarotid glucose-induced norepinephrine response and the development of diet-induced obesity. Int J Obes 1992;16:451–457.

[166] Levin BE, Planas B. Defective glucoregulation of brain α_2-adrenoceptors in obesity-prone rats. Am J Physiol 1993;264:R305–R311.

[167] Dunn-Meynell AA, Govek E, Levin BE. Intracarotid glucose infusions selectively increase Fos-like immunoreactivity in paraventricular, ventromedial and dorsomedial nuclei neurons. Brain Res 1997;748:100–106.

[168] Levin BE, Dunn-Meynell AA. In vivo and in vitro regulation of [3H]glyburide binding to brain sulfonylurea receptors in obesity-prone and resistant rats by glucose. Brain Res 1997;776(1–2):146–153.

[169] Levin BE, Govek EK, Dunn-Meynell AA. Reduced glucose-induced neuronal activation in the hypothalamus of diet-induced obese rats. Brain Res 1998;808:317–319.

[170] Tkacs NC, Levin BE. Obesity-prone rats have pre-existing defects in their counterregulatory response to insulin-induced hypoglycemia. Am J Physiol 2004;287:R1110–R1115.

[171] Levin BE, Triscari J, Sullivan AC. Relationship between sympathetic activity and diet-induced obesity in two rat strains. Am J Physiol 1983;245:R367–R371.

[172] Hill JO, Dorton J, Sykes MN, Digirolamo M. Reversal of dietary obesity is influenced by its duration and severity. Int J Obes 1989;13:711–722.

[173] Knittle JL, Hirsch J. Effect of early nutrition on the development of rat epididymal fat pads: Cellularity and metabolism. J Clin Invest 1968;47(9):2091–2098.

[174] Faust IM, Johnson PR, Hirsch J. Long-term effects of early nutritional experience on the development of obesity in the rat. J Nutr 1980;110:2027–2034.

[175] Levin BE. Diet cycling and age alter weight gain and insulin levels in rats. Am J Physiol 1994; 267:R527–R535.

[176] Levin BE, Dunn-Meynell AA. Maternal obesity alters adiposity and monoamine function in genetically predisposed offspring. Am J Physiol 2002;283:R1087–R1093.

[177] Heidel E, Plagemann A, Davidowa H. Increased response to NPY of hypothalamic VMN neurons in postnatally overfed juvenile rats. Neuroreport 1999;10:1827–1831.

[178] Plagemann A, Rittel F, Waas T, Harder T, Rohde W. Cholecystokinin-8S levels in discrete hypothalamic nuclei of weanling rats exposed to maternal protein malnutrition. Regul Pept 1999;85(2–3):109–113.

[179] Plagemann A, Waas T, Harder T, Rittel F, Ziska T, Rohde W. Hypothalamic neuropeptide Y levels in weaning offspring of low-protein malnourished mother rats. Neuropeptides 2000;34:1–6.

[180] Davidowa H, Plagemann A. Different responses of ventromedial hypothalamic neurons to leptin in normal and early postnatally overfed rats. Neurosci Lett 2000;293(1):21–24.

[181] Gale SK, Van Itallie TB, Faust IM. Effects of palatable diets on body weight and adipose tissue cellularity in the adult obese female Zucker rat (fa/fa). Metab Clin Exp 1981; 30(2):105–110.

[182] Bray GA, Lee M, Bray TL. Weight gain of rats fed medium-chain triglycerides is less than rats fed long-chain triglycerides. Int J Obes 1980;4(1):27–32.

[183] Mayer J. Glucostatic mechanism of regulation of food intake. N Engl J Med 1953;249: 13–16.

[184] Stubbs RJ, O'Reilly LM. Carbohydrate and fat metabolism, appetite, and feeding behavior in humans. In: Berthoud H-R, Seeley RJ, eds. Neural and Metabolic Control of Macronutrient Intake. Boca Raton: CRC Press, 2000;165–188.

[185] Raben A, Holst JJ, Christensen NJ, Astrup A. Determinants of postprandial appetite sensations: Macronutrient intake and glucose metabolism. Int J Obes Relat Metab Disord 1996;20(2):161–169.

[186] Campfield LA, Smith FJ. Functional coupling between transient declines in blood glucose and feeding behavior: Temporal relationships. Brain Res Bull 1986;17:427–433.

[187] Campfield LA, Smith FJ, Rosenbaum M, Hirsch J. Human eating: Evidence for a physiological basis using a modified paradigm. Neurosci Biobehav Rev 1996;20(1):133–137.

[188] Stubbs RJ, Harbron CG, Murgatroyd PR, Prentice AM. Covert manipulation of dietary fat and energy density: Effect on substrate flux and food intake in men eating ad libitum. Am J Clin Nutr 1995;62(2):316–329.

[189] Kasai M, Nosaka N, Maki H, et al. Comparison of diet-induced thermogenesis of foods containing medium- versus long-chain triacylglycerols. J Nutr Sci Vitaminol (Tokyo) 2002;48(6):536–540.

[190] St-Onge MP, Ross R, Parsons WD, Jones PJ. Medium-chain triglycerides increase energy expenditure and decrease adiposity in overweight men. Obes Res 2003;11(3):395–402.

[191] Noguchi O, Takeuchi H, Kubota F, Tsuji H, Aoyama T. Larger diet-induced thermogenesis and less body fat accumulation in rats fed medium-chain triacylglycerols than in those fed long-chain triacylglycerols. J Nutr Sci Vitaminol (Tokyo) 2002;48(6):524–529.

[192] St-Onge MP, Bourque C, Jones PJ, Ross R, Parsons WE. Medium- versus long-chain triglycerides for 27 days increases fat oxidation and energy expenditure without resulting in changes in body composition in overweight women. Int J Obes Relat Metab Disord 2003;27(1):95–102.

[193] Flatt JP. Influence of body composition on food intake. In: Allen L, King J, Lonnerdal B, eds. Nutrient Regulation During Pregnancy, Lactation and Growth. New York: Plenum Press, 1994;27–44.

[194] Ramirez I, Tordoff MG, Friedman MI. Dietary hyperphagia and obesity: What causes them? Physiol Behav 1989;45(1):163–168.

[195] Nicolaidis S, Even P. Metabolic rate and feeding behavior. Ann NY Acad Sci 1989; 575:86–104.

[196] Stubbs RJ, Ritz P, Coward WA, Prentice AM. Covert manipulation of the ratio of dietary fat to carbohydrate and energy density: Effect on food intake and energy balance in free-living men eating ad libitum. Am J Clin Nutr 1995;62(2):330–337.

[197] Himms-Hagen J. Role of brown adipose tissue thermogenesis in control of thermoregulatory feeding in rats: A new hypothesis that links thermostatic and glucostatic hypotheses for control of food intake. Proc Soc Exp Biol Med 1995;208(2):159–169.

[198] Schwartz GJ, Moran TH. Leptin and neuropeptide Y have opposing modulatory effects on nucleus of the solitary tract neurophysiological responses to gastric loads: Implications for the control of food intake. Endocrinology 2002;143(10):3779–3784.

[199] Friedman MI, Harris RB, Ji H, Ramirez I, Tordoff MG. Fatty acid oxidation affects food intake by altering hepatic energy status. Am J Physiol 1999;276(4 Pt 2):R1046–R1053.

[200] Levin BE, Dunn-Meynell AA. Defense of body weight depends on dietary composition and palatability in rats with diet-induced obesity. Am J Physiol 2002;282:R46–R54.

[201] Louis-Sylvestre J, Giachetti I, Le Magnen J. Sensory versus dietary factors in cafeteria-induced overweight. Physiol Behav 1984;32(6):901–905.

[202] Rolls BA, van Duijvenvoorde PM, Rowe EA. Variety in the diet enhances intake in a meal and contributes to the development of obesity in the rat. Physiol Behav 1983;31:21–27.

[203] Armitage G, Hervey GR, Rolls BA, Rowe EA, Tobin G. The effects of supplementation of the diet with highly palatable foods upon energy balance in the rat. J Physiol (Lond) 1983;342:229–251.

[204] Milam KM, Keesey RE, Stern JS. Body composition and adiposity in LH-lesioned and pair-fed obese Zucker rats. Am J Physiol 1982;242:E437–E444.

[205] Lucas F, Ackroff K, Sclafani A. Dietary fat-induced hyperphagia in rats as a function of fat type and physical form. Physiol Behav 1989;45(5):937–946.

[206] Winkelstein ML, Feldman RH. Psychosocial predictors of consumption of sweets following smoking cessation. Res Nurs Health 1993;16(2):97–105.

[207] Glanz K, Kristal AR, Sorensen G, Palombo R, Heimendinger J, Probart C. Development and validation of measures of psychosocial factors influencing fat- and fiber-related dietary behavior. Prev Med 1993;22(3):373–387.

[208] Levin BE, Routh VH, Dunn-Meynell AA. Glucosensing neurons in the central nervous system. In: Berthoud H-R, Seeley RJ, eds. Neural and Metabolic Control of Macronutrient Intake. NY: CRC Press, 1999;325–337.

[209] Kelley AE, Bless EP, Swanson CJ. Investigation of the effects of opiate antagonists infused into the nucleus accumbens on feeding and sucrose drinking in rats. J Pharmacol Exp Ther 1996;278(3):1499–1507.

[210] Giraudo SQ, Billington CJ, Levine AS. Effects of the opioid antagonist naltrexone on feeding induced by DAMGO in the central nucleus of the amygdala and in the paraventricular nucleus in the rat. Brain Res 1998;782(1–2):18–23.

[211] Glass MJ, Billington CJ, Levine AS. Naltrexone administered to central nucleus of amygdala or PVN: Neural dissociation of diet and energy. Am J Physiol 2000;279(1):R86–R92.

[212] Pomonis JD, Jewett DC, Kotz CM, Briggs JE, Billington CJ, Levine AS. Sucrose consumption increases naloxone-induced c-Fos immunoreactivity in limbic forebrain. Am J Physiol 2000;278(3):R712–R719.

[213] Levin BE, Dunn-Meynell AA. Sibutramine alters the central mechanisms regulating the defended body weight in diet-induced obese rats. Am J Physiol 2000;279:R2222–R2228.

[214] Levitsky DA, Strupp BJ, Lupoli J. Tolerance to anorectic drugs: Pharmacological or artifactual. Pharm Biochem Behav 1981;14(5):661–667.

[215] Stunkard AJ. Anorectic agents lower a body weight set point. Life Sci 1982;30:2043–2055.

[216] Fantino M, Faion F, Rolland Y. Effect of dexfenfluramine on body weight set-point: Study in the rat with hoarding behaviour. Appetite 1986;7(Suppl):115–126.

[217] Hoffman-Goetz L, MacDonald MA. Effect of treadmill exercise on food intake and body weight in lean and obese rats. Physiol Behav 1983;31(3):343–346.

[218] Levin BE, Dunn-Meynell AA. Differential effects of exercise on body weight gain in obesity-prone and -resistant rats. Int J Obes 2005; in press.

[219] Bi S, Scott KA, Hyun J, Ladenheim EE, Moran TH. Running wheel activity prevents hyperphagia and obesity in OLETF rats: Role of hypothalamic signaling. Endocrinology 2005;146(4):1676–1685.

[220] King NA, Lluch A, Stubbs RJ, Blundell JE. High dose exercise does not increase hunger or energy intake in free living males. Eur J Clin Nutr 1997;51(7):478–483.

[221] Lluch A, King NA, Blundell JE. No energy compensation at the meal following exercise in dietary restrained and unrestrained women. Br J Nutr 2000;84(2):219–225.

[222] Patterson C, Levin BE. Post-weaning exercise prevents obesity in obesity-prone rats even after exercise termination. Obes Res 2004;12(Suppl):A22.

[223] Wing RR, Hill JO. Successful weight loss maintenance. Annu Rev Nutr 2003;21:323–341.

[224] Wyatt HR, Grunwald GK, Seagle HM, et al. Resting energy expenditure in reduced-obese subjects in the National Weight Control Registry. Am J Clin Nutr 1999;69:1189–1193.

[225] Klem ML, Wing RR, Chang CC, et al. A case-control study of successful maintenance of a substantial weight loss: Individuals who lost weight through surgery versus those who lost weight through non-surgical means. Int J Obes Relat Metab Disord 2000;24(5):573–579.

[226] Clegg DJ, Riedy CA, Smith KA, Benoit SC, Woods SC. Differential sensitivity to central leptin and insulin in male and female rats. Diabetes 2003;52(3):682–687.

Chapter 6

Current Views of the Fat Cell as an Endocrine Cell: Lipotoxicity

Tamara Tchkonia, Barbara E. Corkey and James L. Kirkland

Obesity Center, Evans Department of Medicine, Boston University, 650 Albany St., Boston, MA 02118, USA

1. INTRODUCTION

Lipotoxicity can be defined as lipid-induced metabolic damage [1]. It occurs when lipid uptake exceeds capacity to store lipids and lipid oxidative capacity [2]. The principal function of adipose tissue is to store energy, and lipids are a particularly efficient form in which to store energy because of their high caloric density. However, lipids can be cytotoxic and nonadipose tissues have limited capacity to store lipids [3]. Fat tissue is protected against lipotoxicity, but if fat tissue function becomes dysregulated, lipotoxicity in other tissues can ensue. Fatty acids (FAs), the essential role of which is to serve as fuels and to form phospholipid bilayers and phospholipid messengers, are particularly damaging to nonadipose tissues when present in excess [4, 5]. The causes, mechanisms, and consequences of lipotoxicity are considered, with particular regard to the role of adipose tissue in lipotoxicity in other tissues and to possible reasons why adipose tissue is resistant to lipotoxicity.

2. FUNCTIONS OF FAT TISSUE

In addition to storing energy, fat tissue has important immune, endocrine and homeostatic, regenerative, mechanical, and thermal functions. Fat tissue defends against bacterial and fungal infection, as well as tissue injury. To do so, it produces a number of cytokines, chemokines, and hemostatic factors. Indeed, preadipocytes, which account for 15% to 50% of the cells in fat tissue, have gene expression profiles closer to those of macrophages than fat cells [6].

FAs may play a larger than generally recognized role in the defensive function of fat tissue. While there is a lack of information about local FA concentrations in fat tissue, concentrations are likely very high near fat cells, particularly during lipolysis. Direct measurements of FA concentrations adjacent to fat cells are not available. However, the decrease in intracellular pH that accompanies FA transfer across fat cell membranes following induction of lipolysis with isoproterenol or forskolin is as high as that which occurs when cells are exposed to 65 μM oleic acid without albumin (see Figures 1 and 2 in [7]). This suggests that FA concentrations in the immediate vicinity of fat cells could reach levels equivalent to the mid-millimolar range in the presence of physiological albumin concentrations. These levels are lethal to most types of cells. Much lower concentrations are effective in killing *Helicobacter pylori* [8], pneumococcus [9], *Mycobacterium avium* [10], and tuberculosis [11]. Somehow, preadipocytes and fat cells are resistant to these high local FA concentrations. Thus, fat tissue, which is located under the skin and around viscera at points susceptible to invasion by microorganisms, produces both FAs and inflammatory mediators that protect against infection. Indeed, bacterial or fungal infections of fat tissue are rare. Thus, lipotoxicity appears to have been adapted by fat tissue as a defense mechanism. Further, fat cells can use the lipotoxic effects of FAs to regulate function of other cells. For example, human fat cells can release sufficient polyunsaturated FAs in bone marrow to inhibit osteoblastic proliferation without inducing apoptosis [12].

The homeostatic, paracrine, and endocrine functions of adipose tissue are, in part, related to its immune function. Indeed, many of the endocrine and paracrine factors released by adipose tissue with metabolic effects are cytokines (e.g., leptin), while others are lipids. Fat tissue can exert endocrine control over other tissues in a number of ways. It has a traditional endocrine function through releasing protein hormones and processing steroids that act at a distance from fat tissue. Fat cells can also regulate function of other tissues in a nontraditional endocrine manner by taking up residence in nonadipose tissues and exerting effects by producing paracrine factors and lipids. Fat cells can release or fail to remove metabolites, including lipids, that impact function of other tissues. When fat cell numbers increase or their function is dysregulated, they could conceivably contribute to dysfunction of other tissues through lipotoxicity.

3.   CONDITIONS ASSOCIATED WITH LIPOTOXICITY

Several conditions, including obesity, diabetes, the metabolic syndrome, aging, lipodystrophies, and certain drugs have been associated with lipotoxicity in pancreatic β-cells, skeletal muscle, cardiac muscle, hepatocytes, and osteoblasts. Other tissues are likely affected analogously.

Fat tissue is the repository of surplus lipid. In otherwise normal rats, a 60% fat diet for 8 weeks causes a 150% increase in body fat, but only a small increase in pancreatic, liver, heart, and skeletal muscle fat [5]. However, some individuals with obesity, particularly massive obesity, develop lipid accumulation in nonadipose tissues (a sign that lipotoxicity may be occurring). Hepatic, cardiac, skeletal muscle, and pancreatic steatosis have been found in *ob/ob* and *db/db* mice and *fa/fa* rats, which have obesity together with increased appetite, hyperlipidemia, and increased blood free FAs (FFAs) [2, 5, 13]. Obese human subjects can have increased intramyocellular lipid in skeletal muscle [14], increased myocardial lipid by positron emission tomography (PET) scanning [15, 16], and hepatic steatosis [1] associated with dysfunction in each of these tissues. Indeed, cardiac triglyceride (TG) accumulation appears to be an early metabolic marker of cardiac dysfunction in obese subjects [15]. Intramyocardial TG overload occurs in approximately 30% of patients with nonischemic heart failure [13]. Why some, but not all, obese subjects develop lipotoxicity in nonadipose tissues is a potentially illuminating issue that remains to be explained. Among the factors that could account for this are dyslipidemia, genetic traits, altered regional fat distribution, fat tissue dysfunction, aging, extent of adipokine and inflammatory response, hormonal status, coexisting diseases, and activity.

As with obesity, diabetes and insulin resistance are associated with lipid accumulation, cytotoxicity, and dysfunction in a number of tissues. For example, proton magnetic resonance studies suggest that increased intramyocellular lipid content is associated with reduced insulin sensitivity in healthy humans [17]. Type 2 diabetes is associated with increased FA uptake into cardiac myocytes and mitochondria, altered mitochondrial function, and decreased cardiac contractility [2]. Lipotoxicity may be an early event in type 2 diabetes, because inhibiting lipolysis, which results in reduced fasting plasma FFA (but no change in adipokines) improves insulin sensitivity in subjects predisposed to develop diabetes [18]. Of course, obesity and insulin resistance are linked and are components of the metabolic syndrome. The failure of antilipotoxic protection associated with obesity and insulin resistance may even be a cause of the metabolic syndrome [1].

Defective adipose tissue may promote lipotoxicity in peripheral tissues and be a key link among obesity, insulin resistance, and type 2 diabetes [19]. This is highlighted by the observations that aging and congenital lipodystrophies, conditions associated with altered fat tissue function, are themselves associated with the metabolic syndrome and accumulation of lipid associated with dysfunction of nonadipose tissues [5, 20–22]. Congenital lipodystrophies are the most severe of lipotoxic diseases, with little adipose tissue in which to store lipid, low adiponectin and leptin, hyperlipidemia, cardiomyopathy, diabetes, and liver steatosis [5, 23]. Certain drugs associated with fat tissue redistribution and dysfunction are also associated with lipotoxicity. Glucocorticoids cause lipotoxicity with diabetes, steatosis, and hyperlipidemia in rodents [24]. HIV protease inhibitors impede adipogenesis [25] and result in fat redistribution, cardiomyopathy, and diabetes in some patients [26].

4.   MECHANISMS OF LIPOTOXICITY

Several mechanisms probably contribute to the cytotoxicity associated with lipid accumulation in nonadipose tissues. These include increased lipid synthesis, detergent effects on membranes, increased lipolysis or reduced ability to suppress lipolysis in adjacent lipid-containing cells, β-oxidation of FAs, reactive oxygen species (ROS) generation, lipid peroxides, effects on protein kinase B (PKB) and PKC activity, ceramide, stimulation of apoptotic or inhibition of antiapoptotic pathways, necrosis, and promotion of inflammatory cytokine release.

Under most conditions, extensive lipid storage and synthesis, particularly of TGs, is restricted to adipose cells, with smaller amounts being made by liver, muscle, myelin-forming, and steroidogenic cells. Under certain conditions, lipotoxicity can occur in nonadipose cells when lipid synthesis is increased. For example, overexpressing acyl coenzyme A (CoA) synthase (ACS) in cardiomyocytes can induce lipotoxic cardiomyopathy [27]. ACS increases FA import (Figure 1), leading to lipid accumulation with apoptosis, myofiber disorganization, interstitial fibrosis, left ventricular dysfunction, and dilated cardiomyopathy [27]. Decreased ability to suppress lipolysis may contribute to increased local FA concentrations and lipotoxicity. Diabetes and obesity with insulin resistance lead to decreased ability to suppress lipolysis [28] and are associated with lipotoxicity. Thus, increased production or release of FA by cells can contribute to lipotoxicity.

Decreased FA β-oxidation may contribute to lipotoxicity by decreasing removal of cytotoxic FA, while increased β-oxidation may raise production of cytotoxic ROS. Impaired β-oxidation may contribute to increased intramyocellular lipid in obesity and diabetes [29, 30]. Impeding β-oxidation (e.g., by inhibiting ACC activity; Figure 1) can increase levels of potentially lipotoxic nonoxidative metabolites of FAs [5]. Fatty acyl CoA accumulation might be the main factor that leads to cardiac lipotoxicity [31]. Leptin, which increases FA oxidation [32], protects against lipotoxicity in lipodystrophy [33–35]. Thus, reduced β-oxidation may contribute to lipotoxicity. On the other hand, increased β-oxidation can result in ROS generation and lipotoxicity, with the impaired β-oxidation in diabetes and obesity being a compensatory response to protect against excess ROS production [2, 36]. Increasing FA abundance can itself result in increased β-oxidation, possibly through FA binding to peroxisome proliferator activated receptors (PPARs), leading to increased CPT-1 activity and FA oxidation that exceeds energy needs [2, 5, 37] (Figure 1). Indeed, FA oxidation is increased in hearts of obese *db/db* and *ob/ob* animals [38, 39] and cardiac PPARα [13] and PPARγ coactivator-1α (PGC-1α) [40] are increased in diabetes. ROS generation may contribute to palmitate-induced cell death [41]. Fluorescence of an oxidant-sensitive probe is increased

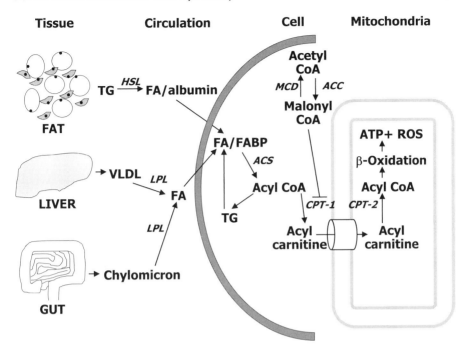

Figure 1. Fatty acid utilization pathways. Triglycerides (TGs) absorbed by the gut circulate as chylomicrons and TGs exported by the liver as lipoproteins. Fatty acids (FAs) released by hormone-sensitive lipase-catalyzed hydrolysis of TGs, circulate as complexes with albumin. TG is hydrolyzed by lipoprotein lipase (LPL) to FA near cell surfaces. FAs diffuse across the cell membrane and are complexed to FA binding proteins (FABP) in the cytosol. Acyl-CoA synthetases (ACS) convert FA to fatty acyl-CoA (acyl CoA). Acyl CoA, in turn, can be incorporated into intracellular TGs or converted into acyl carnitine by carnitine palmitoyl transferase-1 (CPT-1) located in the outer mitochondrial membrane. CPT-1 can be inhibited by malonyl CoA, the concentration of which is determined by a balance between synthesis from acetyl-CoA by acetyl-CoA carboxylase (ACC) and degradation by malonyl CoA decarboxylase (MCD). Once generated by CPT-1, acyl carnitine is transferred into mitochondria by a translocase. After conversion back into acyl CoA by CPT-2 (located in the inner mitochondrial membrane), acyl groups undergo β-oxidation and energy production that entails generation of reactive oxygen species (ROS). PPARα increases ACS (resulting in increased acetyl CoA), MCD (resulting in decreased malonyl CoA), and CPT-1 (enhancing β-oxidation).

by palmitate exposure. Palmitate-induced apoptosis can be blocked by compounds that scavenge reactive intermediates. Thus, increases or decreases in FA β-oxidation can set off events that culminate in cell death.

These findings suggest that lipotoxicity arises from a constellation of cytotoxic mechanisms and is not a single, unified process. This contention is underscored by the observations that such diverse processes as accumulation of peroxidized FA (as a result of increased ROS due to β-oxidation or increased presence of lipid susceptible to peroxidation [2, 42–44]), inhibition of protein kinase B45 or induction or inhibition of certain protein kinase C isoforms by FAs [46–48], and ceramide accumulation (in palmitate- but not oleate-induced lipotoxicity [1, 27, 41, 49, 50] can be involved in cytotoxic effects of FAs.

Exogenous FAs can cause apoptosis within hours in cultured cells [51]. Palmitic acid is a particularly potent apoptosis inducer [51]. Indeed, saturated FAs are generally more lipotoxic than unsaturated FA: excess palmitic acid is more lipotoxic than oleic acid in a number of cell types [3, 41, 50, 52–55]. This has been attributed to generation of specific proapoptotic lipid species or signaling molecules that may vary across cell types: ROS [41], ceramide [56], and nitric oxide [57], decreases in phosphatidylinositol-3-kinase [54] as well as primary effects on mitochondrial structure or function [58]. Exogenous or endogenously generated unsaturated FAs, such as oleate, can rescue palmitate-induced apoptosis by promoting palmitate incorporation into TGs in Chinese hamster ovary (CHO) cells [3]. In cells in which activity of stearoyl-CoA desaturase 1 (SCD1), which catalyzes desaturation of palmitate, is increased, TG accumulation after exposure to palmitate also increases. This suggests that endogenously produced unsaturated FAs can promote TG accumulation. Further, by increasing SCD1 activity, less apoptosis occurs following palmitate exposure. Thus, enhancing ability to synthesize TGs can protect against development of lipotoxicity. Unsaturated FAs reduce lipotoxicity by increasing incorporation of saturated FAs into TGs.

Long-chain FA can suppress Bcl2, an antiapoptotic factor, leading to increased susceptibility to apoptosis in pancreatic cells [59]. Activity of serine/threonine protein phosphatase type 2C is stimulated by certain unsaturated FAs, including oleic acid, and this enzyme dephosphorylates Bad, resulting in increased apoptosis in human umbilical vein endothelial, rat cortical and hippocampal, and human neuroblastoma SH-SY5Y cells [60, 61]. Palmitate and, to a lesser extent, oleate can induce apoptosis in pancreatic β-cells [62]. Both FAs induce endoplasmic reticulum stress response elements (C/EBP homologous protein, activating transcription factor-4 and -6, and immunoglobulin heavy chain binding protein mRNAs and alternative splicing of X-box binding protein-1), but not NFκB. Thus, FFAs can cause apoptosis by activating ER stress responses through an NFκB- and nitric oxide-independent mechanism. In endothelial cells, palmitate is also more effective than oleate in inducing apoptosis, but NO synthase is increased by FA in these cells [63]. Also, elevated FFAs can cause apoptosis of β-cells partly as a result of ceramide generation [50, 64]. Again, cytotoxicity of palmitate is higher than oleate under these conditions. In CHO cells, palmitate, but not oleate, can induce apoptosis through the generation of ROS independently of ceramide synthesis [41]. Thus, FA can cause apoptosis in multiple cell types through diverse mechanisms.

TGs can also cause cell death, in some cases by necrosis rather than apoptosis. In macrophages, exposure to TGs under conditions in which no FFAs were detectable caused cell death in a dose-dependent fashion without an increase in caspase-3 activity [51]. Indeed, caspase-3 activity was reduced in the presence of TGs. Cell death was associated with increased ROS generation by mitochondrial complex 1. Thus, although TGs induce less lipotoxicity than FFAs, they are not completely neutral. The processes through which TGs mediate changes in cell function and death appear to be distinct from those of FAs.

5. INHERENT PROPERTIES OF CELLS CONTRIBUTE TO SUSCEPTIBILITY TO LIPOTOXICITY

Different cell types vary in susceptibility to lipotoxicity (e.g., pancreatic β-cells compared to other pancreatic cell types, or fat cells compared to hepatocytes). This is compatible with the contention that susceptibility to lipotoxicity is partly determined by inherent properties of cells. Studies of effects of aging also support this contention. Dysfunctional cells containing lipid can accumulate with aging in various tissues such as muscle, liver, and bone marrow [20]. Even preadipocytes isolated from animals of different ages maintained for several cell generations under identical culture conditions become increasingly susceptible to FA-induced apoptosis with increasing age [65], pointing to a predisposition to lipotoxicity caused by inherent changes in cell function. With aging, progenitors of a variety of mesenchymal cell types (e.g., muscle satellite cells, osteoblasts) accumulate lipid, express some markers associated with fat cells such as PPARγ2 or FA binding protein 4 (aP2), and continue to express some transcription factors and markers characteristic of their own cells type, but do not develop into functional differentiated cells. This occurs even when these progenitors are maintained under identical culture conditions without exposure to any of the changes in circulating lipids, hormones, or paracrine factors that may occur with aging. Although these adipocyte-like cells contain lipid and are dysfunctional, it is not clear if they really result from lipotoxicity or changes in transcription factor expression related to cell autonomous aging events.

6. ASSOCIATION BETWEEN LIPIDS AND INFLAMMATORY RESPONSES

In addition to causing cytotoxicity directly, lipids can induce immune responses that amplify extent of tissue damage. FAs regulate macrophage gene expression and can induce expression of inflammatory cytokines in macrophages [11, 66]. Given the close relationship between preadipocytes and macrophages, and because inflammatory cytokine expression increases in obesity, it would not be surprising if FAs, particularly saturated FAs, elicited increased inflammatory cytokine expression in adipose tissue with an impact on other organs.

7. MECHANISMS OF DEFENSE AGAINST LIPOTOXICITY

Tissues employ a variety of strategies for protection from the lipotoxic effects of lipids. Lipid depletion is effective in protecting cells from lipotoxicity. For example, lipid depletion protects pancreatic β-cells from apoptotic effects of cytokines [67]. Depletion of intramyocellular lipid is associated with improved insulin sensitivity, reduced ACC mRNA, and increased GLUT4 expression [68]. Overexpression of apolipoprotein B leads to a reduction in cardiac TG stores and increased TG secretion [69, 70], but it is important to acknowledge that lipoprotein secretion has not been demonstrated in cardiac tissue of wild type mice [2]. Insulin can induce lipid accumulation acutely and through up regulating SREBP-1c, which induces lipogenic enzyme expression [71]. Paradoxically, insulin resistance may protect against lipid accumulation, because excluding glucose from cells reduces glucose-derived lipogenesis. Thus, mechanisms that can potentially defend against lipotoxicity include lipoprotein secretion (in cells containing microsomal TG transfer protein), FA export, and insulin resistance.

Control of circulating lipids is another defense against lipotoxicity. While diabetes and obesity can result in increased plasma FAs [72, 73], fasting FFAs are not consistently increased in obese subjects [74], although marked variations in plasma FFAs occur in response to feeding and fasting. FFAs might be elevated at night or integrated basal FFA levels may be higher in obese subjects with the metabolic syndrome than in lean subjects, an area warranting further study. Also, increased circulating lipoproteins and *de novo* lipogenesis from glucose may predispose to lipotoxicity. However, the fact that TG content in cell types other than adipocytes remains within a very narrow range, despite excess caloric intake sufficient to increase fat cell TGs, is consistent with a system of FA homeostasis to protect against lipotoxicity [75]. Normally rats can tolerate a 60% fat diet because 96% of surplus fat is deposited in adipocytes [42].

Although TGs can induce cell necrosis, TGs are less cytotoxic than FAs [3, 50]. While TG accumulation is an indicator of ectopic lipid deposition, storage as TG is probably the least toxic means for sequestering surplus lipids. However, intracellular TG can become part of the problem. Intracellular TG is a potential source of FAs in excess of oxidative needs and can contribute to an increase in the pool of FA CoA, a substrate and regulator of many pathways of nonoxidative FA metabolism. Of nonadipocytes, liver and muscle have highest tolerance to surplus TG: liver can export surplus TG as very low density lipoprotein (VLDL), while muscle can β-oxidize lipid. Also, fat cells present in nonadipose tissues may actually protect those tissues from lipotoxicity by storing or processing excess FAs locally.

Exercise is associated with protection against potentially adverse effects of intramyocellular lipid [76]. Endurance training results in increased intramyocellular lipid despite increased β-oxidation. In obesity and diabetes, increased intramyocellular TG correlates with insulin resistance and is associated with increased lipid peroxidation, but not in endurance-trained subjects [43]. This suggests that endurance training increases intramyocellular antioxidant enzyme activity. Further, increased intramyocellular TG may be a constantly utilized source of energy for ATP production in endurance-trained subjects, while in obese subjects, intramyocellular TG may be stored but not mobilized. Thus, intramyocellular TG accumulation does not necessarily indicate lipotoxicity.

Adiponectin and leptin can defend against cytotoxic effects of lipids. Adiponectin protects against metabolic syndrome [77–80]. It increases AMP-activated protein kinase (AMPK) activity and enhances FA oxidation [81]. Leptin also increases AMPK activity [82] and FA oxidation [32]. In obese, leptin-deficient Zucker rats, adenoviral overexpression of leptin in the liver protects from hepatic fat accumulation and hypertriglyceridemia [32]. Thus, leptin and other factors produced by subcutaneous fat may protect against lipotoxicity [1]. Indeed, increased leptin or transplantation of normal fat ameliorates the lipotoxicity caused by lipodystrophy: leptin reduces the steatosis and diabetes of lipodystrophy in mice and humans [33–35]. Infection with an adenovirus that increases circulating leptin improves lipotoxic cardiomyopathy and decreases blood FA and TG, elevates cardiac expression of anti-apoptotic Bcl2, and decreases expression of proapoptotic Bax [83]. In addition to increasing AMPK, high levels of leptin reduce lipogenic transcription factor expression (SREBP-1C in liver and PPARγ [and ACC and FAS] in fat), increase PGC-1α (increasing numbers of mitochondria) [42]), and prevent the FA-mediated decline in Bcl2 [59]. Thus, the increase in leptin or other adipokines in diet-induced obesity may protect against lipotoxicity in nonadipose tissues, although resistance to effects of these adipokines may eventually develop, as occurs with leptin.

AMPK activation decreases ACC activity, reducing malonyl CoA, resulting in increased CPT1 activity and β-oxidation (Figure 1). AMP kinase activating agents (leptin [82, 84, 85], adiponectin [84], thiazolidinediones [86], metformin [87], and 5-aminoimidazole 4-carboxamide 1-β-D-ribofuranoside AICAR [88, 89]) decrease lipotoxicity. AMP kinase activation reduces the diabetes and ectopic lipid accumulation that occur in Zucker rats [89]. Thus,

AMP kinase appears to have an important role in the lipotoxicity associated with obesity and fat tissue dysfunction.

Despite the importance of adipokines in the genesis of some forms of lipotoxicity, lipotoxicity can occur independently of altered adipokine levels. Transgenic mice with muscle- or liver-specific overexpression of lipoprotein lipase have increased muscle and liver TG content and insulin resistance because of altered insulin signaling [90]. These defects in insulin action are associated with increases in diacylglycerol, fatty acyl CoA, and ceramides. Thus, increased TG synthesis can cause accumulation of intracellular FA-derived metabolites and insulin resistance through alterations in insulin signaling independently of circulating adipokines.

Exogenous or endogenously generated unsaturated FA can rescue palmitate-induced apoptosis in CHO cells [3]. Oleate promotes palmitate incorporation into TG and prevents increased ROS and ceramide generation resulting from palmitate. In cells with increased stearoyl-CoA desaturase 1 (SCD1), TG accumulation is increased in the presence of palmitate, suggesting that endogenously produced unsaturated FAs can promote TG accumulation. These cells are resistant to palmitate-induced apoptosis. Thus, generation of unsaturated FAs can protect against lipotoxicity by increasing incorporation of saturated FAs into TGs.

Other mechanisms may also provide protection from lipotoxicity. For example, removal of ceramide can reduce lipotoxicity. Ceramide is formed by the condensation of palmitoyl CoA and serine, catalyzed by serine palmitoyl transferase (SPT [91]). Reducing palmitoyl CoA and SPT decreases apoptosis in pancreatic islets. Caloric restriction and thiazolidinediones reduce SPT activity and lead to protection from apoptosis [5]. Sirtuins, which promote fat mobilization [92] and are activated by dietary flavinoids, may turn out to be involved in protection from lipotoxicity. In pancreatic β-cells, PKB activation can prevent apoptosis through inhibition of the proapoptotic proteins glycogen synthase kinase-$3\alpha/\beta$, FoxO1, and p53 [45].

8.   PREADIPOCYTES AND FAT CELLS ARE MORE RESISTANT THAN OTHER CELL TYPES TO FA

Defenses against lipotoxicity are best developed in adipose tissue. Nonadipose tissues have very limited capacity to store lipids [3]. Lipotoxicity does not seem to occur in fat tissue itself [93], at least under most conditions. Preadipocytes, which account for 15% to 50% of the cells in fat tissue, are resistant to levels of FAs that would destroy other cell types. 3T3-L1 cells are resistant to 1.5 mM palmitic acid [93]. Fat cells themselves are resistant to FA. Treatment of collagenase-isolated rat epididymal adipocytes for up to 24 hours with 1.5 mM oleate or palmitate at an FFA: albumin ratio of 2.5:1 results in no significant effects on IRS-1, PI3 kinase, PKB, phosphorylated PKB, GLUT4, insulin-stimulated glucose uptake, or basal or cAMP-stimulated lipolysis or inhibition of lipolysis by insulin [93].

How do preadipocytes and fat cells protect themselves against the consequences of exposure to very high concentrations of FAs? Very few data are available about this. Possible mechanisms include the following. Fat cells express abundant aP2 and other FA-binding proteins, which may provide protection against high intracellular levels of FAs and their metabolites. Long-chain FAs induce preadipocyte aP2 expression [94]. aP2 and other intracellular lipid-binding proteins may also function as lipid chaperones, facilitating the movement of FA out of fat cells [95]. Fat cells likely have well developed antiapoptotic mechanisms, because there are high local concentrations of tumor necrosis factor-alpha (TNF-α) and interleukin-6 (IL-6) in adipose tissue that they must defend themselves against. Fat tissue turns over at a greater rate than generally appreciated—with fat cell numbers increasing throughout life in some fat depots [96], permitting replacement of damaged cells. There is a large pool of fat cell progenitors that can replace damaged adipocytes. Fat cells have highly developed machinery to esterify potentially lipotoxic FAs into TGs. Also, β-oxidation occurs in fat cells, providing another means to dispose of acyl-CoA. Further, fat cells are resistant to potentially high levels of ROS resulting from FAs. Interestingly, the dicarboxylate carrier is expressed at higher levels in adipocytes than in any other cell type [97]. Overexpression of the mitochondrial dicarboxylate carrier leads to hyperpolarization of the mitochondrial membrane, resulting in increased ROS formation [98]. Exposure of primary rat adipocytes to hyperglycemic conditions *in vitro* reduces insulin sensitivity and increases ROS levels [99]. Adipocytes isolated from mice fed high-fat have significantly elevated ROS [100]. ROS are increased in primary adipocytes isolated from mice exposed to nutrient excess *in vivo* [98]. Further, differentiation of murine 3T3-L1 preadipocytes into adipocytes is associated with the acquisition of apoptotic resistance accompanied by upregulation of cell survival genes even under conditions in which ROS production is increased [101]. Thus, ROS in fat cells may be high and these cells appear to have well developed mechanisms to resist ROS damage.

There may be situations in which even cells in fat tissue become paradoxically susceptible to lipotoxicity. An example of this is the increasing susceptibility of preadipocytes to apoptosis induced by FA with aging [65]. Perhaps other disease states, such as fat redistribution and the metabolic syndrome associated with HIV protease inhibitors that interfere with adipogenesis, may also prove to involve this hypothetical mechanism. Such processes could set up a cycle of lipotoxicity in fat tissue (Figure 2), with FA contributing to preadipocyte dysfunction, impeding adipogenesis with failure to store FAs as

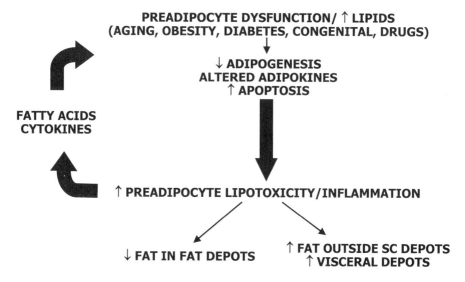

Figure 2. Hypothetical lipotoxicity cycle in fat tissue. Fat cells and preadipocytes presumably have stronger defenses against lipotoxic effects of potentially high local FA concentrations and flux than cells in other tissues. Should these defenses (including capacity to undergo adipogenesis, FA binding proteins, β-oxidation, mechanisms to remove reactive oxygen species, resistance to apoptosis) fail, a cycle of reduced FA removal leading to more damage, resulting in further reduction in capacity to remove FA could ensue. This could contribute to increased fat tissue inflammatory cytokine generation and reduced capacity to store FA as TG, with spillover into nonadipose tissues and other fat depots.

TGs, leading to further increases in FAs, compounding fat tissue dysfunction and causing reduced adiponectin and leptin production and increased inflammatory cytokine generation.

9.   SUMMARY

Lipotoxicity, defined as lipid-induced metabolic damage, occurs when net capacity to store and utilize lipids is exceeded. In diabetes, obesity, the metabolic syndrome, lipodystrophies, aging, and other conditions, lipotoxicity can result in systemic dysfunction. However, lipotoxicity can be adaptive, possibly providing defense against infection and accumulation of dysfunctional cells. Fatty acids are more lipotoxic than triglycerides, and different fatty acids vary in extent and mechanisms of lipotoxicity. Lipotoxicity is predisposed to by multiple factors, occurs through diverse mechanisms, and can cause cell removal through apoptosis or necrosis. Fat cells and preadipocytes are particularly resistant. Thus, lipotoxicity is not a single process and can have adaptive as well as detrimental consequences.

10. CONCLUSIONS

Although it is tempting to consider lipotoxicity to be a single process, this is probably simplistic. A diversity of triggers and pathways can lead to the lipid accumulation and cell death that are features of lipotoxicity. With respect to triggers, increased external lipid concentrations, decreased adiponectin or leptin, increased glucocorticoids, and intracellular processes, such as mitochondrial dysfunction with aging, may all predispose to lipotoxic cell death. None of these processes appears to be uniformly required for intracellular lipid accumulation and then cell death to occur. With respect to pathways involved, increases as well as decreases in FA β-oxidation, depending on cellular context, have been associated with mechanisms culminating in cell death. Accumulation of ceramide, which is likely important in the lipotoxicity resulting specifically from palmitic acid exposure, is much less likely to be a key factor in the lipotoxicity resulting from oleic acid. Deficiency of adiponectin or leptin may predispose to lipotoxicity, but lipotoxicity can occur without this, for example, in the setting of increased lipoprotein lipase activity. Even the mechanisms of cell death resulting from exposure to increased concentrations of various types of lipids differ: FAs are associated with apoptosis while TGs induce necrotic cell death. Thus, lipotoxicity is a group of processes predisposing to cell death through diverse triggers and pathways. A search for a unifying mechanism leading to cell death from lipids in all tissues is unlikely to be revealing. Although description of the diverse mechanisms resulting in cell death due to lipids is important, it is even more important to understand the tissue- and situation-specific processes that defend against cell death in order to devise specific therapies.

Lipotoxicity is not uniformly detrimental. It can be an adaptive process that removes dysfunctional cells or invading organisms, provides a means for regulating tissue development (e.g., osteoprogenitor function), and defends against overshoot effects of chronically high insulin levels by contributing to insulin resistance. The high FA levels likely present in fat tissue have been incorporated into its metabolic storage, regulatory, and immune roles. Obesity, a state rarely found in nature, and other types of fat tissue dysfunction may subvert these normal responses, resulting in lipotoxicity in fat and other tissues. The metabolic syndrome might be a particularly extreme example of this.

Thus, lipotoxicity is not a single process with uniformly destructive effects. The extent of lipotoxicity is predisposed to by multiple factors (including type of lipid, cellular context, inflammatory cytokines, hormonal status, drugs), proceeds through diverse mechanisms, and can have beneficial as well as destructive consequences.

ACKNOWLEDGMENTS

The authors are grateful for the assistance of J. Armstrong. This work was funded by NIH grants DK56891 and 13925 (JLK) and DK35914, 46200, and 56690 (BEC).

REFERENCES

[1] Unger RH. Longevity, lipotoxicity and leptin: The adipocyte defense against feasting and famine. Biochimie 2005;87:57–64.

[2] Carley AN, Severson DL. Fatty acid metabolism is enhanced in type 2 diabetic hearts. Biochim Biophys Acta 2005;1734:112–126.

[3] Listenberger LL, Han H, Lewis SE, et al. Triglyceride accumulation protects against fatty acid-induced lipotoxicity. Proc Natl Acad Sci USA 2003;100:3077–3082.

[4] DeFronzo RA. Dysfunctional fat cells, lipotoxicity and type 2 diabetes. Int J Clin Pract 2004;(Suppl):9–21.

[5] Unger RH. Lipotoxic diseases. Annu Rev Med 2002;53:319–336.

[6] Charriere G, Cousin B, Arnaud E, et al. Preadipocyte conversion to macrophage. J Biol Chem 2003;278:9850–9855.

[7] Civelek VN, Hamilton JA, Tornheim K, et al. Intracellular pH in adipocytes: Effects of free fatty acid diffusion across the plasma membrane, lipolytic agonists, and insulin. Proc Natl Acad Sci USA 1996;93:10139–10144.

[8] Petschow BW, Batema RP, Ford LL., Susceptibility of *Helicobacter pylori* to bactericidal properties of medium-chain monoglycerides and free fatty acids. Antimicrob Agents Chemother 1996;40:302–306.

[9] Coonrod JD. Role of surfactant free fatty acids in antimicrobial defenses. Eur J Resp Dis 1987;153(Suppl):209–214.

[10] Akaki T, Sato K, Shimizu T, et al. Effector molecules in expression of the antimicrobial activity of macrophages against *Mycobacterium avium* complex: Roles of reactive nitrogen intermediates, reactive oxygen intermediates, and free fatty acids. J Leukoc Biol 1997;62:795–804.

[11] Akaki T, Tomioka H, Shimizu T, et al. Comparative roles of free fatty acids with reactive nitrogen intermediates and reactive oxygen intermediates in expression of the antimicrobial activity of macrophages against *Mycobacterium tuberculosis*. Clin Exp Immunol 2000;121:302–310.

[12] Maurin AC, Chavassieux PM, Vericel E, et al. Role of polyunsaturated fatty acids in the inhibitory effect of human adipocytes on osteoblastic proliferation. Bone 2002;31:260–266.

[13] Sharma S, Adrogue JV, Golfman L, et al. Intramyocardial lipid accumulation in the failing human heart resembles the lipotoxic rat heart. FASEB J 2004;18:1692–1700.

[14] Goodpaster BH, Theriault R, Watkins SC, et al. Intramuscular lipid content is increased in obesity and decreased by weight loss. Metabolism 2000;49:467–472.

[15] Szczepaniak LS, Dobbins RL, Metzger GJ, et al. Myocardial triglycerides and systolic function in humans: In vivo evaluation by localized proton spectroscopy and cardiac imaging. Magn Reson Med 2003;49:417–423.

[16] Peterson LR, Herrero P, Schechtman KB, et al. Effect of obesity and insulin resistance on myocardial substrate metabolism and efficiency in young women. Circulation 2004;109:2191–2196.

[17] Szczepaniak LS, Babcock EE, Schick F, et al. Measurement of intracellular triglyceride stores by H spectroscopy: Validation in vivo. Am J Physiol 1999;276:E977–989.

[18] Bajaj M, Suraamornkul S, Kashyap S, et al. Sustained reduction in plasma free fatty acid concentration improves insulin action without altering plasma adipocytokine levels in subjects with strong family history of type 2 diabetes. J Clin Endocrinol Metab 2004;89:4649–4655.

[19] Lelliott C, Vidal-Puig AJ. Lipotoxicity, an imbalance between lipogenesis de novo and fatty acid oxidation. Int J Obes Relat Metab Disord 2004;28(Suppl 4):S22–S28.

[20] Kirkland JL, Tchkonia T, Pirtskhalava T, et al. Adipogenesis and aging: Does aging make fat go MAD? Exp Gerontol 2002;37:757–767.

[21] Unger RH. Lipid overload and overflow: Metabolic trauma and the metabolic syndrome. Trends Endocrinol Metab 2003;14:398–403.

[22] Rodriguez A, Muller DC, Engelhardt M, et al. Contribution of impaired glucose tolerance in subjects with the metabolic syndrome: Baltimore Longitudinal Study of Aging. Metabolism 2005;54:542–547.

[23] Agarwal AK, Barnes RI, Garg A. Genetic basis of congenital generalized lipodystrophy. Int J Obes Relat Metab Disord 2004;28:336–339.

[24] Ogawa A, Johnson JH, Ohneda M, et al. Roles of insulin resistance and beta-cell dysfunction in dexamethasone-induced diabetes. J Clin Invest 1992;90:497–504.

[25] Dowell P, Flexner C, Kwiterovich PO, et al. Suppression of preadipocyte differentiation and promotion of adipocyte death by HIV protease inhibitors. J Biol Chem 2000;275:41325–41332.

[26] Grinspoon SK. Metabolic syndrome and cardiovascular disease in patients with human immunodeficiency virus. Am J Med 2005;118(Suppl 2):23S–28S.

[27] Chiu HC, Kovacs A, Ford DA, et al. A novel mouse model of lipotoxic cardiomyopathy. J Clin Invest 2001;107:813–822.

[28] Felber JP, Ferrannini E, Golay A, et al. Role of lipid oxidation in pathogenesis of insulin resistance of obesity and type II diabetes. Diabetes 1987;36:1341–1350.

[29] Kelley DE, Goodpaster B, Wing RR, et al. Skeletal muscle fatty acid metabolism in association with insulin resistance, obesity, and weight loss. Am J Physiol 1999;277:E1130–E1141.

[30] Kelley DE, Goodpaster BH. Skeletal muscle triglyceride. An aspect of regional adiposity and insulin resistance. Diab Care 2001;24:933–941.

[31] Jagasia D, McNulty PH. Diabetes mellitus and heart failure. Congest Heart Fail 2003;9:133–139.

[32] Lee Y, Wang MY, Kakuma T, et al. Liporegulation in diet-induced obesity. The antisteatotic role of hyperleptinemia. J Biol Chem 2001;276:5629–5635.

[33] Shimomura I, Hammer RE, Ikemoto S, et al. Leptin reverses insulin resistance and diabetes mellitus in mice with congenital lipodystrophy. Nature 1999;401:73–76.

[34] Oral EA, Simha V, Ruiz E, et al. Leptin-replacement therapy for lipodystrophy. New Engl J Med 2002;346:570–578.

[35] Gavrilova B, Marcus-Samuels B, Graham D, et al. Surgical implantation of adipose tissue reverses diabetes in lipoatrophic mice. J Clin Invest 2000;105:271–278.

[36] Schrauwen P, Hesselink MK. Oxidative capacity, lipotoxicity, and mitochondrial damage in type 2 diabetes. Diabetes 2004;53:1412–1417.

[37] McGarry JD, Dobbins RL. Fatty acids, lipotoxicity and insulin secretion. Diabetologia 1999;42:128–138.

[38] Mazumder PK, O'Neill BT, Roberts MW, et al. Impaired cardiac efficiency and increased fatty acid oxidation in insulin-resistant ob/ob mouse hearts. Diabetes 2004;53:2366–2374.

[39] Carley AN, Semeniuk LM, Shimoni Y, et al. Treatment of type 2 diabetic db/db mice with a novel PPARgamma agonist improves cardiac metabolism but not contractile function. Am J Physiol 2004;286:E449–E455.

[40] Finck BN, Lehman JJ, Leone TC, et al. The cardiac phenotype induced by PPARalpha overexpression mimics that caused by diabetes mellitus. J Clin Invest 2002;109:121–130.

[41] Listenberger LL, Ory DS, Schaffer JE. Palmitate-induced apoptosis can occur through a ceramide-independent pathway. J Biol Chem 2001;276:14890–14895.

[42] Unger RH. The physiology of cellular liporegulation. Annu Rev Physiol 2003;65:333–347.

[43] Russell AP, Gastaldi G, Bobbioni-Harsch E, et al. Lipid peroxidation in skeletal muscle of obese as compared to endurance-trained humans: A case of good vs. bad lipids? FEBS Lett 2003;551:104–106.

[44] MacDonald GA, Bridle KR, Ward PJ, et al. Lipid peroxidation in hepatic steatosis in humans is associated with hepatic fibrosis and occurs predominately in acinar zone 3. J Gastroenterol Hepatol 2001;16:599–606.

[45] Wrede CE, Dickson LM, Lingohr MK, et al. Protein kinase B/Akt prevents fatty acid-induced apoptosis in pancreatic beta-cells (INS-1). J Biol Chem 2002;277:49676–49684.

[46] Yaney GC, Korchak HM, Corkey BE. Long-chain acyl CoA regulation of protein kinase C and fatty acid potentiation of glucose-stimulated insulin secretion in clonal beta-cells. Endocrinology 2000;141:1989–1998.

[47] Griffin ME, Marcucci MJ, Cline GW, et al. Free fatty acid-induced insulin resistance is associated with activation of protein kinase C theta and alterations in the insulin signaling cascade. Diabetes 1999;48:1270–1274.

[48] Kim YB, Shulman GI, Kahn BB. Fatty acid infusion selectively impairs insulin action on Akt1 and protein kinase C lambda/zeta but not on glycogen synthase kinase-3. J Biol Chem 2002;277:32915–32922.

[49] Shimabukuro M, Zhou YT, Levi M, et al. Fatty acid-induced beta cell apoptosis: A link between obesity and diabetes. Proc Natl Acad Sci USA 1998;95:2498–2502.

[50] Cnop M, Hannaert JC, Hoorens A, et al. Inverse relationship between cytotoxicity of free fatty acids in pancreatic islet cells and cellular triglyceride accumulation. Diabetes 2001;50:1771–1777.

[51] Aronis A, Madar Z, Tirosh O. Mechanism underlying oxidative stress-mediated lipotoxicity: Exposure of J774.2 macrophages to triacylglycerols facilitates mitochondrial reactive oxygen species production and cellular necrosis. Free Radical Biol Med 2005;38:1221–1230.

[52] de Vries JE, Vork MM, Roemen TH, et al. Saturated but not mono-unsaturated fatty acids induce apoptotic cell death in neonatal rat ventricular myocytes. J Lipid Res 1997; 38:1384–1394.

[53] Maedler K, Spinas GA, Dyntar D, et al. Distinct effects of saturated and monounsaturated fatty acids on beta-cell turnover and function. Diabetes 2001;50:69–76.

[54] Hardy S, Langelier Y, Prentki M. Oleate activates phosphatidylinositol 3-kinase and promotes proliferation and reduces apoptosis of MDA-MB-231 breast cancer cells, whereas palmitate has opposite effects. 2000;60:6353–6358.

[55] Paumen MB, Ishida Y, Muramatsu M, et al. Inhibition of carnitine palmitoyltransferase I augments sphingolipid synthesis and palmitate-induced apoptosis. J Biol Chem 1997; 272:3324–3329.

[56] Shimabukuro M, Higa M, Zhou YT, et al. Lipoapoptosis in beta-cells of obese prediabetic fa/fa rats. Role of serine palmitoyltransferase overexpression. J Biol Chem 1998; 273:32487–32490.

[57] Shimabukuro M, Ohneda M, Lee Y, et al. Role of nitric oxide in obesity-induced beta cell disease. J Clin Invest 1997;100:290–295.

[58] Ostrander DB, Sparagna GC, Amoscato AA, et al. Decreased cardiolipin synthesis corresponds with cytochrome c release in palmitate-induced cardiomyocyte apoptosis. J Biol Chem 2001;276:38061–38067.

[59] Shimabukuro M, Wang MY, Zhou YT, et al. Protection against lipoapoptosis of beta cells through leptin-dependent maintenance of Bcl-2 expression. Proc Natl Acad Sci USA 1998;95:9558–9561.

[60] Hufnagel B, Dworak M, Soufi M, et al. Unsaturated fatty acids isolated from human lipoproteins activate protein phosphatase type 2Cbeta and induce apoptosis in endothelial cells. Atherosclerosis 2005;180:245–254.

[61] Zhu Y, Schwarz S, Ahlemeyer B, et al. Oleic acid causes apoptosis and dephosphorylates Bad. Neurochem Int 2005;46:127–135.

[62] Kharroubi I, Ladriere L, Cardozo AK, et al. Free fatty acids and cytokines induce pancreatic beta-cell apoptosis by different mechanisms: Role of nuclear factor-kappaB and endoplasmic reticulum stress. Endocrinology 2004;145:5087–5096.

[63] Artwohl M, Roden M, Waldhausl W, et al. Free fatty acids trigger apoptosis and inhibit cell cycle progression in human vascular endothelial cells. FASEB J 2003;18:146–148.

[64] Lupi R, Dotta F, Marselli L, et al. Prolonged exposure to free fatty acids has cytostatic and pro-apoptotic effects on human pancreatic islets: Evidence that beta-cell death is caspase mediated, partially dependent on ceramide pathway, and Bcl-2 regulated. Diabetes 2002;51:1437–1442.

[65] Guo W, Pirtskhalava T, Tchkonia T, et al. Aging results in paradoxical susceptibility of fat cell progenitors to lipotoxicity. Obesity Res 2004;12(Suppl):A31.

[66] Chawla A, Lee CH, Barak Y, et al. PPAR delta is a very low-density lipoprotein sensor in macrophages. Proc Natl Acad Sci USA 2003;100:1268–1273.

[67] Shimabukuro M, Koyama K, Lee Y, et al. Leptin- or troglitazone-induced lipopeniaprotects islets frominterleukin 1beta toxicity. J Clin Invest 1997;100:1750–1754.

[68] Manco M, Calvani M, Mingrone G. Effects of dietary fatty acids on insulin sensitivity and secretion. Diabetes Obes Metab 2004;6:402–413.

[69] Nielsen LB, Bartels ED, Bollano E. Overexpression of apolipoprotein B in the heart impedes cardiac triglyceride accumulation and development of cardiac dysfunction in diabetic mice. J Biol Chem 2002;277:27014–27020.

[70] Yokoyama M, Yagyu H, Hu Y, et al. Apolipoprotein B production reduces lipotoxic cardiomyopathy: Studies in heart-specific lipoprotein lipase transgenic mouse. J Biol Chem 2004;279:4204–4211.

[71] Foufelle F, Ferre P. New perspectives in the regulation of hepatic glycolytic and lipogenic genes by insulin and glucose: A role for the transcription factor sterol regulatory element binding protein-1c. Biochem J 2002;366(Pt 2):377–391.

[72] Gordon E. Non-esterified fatty acids in the blood of obese and lean subjects. Am J Clin Nutr 1960;8:740–747.

[73] Reaven GM, Hollenbeck C, Jeng CY, et al. Measurement of plasma glucose, free fatty acid, lactate, and insulin for 24 h in patients with NIDDM. Diabetes 1988;37:1020–1024.

[74] Maslowska M, Vu H, Phelis S, et al. Plasma acylation stimulating protein, adipsin and lipids in non-obese and obese populations. Eur J Clin Invest 1999;29:679–686.

[75] Unger RH, Orci L. Lipotoxic diseases of nonadipose tissues in obesity. Int J Obes Relat Metab Disord 2000;24(Suppl 4):S28–S32.

[76] Goodpaster BH, He J, Watkins S, et al. Skeletal muscle lipid content and insulin resistance: Evidence for a paradox in endurance-trained athletes. J Clin Endocrinol Metab 2001;86:5755–5761.

[77] Combs TP, Wagner JA, Berger J, et al. Induction of adipocyte complement-related protein of 30 kilodaltons by PPARgamma agonists: A potential mechanism of insulin sensitization. Endocrinology 2002;143:998–1007.

[78] Addy CL, Gavrila A, Tsiodras S, et al. Hypoadiponectinemia is associated with insulin resistance, hypertriglyceridemia, and fat redistribution in human immunodeficiency virus-infected patients treated with highly active antiretroviral therapy. J Clin Endocrinol Metab 2003;88:627–636.

[79] Thamer C, Machann J, Tschritter O, et al. Relationship between serum adiponectin concentration and intramyocellular lipid stores in humans. Horm Metab Res 2002;34:646–649.

[80] Lindsay RS, Funahashi T, Hanson RL, et al. Adiponectin and development of type 2 diabetes in the Pima Indian population. Lancet 2002;360:57–58.

[81] Tomas E, Tsao TS, Saha AK, et al. Enhanced muscle fat oxidation and glucose transport by ACRP30 globular domain: Acetyl-CoA carboxylase inhibition and AMP-activated protein kinase activation. Proc Natl Acad Sci USA 2002;99:16309–16313.

[82] Minokoshi Y, Kim Y, Peroni O, et al. Leptin stimulates fatty acid oxidation by activating AMP-activated protein kinase. Nature 2002;415:339–343.

[83] Lee Y, Naseem RH, Duplomb L, et al. Hyperleptinemia prevents lipotoxic cardiomyopathy in acyl CoA synthase transgenic mice. Proc Natl Acad Sci USA 2004;101(37):13624–13629.

[84] Tomas E, Kelly M, Xiang X, et al. Metabolic and hormonal interactions between muscle and adipose tissue. Proc Nutr Soc 2004;63:381–385.

[85] Minokoshi Y, Kahn BB. Role of AMP-activated protein kinase in leptin-induced fatty acid oxidation in muscle. Biochem Soc Trans 2003;31(Pt 1):196–201.

[86] Saha AK, Avilucea PR, Ye JM, et al. Pioglitazone treatment activates AMP-activated protein kinase in rat liver and adipose tissue in vivo. Biochem Biophys Res Commun 2004;314:580–585.

[87] Fryer LG, Parbu-Patel A, Carling D. The anti-diabetic drugs rosiglitazone and metformin stimulate AMP-activated protein kinase through distinct signaling pathways. J Biol Chem 2002;277:25226–25232.

[88] Iglesias MA, Ye JM, Frangioudakis G, et al. AICAR administration causes an apparent enhancement of muscle and liver insulin action in insulin-resistant high-fat-fed rats. Diabetes 2002;51:2886–2894.

[89] Yu X, McCorkle S, Wang M, et al. Leptinomimetic effects of the AMP kinase activator AICAR in leptin-resistant rats: Prevention of diabetes and ectopic lipid deposition. Diabetologia 2004;47:2012–2021.

[90] Kim JK, Fillmore JJ, Chen Y, et al. Tissue-specific overexpression of lipoprotein lipase causes tissue-specific insulin resistance. Proc Natl Acad Sci USA 2001;98:7522–7527.

[91] Hanada K. Serine palmitoyltransferase, a key enzyme of sphingolipid metabolism. Biochim Biophys Acta 2003;1632:16–30.

[92] Picard F, Kurtev M, Chung N, et al. Sirt1 promotes fat mobilization in white adipocytes by repressing PPAR-γ. Nature 2004;430:921.

[93] Lundgren M, Eriksson JW. No *in vitro* effects of fatty acids on glucose uptake, lipolysis or insulin signaling in rat adipocytes. Horm Metab Res 2004;36:203–209.

[94] Grimaldi PA, Knobel SM, Whitesell RR, et al. Induction of aP2 gene expression by non-metabolized long-chain fatty acids. Proc Natl Acad Sci USA 1992;15:10930–10934.

[95] Coe NR, Simpson MA, Bernlohr DA. Targeted disruption of the adipocyte lipid-binding protein (aP2 protein) gene impairs fat cell lipolysis and increases cellular fatty acid levels. J Lipid Res 1999;40:967–972.

[96] Bertrand HA, Masoro EJ, Yu BP. Increasing adipocyte number as the basis for perirenal depot growth in adult rats. Science 1978;201:1234–1235.

[97] Das K, Lewis RY, Combatsiaris TP, et al. Predominant expression of the mitochondrial dicarboxylate carrier in white adipose tissue. Biochem J 1999;344(Pt 2):313–320.

[98] Lin Y, Berg AH, Iyengar P, et al. The hyperglycemia-induced inflammatory response in adipocytes: The role of reactive oxygen species. J Biol Chem 2005;280:4617–4626.

[99] Lu B, Ennis D, Lai R, et al. Enhanced sensitivity of insulin-resistant adipocytes to vanadate is associated with oxidative stress and decreased reduction of vanadate (+5) to vanadyl (+4). J Biol Chem 2001;276:35589–35598.

[100] Talior I, Tennenbaum T, Kuroki T, et al. PKC-delta-dependent activation of oxidative stress in adipocytes of obese and insulin-resistant mice: Role for NADPH oxidase. Am J Physiol 2005;288:E405–E411.

[101] Carriere A, Fernandez Y, Rigoulet M, et al. Inhibition of preadipocyte proliferation by mitochondrial reactive oxygen species. FEBS Lett 2003;550:163–167.

Chapter 7

Ectopic Fat and the Metabolic Syndrome

Frederico G.S. Toledo and David E. Kelley

Division of Endocrinology and Metabolism, Department of Medicine, University of Pittsburgh, School of Medicine, Pittsburgh, PA 15213, USA

1.   INTRODUCTION

It has been long recognized that increased adiposity, especially a predominance of abdominal adiposity, is associated with insulin resistance. A central pattern of obesity is also frequently observed in association with hypertension and a distinct pattern of atherogenic dyslipidemia characterized by elevated serum triglycerides, low high-density lipoprotein (HDL) cholesterol, and small dense low-density lipoprotein (LDL) particles. This cluster of associations is now grouped and recognized as the "metabolic syndrome" [1]. The metabolic syndrome appears to be quite prevalent in the Western world and is estimated to be manifest by nearly one quarter of adults in the US population [2]. Although there is still uncertainty and debate about which is the best set of clinical criteria and diagnostic cutoffs to define the metabolic syndrome, and how these vary according to ethnicity, consensus definitions have been established by the National Cholesterol Education Program [3], the World Health Organization [4], and the International Diabetes Federation.

Despite broad concordance that obesity induces clinically significant insulin resistance, there is the paradox to be considered that nearly two thirds of the adults in the US population are overweight or obese, and yet a substantially lesser fraction manifests the metabolic syndrome. Thus while it is clear that adiposity can be causative of the metabolic syndrome, there is variance in the strength of this link. Central obesity stands as a major risk factor for insulin resistance. Nonetheless, the exact mechanisms by which obesity causes or aggravates insulin resistance are not entirely understood. A predominance of central rather than lower body fat distribution has long been recognized as one important distinction, posited by Vague and colleagues a number of years ago [5], between those who develop the metabolic syndrome compared to those who do not. Another aspect of adiposity that has drawn increasing attention more recently is accumulation of fat within nonadipose organs, notably liver and skeletal muscle, and potentially other organs such as pancreatic islets and myocardium. We review several mechanisms that link obesity with insulin resistance and in particular consider the causes and consequences of fat accretion within liver and skeletal muscle, a manifestation that has been described as "ectopic fat."

The primary storage place for lipids is adipose tissue. *Ectopic*, in Greek, means "out of place." The ectopic fat theory postulates that systemic metabolic repercussions may occur as a result of excessive lipid accumulation in certain metabolically active tissues, most notably those known to be highly insulin-responsive, such as liver and skeletal muscle [6]. However, it should be noted that it is normal for liver and skeletal muscle to contain triglycerides, so the term "ectopic" is somewhat technically imprecise. Rather, in the context of physiopathology the use of the term denotes increased fat content.

2.   CONSEQUENCES OF EXCESS ADIPOSITY TO WHOLE-BODY GLUCOSE HOMEOSTASIS

Insulin resistance is characterized by decreased whole-body glucose disposal, decreased suppression of glucose production, and decreased inhibition of lipolysis, which can be accounted for, respectively, by decreased insulin responsiveness in skeletal muscle, liver, and adipose tissue. Together, these three tissues play a major role in determining whole-body insulin resistance and abnormalities of glucose and lipid homeostasis. What has yet to be fully understood is how these tissues become less responsive to insulin in relation to obesity.

In obesity, insulin resistance in liver and skeletal muscle appears to be strongly linked to mechanisms of lipotoxicity, i.e., impairments in insulin-signaling brought about by excess lipids within hepatocytes or myocytes. One mechanism might be an increased delivery of circulating free fatty acids (FFAs), arising from dysregulation of lipolysis from within the expanded mass of adipose tissue. This would be present both during fasting conditions, but also, and perhaps more importantly, by impaired suppression of plasma FFAs during insulin-stimulated conditions after meal ingestion. Another equally reasonable postulation is that liver and skeletal muscle may become insulin resistant because of intrinsic metabolic derangements in these tissues that confer a relative inability to handle excessive FFA fluxes. These two postulates are not mutually exclusive but could coexist in a feed-forward manner that compounds the risk for insulin resistance. One possibility is that in individuals predisposed to develop insulin resistance, liver and/or skeletal muscle may have a low capacity to metabolize an excessive flux of FFAs [7]. The net effect would be lipid accumulation in these tissues, which would be compounded if flux of FFAs to these tissues is increased above normal rates. Both excess FFA flux or decreased oxidation and metabolism are two mechanisms that may vary in relative contribution in different individuals.

3.   FFA-INDUCED INSULIN RESISTANCE

A rise in plasma FFAs reduces insulin sensitivity in skeletal muscle and liver [8–10]. Plasma FFAs are typically elevated in the insulin resistant individuals, providing liver and skeletal muscle with an increased flux of FFAs. An increased FFA flux to these tissues can induce competition between FFAs and glucose oxidation, resulting in an inhibition of glucose oxidation and secondary inhibition of glycolysis and ultimately glucose uptake, one of the hallmarks of insulin resistance. This specific biochemical model continues to be described as the Randle cycle [9, 11], citing the seminal work of this investigator that was initially described nearly half a century ago. More recent studies indicate that the site of inhibition induced by FFAs in skeletal muscle may be at the step of glucose transport and insulin signaling [12, 13]. Indeed, in addition to providing competing substrate, FFAs are now recognized to interfere with insulin sensitivity by additional mechanisms, such as disruption of intracellular signaling pathways [8, 10, 14–16].

Although the intracellular mechanisms by which FFAs interfere with insulin sensitivity continue to be an important area for investigation, the notion that increased levels of FFAs are important in the genesis of hepatic insulin resistance is well established, and one perspective on this has been refined in the "portal hypothesis," which attempts to explain why visceral adiposity, although generally accounting for just one tenth of overall adiposity, is nonetheless a stronger correlate of insulin resistance than total adiposity. This crux of the portal hypothesis is that increased visceral adiposity leads to excessive FFA flux to the liver. Visceral adipocytes are more insulin resistant than subcutaneous fat adipocytes with regard to suppression of lipolysis [17] and FFAs are released predominantly into the portal circulation. This exposes the liver to high FFA concentrations in those with central obesity. Despite its elegance, this hypothesis has not been proven in humans, largely owing to technical difficulties in sampling blood from the portal vein. Rather it has been suggested that the majority of FFAs entering hepatocytes derive from subcutaneous depots [18]. Alternatively, or in addition, visceral fat may also affect hepatic insulin sensitivity by releasing adipokines into the portal circulation, potentially causing increased hepatic insulin resistance [19]. Although the portal hypothesis may in part explain hepatic insulin resistance and provide a context for understanding the better correlation between central adiposity and insulin resistance, it does not satisfactorily explain by itself all the features of insulin resistance and does not account well for insulin resistance observed in skeletal muscle.

It should be highlighted that an increase in FFA flux to liver and skeletal muscle does not in itself constitute a determinant of insulin resistance in these tissues, unless it results in the accumulation of lipid metabolites in these tissues. Such a notion is consistent with idea of lipotoxicity and is one of the cornerstones of the ectopic fat theory. The ectopic fat theory has emerged as an appealing candidate explanation to integrate obesity, lipotoxicity, and increased FFA fluxes into a cohesive concept responsible for insulin resistance.

4.   ECTOPIC FAT IN SKELETAL MUSCLE AND INSULIN RESISTANCE

Support for the ectopic fat theory has increased in recent years as a result of numerous experimental observations that skeletal muscle and liver have increased intracellular triglyceride in insulin resistant states. In skeletal muscle of individuals with obesity as well as those type 2 diabetes, the intracellular content of lipids is increased [20–23]. This observation suggests that intramyocellular lipid (IMCL) content and insulin resistance are related, which has been further suggested by several more refined experimental observations. First, the magnitude of skeletal muscle lipid accumulation appears to be predictive of the degree of whole-body insulin sensitivity [23, 24]. Second, the skeletal muscle IMCL content of obese individuals, determined by computed tomography (CT) scan attenuation values, is reduced by weight loss in a magnitude that is correlated with the degree of change in whole-body insulin sensitivity [25]. In addition, in some studies muscle CT attenuation predicts insulin resistance when taking into account visceral adiposity and overall adiposity [20]. Similar associations between whole-body insulin resistance and ectopic fat in skeletal muscle have also been extensively reported with ^{1}H nuclear magnetic resonance (NMR) spectroscopy, another method that quantifies IMCL content noninvasively [26–29].

Two important considerations must be discussed about these observations: first, a priori, the association between IMCL and insulin resistance does not necessarily imply causality between these two. It could be easily argued that these are coincidental associations in individuals destined to develop both conditions in parallel. However, data from experimental animal models suggest that a primary increase in IMCL in skeletal muscle can induce insulin resistance in muscle [30–32]. When lipoprotein lipase is specifically overexpressed in skeletal muscle, inducing IMCL accumulation, animals develop insulin resistance in muscle. The second consideration is that although the increased IMCL reflects mostly triglyceride accumulation, it is more likely that one (or many) accompanying lipid or lipid-derived species actually mediate lipotoxicity. Fatty-acyl-CoAs, diacylglycerol, and ceramides have been the most notable candidates. Excellent reviews on this topic have been published recently [8, 33].

5. RELATIONSHIPS BETWEEN ECTOPIC FAT IN LIVER AND INSULIN RESISTANCE

Another very common feature of the ectopic fat syndrome is fatty liver, also known as hepatic steatosis. This entity encompasses a spectrum of pathological abnormalities spanning from fatty liver without inflammation to steatohepatitis, which can ultimately lead to hepatic fibrosis and cirrhosis [34, 35]. Hepatic steatosis, independently of overt inflammation, has been found to be a feature of insulin resistance and the metabolic syndrome [36–39]. Fatty liver is a very frequent finding in T2DM, with estimated prevalence ranging from 21% to 78% [40–42] and is also found in high prevalence among obese individuals [34, 40, 43, 44]. The presence of the metabolic syndrome in nondiabetic individuals increases the likelihood of concomitant steatohepatitis by 3.2-fold [45]. Even in normal weight individuals, the presence of hepatic steatosis seems to be a predictor of characteristic disorders of the metabolic syndrome [46].

The pathogenesis of fat accumulation in the liver is not entirely understood, and multiple risk factors may be involved. Fatty acids are the predominant substrate oxidized by the liver, as oxidation of glucose is much more limited. Increased fatty acid flux to the liver resulting from impaired insulin-suppressed lipolysis in adipose tissue is thought to be a strong contributor to hepatic steatosis [47–51]. In addition, there is also reason to believe that hyperinsulinemia resulting from peripheral and/or hepatic insulin resistance may also contribute to exaggerated lipid accumulation in the liver. The transcriptional factor SREBP-1c (sterol regulatory element-binding protein-1) promotes lipogenesis. Intriguingly, despite insulin resistance within glucose and lipid metabolic pathways, hepatocytes appear to retain responsivity to insulin within SREBP-1c [52]. More evidence for this notion has been found in mice, in which disruption of the classical insulin signaling pathway was established by knocking out the gene encoding for IRS-2 (insulin receptor substrate-2). Paradoxically, the expression of the SREBP-1 gene, a downstream target of insulin was increased and these mice had increased liver triglyceride content [53].

Fatty acid uptake by the liver, in conjunction with hyperinsulinemia, and perhaps accentuated by steatosis, may contribute to the dyslipidemia characteristic of the metabolic syndrome; namely elevated serum triglycerides and low-HDL cholesterol. This dyslipidemia is thought to occur primarily as a result of increased VLDL secretion by the liver [46]. Through the combined action of the enzymes CETP (cholesterol-ester transfer protein) and hepatic lipase, HDL particle clearance increases and results in low HDL cholesterol levels [48, 50]. Small dense LDL particles, which appear to be highly atherogenic, also are formed through the CETP pathway.

The aforementioned mechanisms attempt to explain hepatic fat accumulation as a consequence of insulin resistance in adipose tissue leading to elevated circulating FFA and abnormal fat partitioning. However, one must also consider the possibility that hepatic steatosis contributes to hepatic insulin resistance. Akin to what happens in skeletal muscle, liver-specific overexpression of lipoprotein lipase induces hepatic steatosis without elevated FFAs, and causes hepatic insulin resistance [30]. In humans with T2DM, it was reported that severity of hepatic steatosis is associated with the severity of hepatic insulin resistance, and is a good predictor of the total daily insulin requirement [54]. Also, among nonobese men without T2DM, hepatic steatosis was found to correlate with hepatic insulin resistance, independently of obesity and intraabdominal adiposity [36]. However, in another study in patients with obesity and T2DM, insulin suppression of hepatic glucose production was not different between individuals with or without fatty liver [55].

Another line of evidence to support the notion that hepatic steatosis is associated with the genesis of hepatic insulin resistance originates from the observed insulin-sensitizing properties of thiazolidinediones. Both pioglitazone and rosiglitazone have been shown to decrease hepatic steatosis in association with improvements in hepatic insulin resistance [56, 57]. Drugs in this class act as agonists of the PPAR-γ nuclear receptor, a key transcriptional factor in the differentiation of preadipocytes into adipocytes [58–62]. Therapy with thiazolidinediones increases subcutaneous fat and decreases visceral fat [63–66]. This effect on adipose tissue distribution may explain the amelioration of hepatic insulin resistance and steatosis seen with pharmacotherapy with these drugs.

6.   HUMAN LIPODYSTROPHIC SYNDROMES

The ectopic fat theory is strengthened by observations in patients with lipodystrophic syndromes. Lipodystrophy is a family of syndromes characterized by markedly reduced adipose tissue [67]. Insulin resistance, fatty liver, and T2DM are frequent comorbidities, despite absence of obesity in many cases [67–69]. It is thought that the insufficient mass of adipose tissue predisposes to lipid accumulation in the liver and skeletal muscle, recapitulating the sequence of events of the ectopic fat theory. This notion is supported by transgenic animal models that have had adipose tissue development inhibited, which results in the phenotypes of ectopic fat and diabetes [70–72]. Further, surgical implantation of adipose tissue reverses lipoatrophic diabetes in mice [73]. These experiments, along with the aforementioned observations in humans with lipodystrophy, lend credence to the notion that insufficient subcutaneous fat tissue can contribute to ectopic fat accumulation. It could be argued, however, that these observations do not necessarily prove that abnormal fat partitioning occurs because of an failure of adipocytes to store lipids, because abnormalities in circulating adipokine concentrations could be another plausible explanation. Nevertheless, the lipodystrophic syndromes can be seen as proof-of-concept that a certain amount of functional adipose tissue is crucial for maintenance of insulin sensitivity and lipid buffering.

The observations derived from lipodystrophic syndromes suggest that insufficient fatty acid buffering capacity can be a key contributor to ectopic fat accumulation and raise an intriguing question: is the ectopic fat observed in the metabolic syndrome, obesity and T2DM a result of *functional* impairments in fat storage in adipocytes? A precedent for this idea can be found in the observation that the adipocyte size is positively correlated with hormone-sensitive lipase activity and lipolytic rates [74], which may indicate that larger adipocytes may have reached a state of critical lipid storage capacity. The anticipated consequence of having too many large adipocytes would be a rise in circulating FFAs, which can then be made available for storage as ectopic fat in skeletal muscle, liver, and the β-cells in the pancreas. In other words, obesity may be associated with insulin resistance because the large fat tissue mass may have conceivably approached its maximum potential to sequester lipids. In support of this postulate, a growing body of data suggests that enlarged adipocytes correlate well with insulin resistance [75–78]. *In vitro*, larger adipocytes appear to be less responsive to insulin [79–82] and may represent the phenotype of adipocytes that have failed to proliferate and can then only undergo hypertrophy [6, 83]. Presumably, larger adipocytes become insulin resistant as an adaptation to nutrient excess, and become unable to buffer circulating lipid fluxes. These notions are further supported by the observation that in Pima Indians the best correlation with new-onset type 2 diabetes is the adipocyte size [84].

7. CONCLUDING REMARKS

The ectopic fat theory has gained a significant body of supporting experimental data in the last few years. Yet, much investigational work remains to be done to precisely elucidate the mechanisms by which ectopic fat produce the downstream abnormalities of insulin resistance, hyperglycemia, atherogenic dyslipidemia, and hypertension observed in the metabolic syndrome. Such knowledge is needed not just to further validate the ectopic fat theory, but also to facilitate the design of pharmacological agents that specifically target the pathophysiology of the metabolic syndrome. This is particularly critical because currently there is no commercially available pharmacological treatment that completely reverses the metabolic syndrome, and physicians must rely on multiple drugs to individually treat the multiple abnormalities seen in the metabolic syndrome, i.e., dyslipidemia, hypertension, and insulin resistance. As a result, a significant proportion of the adult population with metabolic syndrome must currently rely on polypharmacy for treatment. In principle, it could be proposed that nonpharmacological treatment by means of weight loss and physical activity is all that is needed to contain the epidemics of obesity and the metabolic syndrome. However, on pragmatic terms, given the formidable challenges of attaining and then sustaining weight loss, there is a need for effective adjunctive pharmacological treatments for obesity and obesity-related insulin resistance.

REFERENCES

[1] Reaven GM. Banting lecture 1988. Role of insulin resistance in human disease. Diabetes 1988;37(12):1595–1607.

[2] Ford ES, Giles WH, Dietz WH. Prevalence of the metabolic syndrome among US adults: Findings from the third National Health and Nutrition Examination Survey. JAMA 2002; 287(3):356–359.

[3] Executive Summary of The Third Report of The National Cholesterol Education Program (NCEP) Expert Panel on Detection, Evaluation, and Treatment of High Blood Cholesterol in Adults (Adult Treatment Panel III). JAMA 2001;285(19):2486–2497.

[4] Alberti KG, Zimmet PZ. Definition, diagnosis and classification of diabetes mellitus and its complications. Part 1: Diagnosis and classification of diabetes mellitus provisional report of a WHO consultation. Diabet Med 1998;15(7):539–553.

[5] Vague J. The degree of masculine differentiation of obesities: A factor determining predisposition to diabetes, atherosclerosis, gout, and uric calculous disease. 1956. Nutrition 1999; 15(1):89–90; discussion 91.

[6] Heilbronn L, Smith SR, Ravussin E. Failure of fat cell proliferation, mitochondrial function and fat oxidation results in ectopic fat storage, insulin resistance and type II diabetes mellitus. Int J Obes Relat Metab Disord 2004;28(Suppl 4):S12–S21.

[7] Toledo FGS, Kelley DE. Mitochondrial dysfunction in the pathogenesis of insulin resistance associated with obesity, diabetes and aging. Current Opinion in Endocrinology and Diabetes 2005;12(12):157–162.

[8] Boden G, Shulman GI. Free fatty acids in obesity and type 2 diabetes: Defining their role in the development of insulin resistance and beta-cell dysfunction. Eur J Clin Invest 2002; 32(Suppl 3):14–23.

[9] Randle PJ. Regulatory interactions between lipids and carbohydrates: The glucose fatty acid cycle after 35 years. Diabetes Metab Rev 1998;14(4):263–283.

[10] Boden G. Effects of free fatty acids (FFA) on glucose metabolism: Significance for insulin resistance and type 2 diabetes. Exp Clin Endocrinol Diabetes 2003;111(3):121–124.

[11] Randle PJ, Garland PB, Hales CN, Newsholme EA. The glucose fatty-acid cycle. Its role in insulin sensitivity and the metabolic disturbances of diabetes mellitus. Lancet 1963;1:785–789.

[12] Shulman GI. Unraveling the cellular mechanism of insulin resistance in humans: New insights from magnetic resonance spectroscopy. Physiology (Bethesda) 2004;19:183–190.

[13] Perseghin G, Petersen K, Shulman GI. Cellular mechanism of insulin resistance: Potential links with inflammation. Int J Obes Relat Metab Disord 2003;27(Suppl 3):S6–S11.

[14] Boden G, Chen X, Ruiz J, White JV, Rossetti L. Mechanisms of fatty acid-induced inhibition of glucose uptake. J Clin Invest 1994;93(6):2438–2446.

[15] Boden G. Free fatty acids (FFA), a link between obesity and insulin resistance. Front Biosci 1998;3:d169–d175.

[16] Lam TK, Carpentier A, Lewis GF, van de Werve G, Fantus IG, Giacca A. Mechanisms of the free fatty acid-induced increase in hepatic glucose production. Am J Physiol Endocrinol Metab 2003;284(5):E863–E873.

[17] Engfeldt P, Arner P. Lipolysis in human adipocytes, effects of cell size, age and of regional differences. Horm Metab Res Suppl 1988;19:26–29.

[18] Nielsen S, Guo Z, Johnson CM, Hensrud DD, Jensen MD. Splanchnic lipolysis in human obesity. J Clin Invest 2004;113(11):1582–1588.

[19] Frayn KN, Karpe F, Fielding BA, Macdonald IA, Coppack SW. Integrative physiology of human adipose tissue. Int J Obes Relat Metab Disord 2003;27(8):875–888.

[20] Goodpaster BH, Thaete FL, Simoneau JA, Kelley DE. Subcutaneous abdominal fat and thigh muscle composition predict insulin sensitivity independently of visceral fat. Diabetes 1997;46(10):1579–1585.

[21] Pan DA, Lillioja S, Kriketos AD, et al. Skeletal muscle triglyceride levels are inversely related to insulin action. Diabetes 1997;46(6):983–988.

[22] Goodpaster BH, Wolf D. Skeletal muscle lipid accumulation in obesity, insulin resistance, and type 2 diabetes. Pediatr Diabetes 2004;5(4):219–226.

[23] Kelley DE, Goodpaster BH. Skeletal muscle triglyceride. An aspect of regional adiposity and insulin resistance. Diabetes Care 2001;24(5):933–941.

[24] Kelley DE, Goodpaster BH, Storlien L. Muscle triglyceride and insulin resistance. Annual Review of Nutrition 2002;22(1):325–346.

[25] Goodpaster BH, Kelley DE, Wing RR, Meier A, Thaete FL. Effects of weight loss on regional fat distribution and insulin sensitivity in obesity. Diabetes 1999;48(4):839–847.

[26] Szczepaniak LS, Babcock EE, Schick F, et al. Measurement of intracellular triglyceride stores by H spectroscopy: Validation in vivo. Am J Physiol 1999;276(5 Pt 1):E977–E989.

[27] Perseghin G, Scifo P, De Cobelli F, et al. Intramyocellular triglyceride content is a determinant of in vivo insulin resistance in humans: A 1H-13C nuclear magnetic resonance spectroscopy assessment in offspring of type 2 diabetic parents. Diabetes 1999;48(8):1600–1606.

[28] Krssak M, Falk Petersen K, Dresner A, et al. Intramyocellular lipid concentrations are correlated with insulin sensitivity in humans: A 1H NMR spectroscopy study. Diabetologia 1999;42(1):113–116.

[29] Kautzky-Willer A, Krssak M, Winzer C, et al. Increased intramyocellular lipid concentration identifies impaired glucose metabolism in women with previous gestational diabetes. Diabetes 2003;52(2):244–251.

[30] Kim JK, Fillmore JJ, Chen Y, et al. Tissue-specific overexpression of lipoprotein lipase causes tissue-specific insulin resistance. Proc Natl Acad Sci USA 2001;98(13):7522–7527.

[31] Pulawa LK, Eckel RH. Overexpression of muscle lipoprotein lipase and insulin sensitivity. Curr Opin Clin Nutr Metab Care 2002;5(5):569–574.

[32] Preiss-Landl K, Zimmermann R, Hammerle G, Zechner R. Lipoprotein lipase: The regulation of tissue specific expression and its role in lipid and energy metabolism. Curr Opin Lipidol 2002;13(5):471–481.

[33] McGarry JD. Banting Lecture 2001: Dysregulation of fatty acid metabolism in the etiology of type 2 diabetes. Diabetes 2002;51(1):7–18.

[34] Angelico F, Del Ben M, Conti R, et al. Non-alcoholic fatty liver syndrome: A hepatic consequence of common metabolic diseases. J Gastroenterol Hepatol 2003;18(5):588–594.

[35] Angulo P. Nonalcoholic fatty liver disease. N Engl J Med 2002;346(16):1221–1231.

[36] Seppala-Lindroos A, Vehkavaara S, Hakkinen AM, et al. Fat accumulation in the liver is associated with defects in insulin suppression of glucose production and serum free fatty acids independent of obesity in normal men. J Clin Endocrinol Metab 2002;87(7):3023–3028.

[37] Goto T, Onuma T, Takebe K, Kral JG. The influence of fatty liver on insulin clearance and insulin resistance in non-diabetic Japanese subjects. Int J Obes Relat Metab Disord 1995;19(12):841–845.

[38] Marceau P, Biron S, Hould FS, et al. Liver pathology and the metabolic syndrome X in severe obesity. J Clin Endocrinol Metab 1999;84(5):1513–1517.

[39] Marchesini G, Brizi M, Bianchi G, et al. Nonalcoholic fatty liver disease: A feature of the metabolic syndrome. Diabetes 2001;50(8):1844–1850.

[40] Adams LA, Angulo P, Lindor KD. Nonalcoholic fatty liver disease. CMAJ 2005;172(7): 899–905.

[41] Kumar KS, Malet PF. Nonalcoholic steatohepatitis. Mayo Clin Proc 2000;75(7):733–739.

[42] Gupte P, Amarapurkar D, Agal S, et al. Non-alcoholic steatohepatitis in type 2 diabetes mellitus. J Gastroenterol Hepatol 2004;19(8):854–858.

[43] Del Gaudio A, Boschi L, Del Gaudio GA, Mastrangelo L, Munari D. Liver damage in obese patients. Obes Surg 2002;12(6):802–804.

[44] Wanless IR, Lentz JS. Fatty liver hepatitis (steatohepatitis) and obesity: An autopsy study with analysis of risk factors. Hepatology 1990;12(5):1106–1110.

[45] Marchesini G, Bugianesi E, Forlani G, et al. Nonalcoholic fatty liver, steatohepatitis, and the metabolic syndrome. Hepatology 2003;37(4):917–923.

[46] Kim HJ, Kim HJ, Lee KE, et al. Metabolic significance of nonalcoholic fatty liver disease in nonobese, nondiabetic adults. Arch Intern Med 2004;164(19):2169–2175.

[47] Lewis GF. Fatty acid regulation of very low density lipoprotein production. Curr Opin Lipidol 1997;8(3):146–153.

[48] Grundy SM. Hypertriglyceridemia, insulin resistance, and the metabolic syndrome. Am J Cardiol 1999;83(9B):25F–29F.

[49] Ginsberg HN. New perspectives on atherogenesis: Role of abnormal triglyceride-rich lipoprotein metabolism. Circulation 2002;106(16):2137–2142.

[50] Goldberg IJ. Clinical review 124: Diabetic dyslipidemia: Causes and consequences. J Clin Endocrinol Metab 2001;86(3):965–971.

[51] Taghibiglou C, Carpentier A, Van Iderstine SC, et al. Mechanisms of hepatic very low density lipoprotein overproduction in insulin resistance. Evidence for enhanced lipoprotein assembly, reduced intracellular ApoB degradation, and increased microsomal triglyceride transfer protein in a fructose-fed hamster model. J Biol Chem 2000;275(12):8416–8425.

[52] Shimomura I, Matsuda M, Hammer RE, Bashmakov Y, Brown MS, Goldstein JL. Decreased IRS-2 and increased SREBP-1c lead to mixed insulin resistance and sensitivity in livers of lipodystrophic and ob/ob mice. Mol Cell 2000;6(1):77–86.

[53] Tobe K, Suzuki R, Aoyama M, et al. Increased expression of the sterol regulatory element-binding protein-1 gene in insulin receptor substrate-2(-/-) mouse liver. J Biol Chem 2001;276(42):38337–38340.

[54] Ryysy L, Hakkinen AM, Goto T, et al. Hepatic fat content and insulin action on free fatty acids and glucose metabolism rather than insulin absorption are associated with insulin requirements during insulin therapy in type 2 diabetic patients. Diabetes 2000;49(5):749–758.

[55] Kelley DE, McKolanis TM, Hegazi RA, Kuller LH, Kalhan SC. Fatty liver in type 2 diabetes mellitus: Relation to regional adiposity, fatty acids, and insulin resistance. Am J Physiol Endocrinol Metab 2003;285(4):E906–E916.

[56] Bajaj M, Suraamornkul S, Pratipanawatr T, et al. Pioglitazone reduces hepatic fat content and augments splanchnic glucose uptake in patients with type 2 diabetes. Diabetes 2003;52(6):1364–1370.

[57] Mayerson AB, Hundal RS, Dufour S, et al. The effects of rosiglitazone on insulin sensitivity, lipolysis, and hepatic and skeletal muscle triglyceride content in patients with type 2 diabetes. Diabetes 2002;51(3):797–802.

[58] Morrison RF, Farmer SR. Hormonal signaling and transcriptional control of adipocyte differentiation. J Nutr 2000;130(12):3116S–3121S.

[59] Ren D, Collingwood TN, Rebar EJ, Wolffe AP, Camp HS. PPARgamma knockdown by engineered transcription factors: Exogenous PPARgamma2 but not PPARgamma1 reactivates adipogenesis. Genes Dev 2002;16(1):27–32.

[60] Tontonoz P, Hu E, Spiegelman BM. Stimulation of adipogenesis in fibroblasts by PPAR gamma 2, a lipid-activated transcription factor. Cell 1994;79(7):1147–1156.

[61] Fajas L, Fruchart JC, Auwerx J. Transcriptional control of adipogenesis. Curr Opin Cell Biol 1998;10(2):165–173.

[62] Loftus TM, Lane MD. Modulating the transcriptional control of adipogenesis. Curr Opin Genet Dev 1997;7(5):603–608.

[63] Miyazaki Y, Mahankali A, Matsuda M, et al. Effect of pioglitazone on abdominal fat distribution and insulin sensitivity in type 2 diabetic patients. J Clin Endocrinol Metab 2002;87(6):2784–2791.

[64] Miyazaki Y, Mahankali A, Matsuda M, et al. Improved glycemic control and enhanced insulin sensitivity in type 2 diabetic subjects treated with pioglitazone. Diabetes Care 2001;24(4):710–719.

[65] Miyazaki Y, Glass L, Triplitt C, et al. Effect of rosiglitazone on glucose and non-esterified fatty acid metabolism in type II diabetic patients. Diabetologia 2001;44(12):2210–2219.

[66] Mori Y, Murakawa Y, Okada K, et al. Effect of troglitazone on body fat distribution in type 2 diabetic patients. Diabetes Care 1999;22(6):908–912.

[67] Garg A. Acquired and inherited lipodystrophies. N Engl J Med 2004;350(12):1220–1234.

[68] Oral EA, Simha V, Ruiz E, et al. Leptin-replacement therapy for lipodystrophy. N Engl J Med 2002;346(8):570–578.

[69] Robbins DC, Horton ES, Tulp O, Sims EA. Familial partial lipodystrophy: Complications of obesity in the non-obese? Metabolism 1982;31(5):445–452.

[70] Reitman ML, Mason MM, Moitra J, et al. Transgenic mice lacking white fat: Models for understanding human lipoatrophic diabetes. Ann NY Acad Sci 1999;892:289–296.

[71] Shimomura I, Hammer RE, Ikemoto S, Brown MS, Goldstein JL. Leptin reverses insulin resistance and diabetes mellitus in mice with congenital lipodystrophy. Nature 1999;401(6748):73–76.

[72] Petersen KF, Oral EA, Dufour S, Befroy D, Ariyan C, Yu C, et al. Leptin reverses insulin resistance and hepatic steatosis in patients with severe lipodystrophy. J Clin Invest 2002;109(10):1345–1350.

[73] Gavrilova O, Marcus-Samuels B, Graham D, et al. Surgical implantation of adipose tissue reverses diabetes in lipoatrophic mice. J Clin Invest 2000;105(3):271–278.

[74] Reynisdottir S, Dauzats M, Thorne A, Langin D. Comparison of hormone-sensitive lipase activity in visceral and subcutaneous human adipose tissue. J Clin Endocrinol Metab 1997;82(12):4162–4166.

[75] Weyer C, Foley JE, Bogardus C, Tataranni PA, Pratley RE. Enlarged subcutaneous abdominal adipocyte size, but not obesity itself, predicts type II diabetes independent of insulin resistance. Diabetologia 2000;43(12):1498–1506.

[76] Abbott WG, Thuillez P, Howard BV, et al. Body composition, adipocyte size, free fatty acid concentration, and glucose tolerance in children of diabetic pregnancies. Diabetes 1986;35(10):1077–1080.

[77] Bjorntorp P, Bengtsson C, Blohme G, et al. Adipose tissue fat cell size and number in relation to metabolism in randomly selected middle-aged men and women. Metabolism 1971;20(10):927–935.

[78] Bjorntorp P, Berchtold P, Tibblin G. Insulin secretion in relation to adipose tissue in men. Diabetes 1971;20(2):65–70.

[79] Olefsky JM. Insensitivity of large rat adipocytes to the antilipolytic effects of insulin. J Lipid Res 1977;18(4):459–464.

[80] Czech MP. Cellular basis of insulin insensitivity in large rat adipocytes. J Clin Invest 1976;57(6):1523–1532.

[81] Olefsky JM. Mechanisms of decreased insulin responsiveness of large adipocytes. Endocrinology 1977;100(4):1169–1177.

[82] Karnieli E, Barzilai A, Rafaeloff R, Armoni M. Distribution of glucose transporters in membrane fractions isolated from human adipose cells. Relation to cell size. J Clin Invest 1986;78(4):1051–1055.

[83] Danforth E Jr. Failure of adipocyte differentiation causes type II diabetes mellitus? Nat Genet 2000;26(1):13.

[84] Paolisso G, Tataranni PA, Foley JE, Bogardus C, Howard BV, Ravussin E. A high concentration of fasting plasma non-esterified fatty acids is a risk factor for the development of NIDDM. Diabetologia 1995;38(10):1213–1217.

Chapter 8

Abdominal Obesity and
the Metabolic Syndrome

Jean-Pierre Després[a,b], Isabelle Lemieux[a] and Natalie Alméras[c]

[a]*Québec Heart Institute, Hôpital Laval Research Center, Hôpital Laval, Québec, Québec,
Canada*
[b]*Department of Social and Preventive Medicine, Université Laval, Québec, Québec, Canada*
[c]*Hôpital Laval Research Center, Hôpital Laval, Québec, Québec, Canada*

1.   INTRODUCTION

Despite the fact that the obesity epidemic has received intense media coverage, many physicians still fail to recognize that the rapidly growing prevalence
of type 2 diabetes in their practice is the result of our "toxic" sedentary and
affluent lifestyle that promotes weight gain, obesity, a positive energy balance,
and the progressive development of a dysmetabolic state [1], potentially leading to glucose intolerance and—eventually—outright hyperglycemia. Citing
obesity's key role in the etiology of type 2 diabetes, Zimmet foresaw a rapid
increase in the prevalence of type 2 diabetes worldwide [2, 3]. Unfortunately,
the progression of obesity has been so brisk that the worldwide prevalence of
type 2 diabetes continues to grow at an alarming rate. This phenomenon should
be of great concern to health care providers, as type 2 diabetes has been clearly
linked to major health care expenses [4]. Indeed, it is a major cause of retinopa-
thy causing blindness, of nephropathy leading to end-stage renal disease and
dialysis, as well as of neuropathic complications, which are the leading cause
of amputations [5]. In addition to the microcirculatory damage it causes, type 2
diabetes also plays a key role in atherosclerotic macrovascular disease. For instance, the majority of type 2 diabetic patients will die from cardiovascular
disease [6–8]. It is therefore crucial to diagnose type 2 diabetic patients early
with a view to optimal management of their condition, given that some 10%
of the North American population has this metabolic disease [9]. Further, its
prevalence is largely underestimated, as it has been found to be even more
prevalent in some populations worldwide [2, 3].

Although it has been shown that better glycemic control can reduce the
complications of diabetes related to microcirculatory damage, the benefits of
glycemic control for prevention of coronary heart disease (CHD) in diabetic
patients are modest at best [10, 11]. Although, as a group, type 2 diabetic patients are clearly at higher risk of CHD than the nondiabetic population, recent

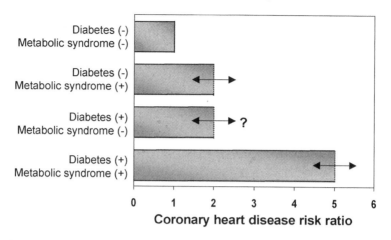

Figure 1. Heterogeneity of coronary heart disease (CHD) risk is associated with the metabolic syndrome and type 2 diabetes. There is considerable evidence that metabolic syndrome features increase CHD risk, even in nondiabetic individuals. Further, studies have shown that CHD risk is heterogeneous in type 2 diabetes. Clearly, type 2 diabetic patients with features of the metabolic syndrome are at the highest risk of CHD. However, debate is currently ongoing as to whether diabetes *per se* (in the absence of the metabolic syndrome) significantly increases CHD risk. These results emphasize the need to watch for factors other than glycemic control in optimally managing CHD risk in type 2 diabetic patients.

studies have shown that type 2 diabetes is a heterogeneous entity: the more abdominally obese type 2 diabetic patients are, the greater is their likelihood of being characterized by the features of the metabolic syndrome [12] and the higher their corresponding CHD risk will be (Figure 1).

The features of the metabolic syndrome may therefore be more important than glycemic control in predicting CHD risk in patients with type 2 diabetes. This finding is consistent with results in nondiabetic subjects indicating that even in the absence of hyperglycemia, nondiabetic, overweight/obese individuals with features of the metabolic syndrome are also characterized by an increased risk for CHD [13–16]. Reaven introduced the concept of an insulin resistance-linked syndrome of abnormalities in 1988 [17] and was the first to suggest that impaired *in vivo* insulin action was central to a cluster of metabolic abnormalities that did not necessarily include classical risk factors such as raised low-density lipoprotein (LDL)-cholesterol, but which was instead characterized by hypertriglyceridemia, low high-density lipoprotein (HDL)-cholesterol, fasting hyperinsulinemia, and elevated blood pressure. At the time, Reaven argued that he could find insulin-resistant subjects among nonobese individuals and therefore did not include obesity as a necessary component of "his" syndrome X (or insulin resistance syndrome [17]). More than two decades before Reaven's landmark conceptual contribution, Crepaldi and colleagues had reported that obesity was often accompanied by hyperinsulinemia, hypertriglyceridemia, and hypertension [18]. In the mid-forties, Jean Vague had suggested that regional body fat distribution—but not obesity *per se*—was the culprit, and he coined the term "android obesity" to describe a form of upper body adiposity most often associated with diabetes and cardiovascular disease [19]. Another pioneer in the history of abdominal obesity was Jeremy Morris, who reported in the mid-1950s that sedentary London bus drivers were at greater risk of CHD compared to more active conductors who had to walk and climb the bus stairs during their shifts [20]. Interestingly, he also reported that higher risk, sedentary bus drivers were substantially more likely to have abdominal obesity (as revealed by the size of their trousers) than lower risk, active bus conductors [21]. This early report is one of the key early findings to link a sedentary lifestyle and abdominal obesity to CHD risk [21]. Later, in the early 1980s, two groups reported almost simultaneously that a high proportion of abdominal fat, expressed as an elevated waist-to-hip ratio, was tied to glucose intolerance, hyperinsulinemia, and hypertriglyceridemia [22, 23]. Investigators in the Gothenburg prospective study published evidence that an elevated waist-to-hip ratio was predictive of an increased risk of ischemic heart disease, independent of body mass index (BMI) [24, 25]. In studying the risk of developing diabetes [26], they also found over the 13 ½ years of study follow-up that an elevated BMI *per se* was not associated with an increased risk of developing the disease. However, being overweight or obese and also having a greater proportion of abdominal fat (as crudely estimated by an elevated waist-to-hip ratio) entailed a 30-fold increase in the risk of developing diabetes [26]. The scientific community studying obesity received these findings with considerable interest. At about the same time, imaging techniques such as computed tomography (CT) began to be used in the field of body composition not only to accurately measure abdominal fat but also to distinguish intraabdominal (visceral) from subcutaneous fat [27, 28]. Since then, numerous studies over the last two decades have clearly indicated that abdominal fat accumulation along with an excess of intraabdominal (or visceral) adipose tissue are predictive of the metabolic syndrome [27, 29–38]. It has also been shown that even individuals of apparently normal weight may nonetheless have excess visceral adipose tissue, placing them at greater risk of a disturbed metabolic profile [37, 39–41].

The metabolic complications associated with obesity and overweight have been extensively studied in the last 20 years. The use of high-precision technologies to measure total body fat and abdominal fat accumulation (e.g., dual-energy x-ray absorptiometry [DEXA], computed tomography, and magnetic resonance imaging) has allowed investigators to conclusively demonstrate that, irrespective of the absence/presence of clinical obesity (BMI above 30 kg/m^2), individuals with a selective excess of intraabdominal or visceral adipose tissue are at a substantially increased risk of developing the cluster of metabolic abnormalities originally described by Reaven [17] as well as being characterized by the features subsequently added to the metabolic syndrome's expanded dysmetabolic profile (hypertriglyceridemia, low HDL-cholesterol, fasting hyperinsulinemia, insulin resistance, elevated apolipoprotein B, small dense LDL, prothrombotic profile, and elevated inflammatory markers) [42].

2. METABOLIC SYNDROME WITHOUT HYPERGLYCEMIA PREDICTS AN INCREASED CHD RISK

We now have evidence that features of the metabolic syndrome commonly found in abdominally obese patients with excess visceral adipose tissue increase CHD risk, even when hyperglycemia is not present. The Québec Cardiovascular Study, a prospective study of middle-aged men in the Québec City Metropolitan Area, has shown that the simultaneous presence of certain metabolic syndrome features—namely fasting hyperinsulinemia (a marker of insulin resistance in nondiabetic individuals), increased apolipoprotein B levels (a marker of atherogenic lipoprotein concentration), and the presence of small LDL particles—substantially increases CHD risk, even in the absence of classical risk factors such as diabetes, raised LDL-cholesterol, hypertension, and smoking [15]. A substantial amount of additional evidence would be required to gauge whether measuring additional metabolic syndrome markers (such as C-reactive protein levels) would further refine our understanding of CHD risk. In this respect, the National Cholesterol Education Program-Adult Treatment Panel III (NCEP-ATP III) criteria are a conceptual leap forward as they include not only aspects of the insulin resistance syndrome (such as triglycerides, HDL-cholesterol, elevated blood pressure, and elevated fasting glucose [as a crude marker of an altered glucose homeostasis likely resulting from an insulin-resistant state]), but also waist circumference as an index of abdominal obesity [43]. The NCEP-ATP III criteria therefore recognize abdominal obesity as a driving force behind the metabolic syndrome's rise to epidemic proportions, a notion that can never be emphasized enough in clinical practice. Studies have consistently shown that individuals meeting the NCEP-ATP III criteria for the metabolic syndrome are at increased relative risk of developing cardiovascular disease [13, 44, 45]. However, this increased relative risk does not necessarily imply a substantial increase in absolute risk, which must be estimated via a global risk algorithm such as the Framingham risk score [46].

3. WHY MEASURE WAIST CIRCUMFERENCE AS WELL AND NOT JUST BMI?

As shown in Figure 2A, population studies have established a fairly strong correlation between BMI and waist girth. The question, then, is why waist cir-

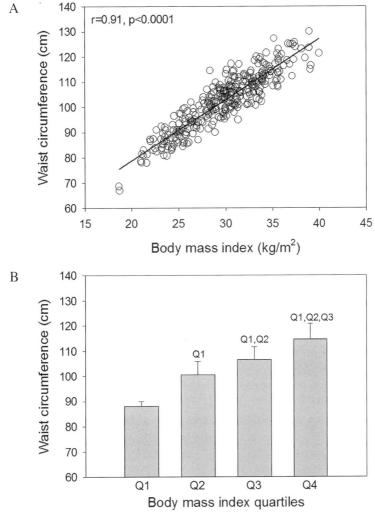

Figure 2. Although there is a highly significant correlation between body mass index (BMI) and waist circumference (upper panel), this correlation is explained by the large variation in BMI values in the samples studied. For instance, standard deviation values for given BMI quartiles (lower panel) clearly show that waist circumference varies substantially per BMI quartile. Waist circumference and BMI are therefore not equivalent in clinical practice. Q1, Q2, Q3: different from the corresponding quartile; $p < 0.0001$. Quartile cutoffs: 25th: 26.62 kg/m^2; 50th: 30.04 kg/m^2; 75th: 32.99 kg/m^2.

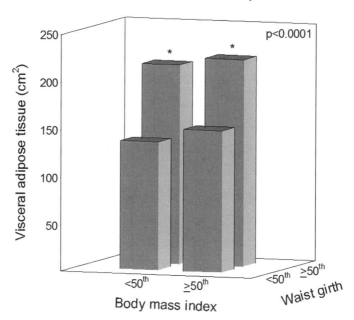

Figure 3. Average cross-sectional areas of visceral adipose tissue measured by computed to-mography (expressed in cm^2) among groups of men stratified according to median body mass index and waist circumference values. For any given BMI subgroup, subjects with a higher waist circumference have a much greater accumulation of visceral adipose tissue than men with lower waist girth values. Body mass index cutoff: 50th: 30.04 kg/m^2; waist circumference cutoff: 50th: 103.5 cm. *Significantly different from individuals with low waist circumference, regardless of BMI.

cumference is preferable to BMI, which is an internationally accepted index of adiposity. Looking further at Figure 2A, the strength of the correlation depends largely on the sample's weight heterogeneity (BMI). Figure 2B shows waist circumference variations for various BMI quartiles, demonstrating that circumference varies considerably for any given BMI quartile. Thus, if waist circumference and BMI do not equally predict the metabolic syndrome, BMI cannot be considered a surrogate for waist girth. This is further supported by Figure 3, which clearly indicates that for any BMI subgroup, subjects with an elevated waist circumference have a much greater accumulation of visceral adipose tissue, a key factor underpinning the dysmetabolic profile associated with abdominal obesity [30–35]. Therefore, waist girth and BMI are not comparable markers of abdominal obesity and do not similarly predict the presence of metabolic complications. In addition, recent findings of the INTERHEART myocardial infarction case-control study have revealed that increased abdominal fat is a key predictor of myocardial infarction, even among individuals with presumably "normal" BMI values [47].

4. ABDOMINAL OBESITY: THE DRIVING FORCE BEHIND THE METABOLIC SYNDROME?

Although rare forms of insulin resistance not accompanied by overweight or obesity can be found in clinical practice [48], clinicians must recognize the pivotal role of abdominal obesity in elevating the metabolic syndrome to the status of an epidemic. Unpublished data from the Québec Health Survey cohort revealed that waist circumference values were markedly elevated among all combinations of NCEP-ATP III criteria that did not include waist circumference (Lemieux I et al., unpublished data). These results clearly indicate that an expanded waistline is the most prevalent form of the metabolic syndrome. Thus, measuring waist circumference is a key step toward identifying individuals likely to have features of the metabolic syndrome.

5. THE METABOLIC SYNDROME: IS WAIST GIRTH SUFFICIENT?

Although we have repeatedly stressed the importance of measuring waist girth, its ability to predict visceral fat accumulation and the presence of the metabolic syndrome is limited. The high waist circumference values often found in very obese premenopausal women provide a telling example of how this measurement can mislead in clinical practice. Though these women may have a substantial accumulation of subcutaneous abdominal fat, they may also have little atherogenic visceral adipose tissue as compared to men [49–51]. To solve this dilemma, we have worked to identify a simple and inexpensive blood marker that could help physicians identify individuals likely to have the atherogenic features of the insulin resistance syndrome. Such a blood marker appears to be fasting plasma triglyceridemia. For example, we have found that middle-aged Caucasian men with both elevated triglyceride concentrations (above 2 mmol/L) and a waist circumference of 90 cm were far more likely (greater than 80% probability) to be characterized by visceral obesity and the metabolic syndrome [52]. Conversely, men with a waist circumference smaller than 90 cm and triglyceride levels under 2 mmol/L were much less likely (about 10% probability) to display features of the metabolic syndrome [52]. We have validated this screening approach in several studies [52–55]. We therefore submit that an elevated waist circumference (as a marker of abdominal obesity) and hypertriglyceridemia (as a crude marker of the dysmetabolic, dyslipidemic profile accompanying abdominal obesity) are the two key variables that should be included in a simple and inexpensive initial screening for individuals at high risk of developing the metabolic syndrome.

6.   ARE NCEP-ATP III CRITERIA VALID IN ALL POPULATIONS?

As a concept, NCEP-ATP III recognizes that some simple clinical markers (including waist circumference) can be used to identify individuals likely to have the metabolic syndrome [43]. Further, studies have shown that individuals who meet these criteria have an increased prevalence or incidence of CHD [13, 44, 45]. However, we do not know whether the NCEP-ATP III cutoffs proposed provide optimal discrimination of CHD risk. Further data must be generated through various cutoffs to verify which values provide optimal sensitivity and specificity in discriminating for clinical events. In addition, it has been shown that susceptibility to visceral fat deposition and the likelihood of developing complications for any given level of abdominal visceral fat can vary by population [56–59]. For instance, African Americans are less likely to accumulate visceral adipose tissue than Caucasians for any given level of total body fat or waist circumference. We had previously reported that the lower susceptibility of African Americans to visceral obesity accounted for their lower triglyceride and apolipoprotein B levels compared to Caucasians [56]. Further proof of the need to develop population-specific cutoffs comes from the Asian population, which develops type 2 diabetes at much lower BMI (and therefore lower waist circumference) values than the Caucasian population [60].

NCEP-ATP III is a remarkable advance in that it provides clinicians with simple syndrome markers whose relationship to CHD risk has been established. However, further study of population differences is clearly warranted to refine NCEP-ATP III criteria and cutoff values for optimal assessment of metabolic syndrome-related risk. This was the rationale underlying the recent International Diabetes Federation (IDF) recommendations on identifying individuals with the metabolic syndrome [61]. In light of evidence that the most prevalent form of the metabolic syndrome is found in patients with abdominal obesity, elevated waist circumference was included as a mandatory criterion in IDF recommendations. Population-specific waist cutoffs for abdominal obesity have also been proposed to reflect population differences in susceptibility to visceral adiposity for a given BMI. However, such criteria should be considered a work in progress, and additional scientific evidence will be necessary to refine screening approaches to optimally discriminate for the metabolic syndrome and the related risk of diabetes and cardiovascular disease in various populations worldwide. Key considerations regarding this process are listed in Table 1.

Table 1. Metabolic syndrome vs. CHD risk: issues

- Impact on heterogeneity of CHD risk in type 2 diabetes
- Impact on CHD risk in the nondiabetic population
- Critical markers (and cutoff values) for identifying and quantifying related CHD risk
- Susceptibility to metabolic syndrome in various populations
- Population differences in susceptibility to visceral adipose tissue deposition
- Population differences in susceptibility to developing complications (type 2 diabetes, CHD) for any given excess of visceral adipose tissue

---

7.   MANAGING CHD RISK IN PATIENTS WITH THE METABOLIC SYNDROME: WHAT SHOULD BE OUR GOAL?

It is clear that features of the metabolic syndrome increase the risk of CHD, whether classical risk factors are present or not [16]. This means that the metabolic syndrome further increases the CHD risk already posed by traditional risk factors such as hypertension, diabetes, elevated LDL-cholesterol, and smoking. These factors must of course be managed in patients with the metabolic syndrome. However, treating them is unlikely to eliminate the risk resulting from the presence of the metabolic syndrome. The findings of the Heart Protection Study (HPS) in diabetic patients provide a simple illustration of this problem. For example, although all diabetic patients benefited from simvastatin therapy in HPS, patients with low HDL-cholesterol levels (presumably resulting from the presence of abdominal obesity and hypertriglyceridemia, the most common form of low HDL-cholesterol in our population) remained at higher risk of CHD events and related mortality than type 2 diabetic patients with normal HDL-cholesterol levels (presumably less abdominally obese and likely to have lower triglyceride levels) [62]. Thus, although it may provide significant clinical benefit, statin therapy in type 2 diabetic patients with low HDL-cholesterol (and presumably the metabolic syndrome) may not normalize their CHD risk if they are abdominally obese and also have features of the metabolic syndrome. It may therefore be necessary to manage other dysmetabolic abnormalities to optimally reduce CHD risk in these high-risk patients. Further study is required to identify which features of the metabolic syndrome should be targeted. This will be a key focus of future studies. Evidence from fibrate trials has suggested that patients with obesity, hypertriglyceridemia, and low HDL-cholesterol (with either hyperinsulinemia or type 2 diabetes) may benefit from fibrate therapy [63–66]. However, recently published results of the long-awaited FIELD trial have failed to confirm this. Further, statin-fibrate combination therapy in very high-risk patients with type 2 diabetes, CHD, and the metabolic syndrome has yet to be tested in large trials for safety and clinical benefits.

It is crucial that physicians stress the importance of weight loss, especially given the spectacular results of Finnish and US diabetes prevention studies demonstrating that small weight loss could afford substantial clinical benefit by preventing or at least delaying by several years the conversion to type 2 diabetes among high-risk obese individuals with glucose intolerance [67, 68]. Whether this finding will prove useful for managing the other features of the metabolic syndrome will likewise have to be tested in clinical trials.

If lifestyle modification cannot successfully spur weight loss and the mobilization of abdominal fat, pharmacotherapy should be considered for high-risk patients with high-risk visceral obesity. The two available weight loss agents approved in clinical practice—sibutramine and orlistat—have both been shown to induce significantly greater weight loss than placebos [69, 70]. With the exception of the XENDOS study [71], which included a subgroup of patients with impaired glucose tolerance, these agents have mostly been tested in low-risk obese women. Trials involving high-risk abdominally obese patients with clinically meaningful outcomes are needed.

Lastly, recent studies have identified the endocannabinoid system as a target for inducing abdominal fat loss and mitigating features of the metabolic syndrome [72, 73]. Blocking CB_1 receptors may therefore be an additional, complementary way to address the root cause of the clustering atherothrombotic–inflammatory and diabetogenic abnormalities of the metabolic syndrome: abdominal obesity. Further trials with hard end points are needed to quantify the clinical benefits of the metabolic improvements observed with this new therapeutic approach.

8.   SUMMARY

Recognition of the metabolic syndrome as a major and prevalent cause of CHD in the NCEP-ATP III guidelines represents a remarkable contribution to preventive medicine by stressing the importance of assessing abdominal obesity in clinical practice. The NCEP-ATP III panel has proposed simple variables to identify individuals who are likely to have features of the metabolic syndrome and who are at increased relative risk of type 2 diabetes and cardiovascular disease. Among the five criteria (waist circumference, triglycerides, HDL-cholesterol, fasting glycemia, blood pressure) proposed to identify metabolic syndrome carriers, the recommendation to measure waist circumference rather than BMI has been a giant conceptual leap forward, as it recognizes abdominal obesity as the most important component of the metabolic syndrome in our affluent, sedentary population. The NCEP-ATP III guidelines have also recognized the value of elevated triglyceride and reduced HDL-cholesterol levels as lipid markers for the presence of an athero-genic "dysmetabolic" profile that adds to the impact of raised plasma LDL-cholesterol levels on the risk of CHD.

Unfortunately, since the publication of the NCEP-ATP III guidelines, clini-cians have often confused the conceptual definition of the metabolic syndrome with the above five criteria, which are intended for use in clinical practice as simple surrogate variables to identify high-risk individuals likely to be charac-terized by abdominal obesity, insulin resistance, and atherogenic dyslipidemia, as well as by a prothrombotic, inflammatory profile that may or may not co-exist with hyperglycemia and/or hypertension (Figure 4). More recently, the recommendations of an IDF working group placed further emphasis on ab-dominal obesity as the most prevalent component of the metabolic syndrome and consequently on the need to first have an elevated waist circumference before being considered at risk of having the metabolic syndrome (Figure 4). Further, in light of compelling evidence that the waist circumference cutoff values proposed by NCEP-ATP III was too high, recent IDF recommendations have reduced the waist girth value to 94 cm in men and 80 cm in women, adding that factors such as ethnicity and age affect the relationship of waist circumference to abdominal visceral fat deposition and related metabolic ab-

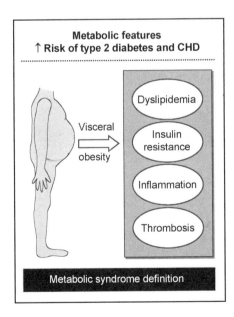
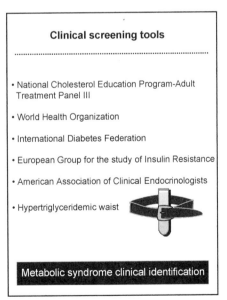

Figure 4. A distinction should be drawn between the metabolic syndrome as a concept and the clinical tools proposed by various organizations/groups to identify patients likely to have the clustering abnormalities of the metabolic syndrome. Careful attention should be paid to this issue so as not to confuse the metabolic syndrome definition with the criteria used for its identification in clinical practice.

normalities. Thus, the mandatory inclusion in the IDF guidelines of elevated waist girth as the initial criterion used to denote likely metabolic syndrome patients marks another step toward developing a simplified approach to identifying these patients in clinical practice. Based on additional work performed by several groups, there is now evidence that the simultaneous presence of elevated waist circumference and fasting triglyceride levels (a condition termed the "hypertriglyceridemic waist") may be initially useful in identifying a subgroup of individuals at high risk of being carriers of the metabolic syndrome (Figure 4). The syndrome features could then be confirmed through additional and more sophisticated metabolic risk marker measurements.

However, given the knowledge gaps in recent IDF recommendations, these new waist circumference criteria should be considered a work in progress. Accordingly, their ability to optimally discriminate for subgroups at high risk of type 2 diabetes or CHD because of the presence of metabolic syndrome features will have to be validated. Finally, based on evidence that both abdominal obesity and related metabolic syndrome features affect the absolute residual CHD risk of patients treated for traditional risk factors, new therapeutic approaches that either modify the visceral obesity phenotype or target abdominal obesity and related metabolic abnormalities may hold out great promise to optimally reduce CHD risk in abdominally obese patients with features of the metabolic syndrome.

ACKNOWLEDGMENTS

The authors of this chapter have been supported by research grants from the Canadian Institutes of Health Research and the Canadian Diabetes Association. Jean-Pierre Després is Scientific Director of the International Chair on Cardiometabolic Risk which is supported by an unrestricted grant from Sanofi Aventis awarded to Université Laval.

REFERENCES

[1] Després JP. Our passive lifestyle, our toxic diet, and the atherogenic/diabetogenic metabolic syndrome: Can we afford to be sedentary and unfit? Circulation 2005;112(4):453–455.

[2] Zimmet P, Shaw J, Murray S, Sicree R. The diabetes epidemic in full flight: Forecasting the future. Diabetes Voice 2003;48:12–16.

[3] Zimmet PZ. Diabetes epidemiology as a tool to trigger diabetes research and care. Diabetologia 1999;42(5):499–518.

[4] Third-Party Reimbursement for Diabetes Care, Self-Management Education, and Supplies. Diabet Care 2006;29(Suppl 1):S68–S69.

[5] He Z, King GL. Microvascular complications of diabetes. Endocrinol Metab Clin North Am 2004;33(1):215–238, xi–xii.

[6] Grundy SM, Benjamin EJ, Burke GL, et al. Diabetes and cardiovascular disease. A statement for healthcare professionals from the American Heart Association. Circulation 1999; 100:1134–1146.

[7] Kaukua J, Turpeinen A, Uusitupa M, Niskanen L. Clustering of cardiovascular risk factors in type 2 diabetes mellitus: Prognostic significance and tracking. Diabetes Obes Metab 2001;3(1):17–23.

[8] Lee WL, Cheung AM, Cape D, Zinman B. Impact of diabetes on coronary artery disease in women and men. Diabet Care 2000;23(7):962–968.

[9] Wild S, Roglic G, Green A, Sicree R, King H. Global prevalence of diabetes: Estimates for the year 2000 and projections for 2030. Diabet Care 2004;27(5):1047–1053.

[10] Intensive blood-glucose control with sulphonylureas or insulin compared with conventional treatment and risk of complications in patients with type 2 diabetes (UKPDS 33). UK Prospective Diabetes Study (UKPDS) Group. Lancet 1998;352(9131):837–853.

[11] Nathan DM, Cleary PA, Backlund JY, et al. Intensive diabetes treatment and cardiovascular disease in patients with type 1 diabetes. N Engl J Med 2005;353(25):2643–2653.

[12] Alexander CM, Landsman PB, Teutsch SM, Haffner SM. NCEP-defined metabolic syndrome, diabetes, and prevalence of coronary heart disease among NHANES III participants age 50 years and older. Diabetes 2003;52:1210–1214.

[13] Lakka HM, Laaksonen DE, Lakka TA, et al. The metabolic syndrome and total and cardiovascular disease mortality in middle-aged men. JAMA 2002;288(21):2709–2716.

[14] Isomaa B, Almgren P, Tuomi T, et al. Cardiovascular morbidity and mortality associated with the metabolic syndrome. Diabet Care 2001;24(4):683–689.

[15] Lamarche B, Tchernof A, Mauriège P, et al. Fasting insulin and apolipoprotein B levels and low-density lipoprotein particle size as risk factors for ischemic heart disease. JAMA 1998;279(24):1955–1961.

[16] Grundy SM, Cleeman JI, Daniels SR, et al. Diagnosis and management of the metabolic syndrome: An American Heart Association/National Heart, Lung, and Blood Institute Scientific Statement. Circulation 2005;112 (17):2735–2752.

[17] Reaven GM. Banting lecture 1988. Role of insulin resistance in human disease. Diabetes 1988;37(12):1595–1607.

[18] Avogaro P, Crepaldi G, Enzi G, Tiengo A. Associazione di iperlipidemia, diabete mellito e obesità di medio grado. Acta Diabetol Lat 1967;4:36–41.

[19] Vague J. Sexual differentiation, a factor affecting the forms of obesity. Presse Méd 1947;30:339–340.

[20] Morris JN, Heady JA, Raffle PA, Roberts CG, Parks JW. Coronary heart-disease and physical activity of work. Lancet 1953;265(6796):1111–1120; concl.

[21] Heady JA, Morris JN, Raffle PA. Physique of London busmen; epidemiology of uniforms. Lancet 1956;271(6942):569–570.

[22] Kissebah AH, Vydelingum N, Murray R, et al. Relation of body fat distribution to metabolic complications of obesity. J Clin Endocrinol Metab 1982;54(2):254–260.

[23] Krotkiewski M, Björntorp P, Sjöström L, Smith U. Impact of obesity on metabolism in men and women. Importance of regional adipose tissue distribution. J Clin Invest 1983;72:1150–1162.

[24] Larsson B, Svardsudd K, Welin L, Wilhelmsen L, Björntorp P, Tibblin G. Abdominal adipose tissue distribution, obesity, and risk of cardiovascular disease and death: 13 year follow-up of participants in the study of men born in 1913. Br Med J 1984;288:1401–1404.

[25] Lapidus L, Bengtsson C, Larsson B, Pennert K, Rybo E, Sjöström L. Distribution of adipose tissue and risk of cardiovascular disease and death: A 12 year follow up of participants in the population study of women in Gothenberg, Sweden. Br Med J 1984;289:1257–1261.

[26] Ohlson LO, Larsson B, Svardsudd K, et al. The influence of body fat distribution on the incidence of diabetes mellitus: 13.5 years of follow-up of the participants in the study of men born in 1913. Diabetes 1985;34:1055–1058.

[27] Fujioka S, Matsuzawa Y, Tokunaga K, Tarui S. Contribution of intra-abdominal fat accumulation to the impairment of glucose and lipid metabolism in human obesity. Metabolism 1987;36(1):54–59.

[28] Sjöström L, Kvist H, Cederblad A, Tylen U. Determination of total adipose tissue and body fat in women by computed tomography, 40K, and tritium. Am J Physiol 1986;250:E736–E745.

[29] Peiris AN, Sothmann MS, Hoffmann RG, et al. Adiposity, fat distribution, and cardiovascular risk. Ann Intern Med 1989;110(11):867–872.

[30] Pascot A, Lemieux I, Prud'homme D, et al. Reduced HDL particle size as an additional feature of the atherogenic dyslipidemia of abdominal obesity. J Lipid Res 2001;42(12):2007–2014.

[31] Pouliot MC, Després JP, Nadeau A, et al. Visceral obesity in men. Associations with glucose tolerance, plasma insulin, and lipoprotein levels. Diabetes 1992;41(7):826–834.

[32] Tchernof A, Lamarche B, Prud'homme D, et al. The dense LDL phenotype. Association with plasma lipoprotein levels, visceral obesity, and hyperinsulinemia in men. Diabet Care 1996;19(6):629–637.

[33] Lemieux I, Pascot A, Prud'homme D, et al. Elevated C-reactive protein: Another component of the atherothrombotic profile of abdominal obesity. Arterioscler Thromb Vasc Biol 2001;21(6):961–967.

[34] Couillard C, Bergeron N, Prud'homme D, et al. Postprandial triglyceride response in visceral obesity in men. Diabetes 1998;47:953–960.

[35] Després JP, Moorjani S, Lupien PJ, Tremblay A, Nadeau A, Bouchard C. Regional distribution of body fat, plasma lipoproteins, and cardiovascular disease. Arteriosclerosis 1990;10(4):497–511.

[36] Després JP, Lemieux I, Prud'homme D. Treatment of obesity: Need to focus on high risk abdominally obese patients. BMJ 2001;322(7288):716–720.

[37] Matsuzawa Y, Shimomura I, Nakamura T, Keno Y, Kotani K, Tokunaga K. Pathophysiology and pathogenesis of visceral fat obesity. Obes Res 1995;3(Suppl 2):187S–194S.

[38] Côté M, Mauriège P, Bergeron J, et al. Adiponectinemia in visceral obesity: Impact on glucose tolerance and plasma lipoprotein and lipid levels in men. J Clin Endocrinol Metab 2005;90(3):1434–1439.

[39] Goodpaster BH, Krishnaswami S, Harris TB, et al. Obesity, regional body fat distribution, and the metabolic syndrome in older men and women. Arch Intern Med 2005;165(7):777–783.

[40] Ruderman N, Chisholm D, Pi-Sunyer X, Schneider S. The metabolically obese, normal-weight individual revisited. Diabetes 1998;47(5):699–713.

[41] Wajchenberg BL. Subcutaneous and visceral adipose tissue: Their relation to the metabolic syndrome. Endocr Rev 2000;21(6):697–738.

[42] Després JP. Is visceral obesity the cause of the metabolic syndrome? Ann Med 2006; 38(1):52–63.

[43] Executive Summary of The Third Report of The National Cholesterol Education Program (NCEP) Expert Panel on Detection, Evaluation, and Treatment of High Blood Cholesterol in Adults (Adult Treatment Panel III). JAMA 2001;285(19):2486–2497.

[44] Wilson PW, D'Agostino RB, Parise H, Sullivan L, Meigs JB. Metabolic syndrome as a precursor of cardiovascular disease and type 2 diabetes mellitus. Circulation 2005;112(20): 3066–3072.

[45] Ford ES. Risks for all-cause mortality, cardiovascular disease, and diabetes associated with the metabolic syndrome: A summary of the evidence. Diabet Care 2005;28(7):1769–1778.

[46] Wilson PW, D'Agostino RB, Levy D, Belanger AM, Silbershatz H, Kannel WB. Prediction of coronary heart disease using risk factor categories. Circulation 1998;97(18):1837–1847.

[47] Yusuf S, Hawken S, Ounpuu S, et al. Obesity and the risk of myocardial infarction in 27,000 participants from 52 countries: A case-control study. Lancet 2005;366(9497): 1640–1649.

[48] Reaven GM. Pathophysiology of insulin resistance in human disease. Physiol Rev 1995;75(3):473–486.

[49] Lemieux S, Prud'homme D, Bouchard C, Tremblay A, Després JP. Sex differences in the relation of visceral adipose tissue accumulation to total body fatness. Am J Clin Nutr 1993;58(4):463–467.

[50] Pouliot MC, Després JP, Lemieux S, et al. Waist circumference and abdominal sagittal diameter: Best simple anthropometric indexes of abdominal visceral adipose tissue accumulation and related cardiovascular risk in men and women. Am J Cardiol 1994;73(7):460–468.

[51] Kuk JL, Lee S, Heymsfield SB, Ross R. Waist circumference and abdominal adipose tissue distribution: Influence of age and sex. Am J Clin Nutr 2005;81(6):1330–1334.

[52] Lemieux I, Pascot A, Couillard C, et al. Hypertriglyceridemic waist. A marker of the atherogenic metabolic triad (hyperinsulinemia, hyperapolipoprotein B, small, dense LDL) in men? Circulation 2000;102:179–184.

[53] Lemieux I, Alméras N, Mauriège P, et al. Prevalence of "hypertriglyceridemic waist" in men who participated in the Quebec Health Survey: Association with atherogenic and diabetogenic metabolic risk factors. Can J Cardiol 2002;18:725–732.

[54] Blackburn P, Lamarche B, Couillard C, et al. Postprandial hyperlipidemia: Another correlate of the "hypertriglyceridemic waist" phenotype in men. Atherosclerosis 2003;171(2):327–336.

[55] St-Pierre J, Lemieux I, Vohl MC, et al. Contribution of abdominal obesity and hypertriglyceridemia to impaired fasting glucose and coronary artery disease. Am J Cardiol 2002;90(1):15–18.

[56] Després JP, Couillard C, Gagnon J, et al. Race, visceral adipose tissue, plasma lipids, and lipoprotein lipase activity in men and women: The Health, Risk Factors, Exercise Training, and Genetics (HERITAGE) family study. Arterioscler Thromb Vasc Biol 2000;20(8):1932–1938.

[57] Lovejoy JC, de la Bretonne JA, Klemperer M, Tulley R. Abdominal fat distribution and metabolic risk factors: Effects of race. Metabolism 1996;45(9):1119–1124.

[58] Albu JB, Murphy L, Frager DH, Johnson JA, Pi-Sunyer FX. Visceral fat and race-dependent health risks in obese nondiabetic premenopausal women. Diabetes 1997;46:456–462.

[59] Conway JM, Chanetsa FF, Wang P. Intrabdominal adipose tissue and anthropometric surrogates in African American women with upper- and lower-body obesity. Am J Clin Nutr 1997;66:1345–1351.

[60] Appropriate body-mass index for Asian populations and its implications for policy and intervention strategies. Lancet 2004;363(9403):157–163.

[61] Alberti KG, Zimmet P, Shaw J. The metabolic syndrome—a new worldwide definition. Lancet 2005;366(9491):1059–1062.

[62] Collins R, Armitage J, Parish S, Sleigh P, Peto R. MRC/BHF Heart Protection Study of cholesterol-lowering with simvastatin in 5963 people with diabetes: A randomised placebo-controlled trial. Lancet 2003;361(9374):2005–2016.

[63] Rubins HB, Robins SJ, Collins D, et al. Diabetes, plasma insulin, and cardiovascular disease: Subgroup analysis from the Department of Veterans Affairs high-density lipoprotein intervention trial (VA-HIT). Arch Intern Med 2002;162:2597–2604.

[64] Després JP, Lemieux I, Robins SJ. Role of fibric acid derivatives in the management of risk factors for coronary heart disease. Drugs 2004;64(19):2177–2198.

[65] Manninen V, Tenkanen L, Koshinen P, et al. Joint effects of serum triglyceride and LDL cholesterol and HDL cholesterol concentrations on coronary heart disease risk in the Helsinki Heart Study: Implications for treatment. Circulation 1992;85:37–45.

[66] Tenenbaum A, Motro M, Fisman EZ, Tanne D, Boyko V, Behar S. Bezafibrate for the secondary prevention of myocardial infarction in patients with metabolic syndrome. Arch Intern Med 2005;165(10):1154–1160.

[67] Tuomilehto J, Lindstrom J, Eriksson JG, et al. Prevention of type 2 diabetes mellitus by changes in lifestyle among subjects with impaired glucose tolerance. N Engl J Med 2001;344(18):1343–1350.

[68] Knowler WC, Barrett-Connor E, Fowler SE, et al. Reduction in the incidence of type 2 diabetes with lifestyle intervention or metformin. N Engl J Med 2002;346(6):393–403.

[69] Sjöström L, Rissanen A, Andersen T, Boldrin M, Golay A, Koppeschaar HP. Randomised placebo-controlled trial of orlistat for weight loss and prevention of weight regain in obese patients. European Multicentre Orlistat Study Group. Lancet 1998;352:167–172.

[70] James WP, Astrup A, Finer N, et al. Effect of sibutramine on weight maintenance after weight loss: A randomised trial. STORM Study Group. Sibutramine Trial of Obesity Reduction and Maintenance. Lancet 2000;356(9248):2119–2125.

[71] Torgerson JS, Hauptman J, Boldrin MN, Sjöström L. XENical in the prevention of diabetes in obese subjects (XENDOS) study: A randomized study of orlistat as an adjunct to lifestyle changes for the prevention of type 2 diabetes in obese patients. Diabet Care 2004;27(1):155–161.

[72] Van Gaal LF, Rissanen AM, Scheen AJ, Ziegler O, Rossner S. Effects of the cannabinoid-1 receptor blocker rimonabant on weight reduction and cardiovascular risk factors in overweight patients: 1-year experience from the RIO-Europe study. Lancet 2005;365(9468): 1389–1397.

[73] Després JP, Golay A, Sjöström L. Effects of rimonabant on metabolic risk factors in overweight patients with dyslipidemia. N Engl J Med 2005;353(20):2121–2134.

Chapter 9

The Problems of Childhood Obesity and the Metabolic Syndrome

Sonia Caprio and Ram Weiss

*Department of Pediatrics and the Children's General Clinical Research Center,
Yale University School of Medicine, New Haven, CT 06520, USA*

1. INTRODUCTION

Obesity has reached epidemic proportions in the United States. The number of overweight and obese youth continues to rise despite national efforts by government officials, academic researchers, and the media to bring attention to this growing health problem. Since 1970, the prevalence of overweight has doubled among children 6 to 11 years of age and tripled among those 12 to 17 years of age [1]. The problem falls disproportionately on African-American and Hispanic children [2]. The Center of Disease Control reports that 21% of African-American and Hispanic children are classified as overweight compared to 12% of non-Hispanic white children [2]. In the United States today, approximately 9 million children older than 6 years of age are considered overweight. Obesity is associated with significant health problems in the pediatric age group and is an important early risk factor for much of adult morbidity and mortality [3]. Between 1979 and 1999, the rates of obesity associated hospital discharge diagnoses, such as sleep apnea and gallbladder disease, and the cost of hospitalization tripled among children 6 to 17 years of age [4]. Recent studies from our group reported that 20% of obese children and adolescents have impaired glucose tolerance (IGT) [5]. IGT is defined as a 2-hour glucose level between 140 and 200 mg/dL on a standard oral glucose tolerance test. Our group has also reported that the prevalence of the metabolic syndrome is high among obese children and adolescents, and it increases with worsening obesity [6]. Notably, we found that biomarkers of an increased risk of adverse cardiovascular outcomes are already present in these youngsters. Likely these comorbidities will persist into adulthood [7, 8]; thus the potential future health care costs associated with pediatric obesity and its comorbidities is staggering. Therefore, it is incumbent on the pediatric community to take the leadership role in prevention and treatment of pediatric obesity.

Here we review the metabolic complications associated with childhood obesity. Particular emphasis is given to the description of studies regarding the prevalence and impact of varying degrees of obesity on the metabolic syndrome in youth and metabolic phenotype of impaired glucose tolerance in childhood obesity.

2.   PREVALENCE OF THE METABOLIC SYNDROME IN CHILDREN AND ADOLESCENTS: IMPACT OF OBESITY

Reaven and colleagues [9] described the link between insulin resistance and hypertension, dyslipidemia, type 2 diabetes, and other metabolic abnormalities in adults in 1988. This constellation of comorbid conditions has become known as the "metabolic syndrome" and is associated with an increased risk of morbidity and mortality from cardiovascular disease [10]. More recent studies suggest that the pathophysiologic defects leading to the development of the metabolic syndrome in adults may begin as early as the intrauterine period [11, 12]. While the concept of the metabolic syndrome was accepted for many years, it was not until 1998 that both the World Health Organization (WHO) [13] and The National Cholesterol Education Program Adult Treatment Panel III (NCEP: ATP III) [14] have formulated definitions. These definitions agree on the essential components, namely obesity, glucose intolerance, hypertension, and dyslipidemia. However, the WHO definition includes impaired glucose tolerance or insulin resistance in contrast in the NCEP: ATP III, in which these criteria are not included. In the United States the prevalence of the metabolic syndrome in adults is 25%, with lower prevalence in African Americans compared to Hispanics and whites [15]. Of note is the fact that the prevalence of the metabolic syndrome is highly age dependent in adults, increasing from approximately 15% in participants aged 20 to 39 years to 50% for those 60 to 69 years of age [16]. In contrast to the vast research in adults, little is known about this important syndrome in children. Indeed, until recently the metabolic syndrome and type 2 diabetes have been considered as diseases of adults. More recently, however, with the increasing rates of childhood obesity, type 2 diabetes and the metabolic syndrome have emerged as new metabolic diseases in pediatrics [17, 18]. Despite the lack of a uniform definition of the syndrome in pediatrics, population studies indicated that the overall prevalence is low in children and adolescents (approximately 4%) when compared to adults. Using data collected between 1988 and 1994 on a nationally representative sample of US adolescents (National Health and Nutrition Examination Survey III [NHANES III]), Cook et al. [19] reported a prevalence of the metabolic syndrome of 6.8% in overweight and 28.7% in obese adolescents. However, these rates may underestimate the current magnitude of the problem, in view of the growing epidemic of obesity in children and adolescents. It is also important to note that the degree, as well as the prevalence, of childhood obesity has been increasing over time. Cruz and colleagues [20] developed a pediatric definition of the metabolic syndrome based on the ATP III guidelines as a model and reported that 30% of overweight Hispanic children, with a family history for type 2 diabetes, have the metabolic syndrome.

To begin assessing the impact of varying degrees of obesity on the prevalence of the metabolic syndrome in children and adolescents, we recently completed a cross-sectional analysis of our cohort of obese youth [6]. The cohort consisted of 439 children and adolescents. Eligibility criteria included age between 4 and 20 years, body mass index (BMI) greater than 97th percentile for age and gender, and otherwise healthy status. Exclusion criteria were known diabetes or taking any medication that alters blood pressure, glucose, or lipid metabolism. Twenty nonobese (BMI < 85th%) and 31 overweight (85th% $>$ BMI < 97th%) siblings of obese subjects were recruited to serve as comparison groups. All subjects underwent a standard 75-g oral glucose test. We further divided the obese children to moderately obese (BMI z-score < 2.5) and severely obese (BMI z-score > 2.5). Baseline measures included plasma lipids, C-reactive protein (CRP), interleukin-6 (IL-6), and adiponectin levels. In our study we used age-, gender-, and ethnicity-specific criteria. Insulin sensitivity was determined by the homeostatic model assessment (HOMA-IR).

The adverse impact of increasing degrees of obesity on components of the MS is summarized in Table 1. Specifically, fasting glucose levels, fasting insulin, HOMA-IR, systolic blood pressure, triglycerides, CRP, IL-6, and prevalence of impaired glucose tolerance (IGT) increased significantly with increasing degree of obesity, while HDL-cholesterol and adiponectin levels decreased with increasing obesity. The moderately and severely obese African-American subjects had lower triglycerides and higher HDL-cholesterol as compared to their Caucasian and Hispanic counterparts. Prevalence of IGT increased with the degree of obesity in all ethnicities. It is of note that the significance of these trends persisted after adjustment for gender, pubertal status, and ethnicity.

The prevalence of the metabolic syndrome increased with severity of obesity and reached 50% in severely obese youngsters. Each half unit increase in BMI was associated with an increase in the risk of the metabolic syndrome in overweight and obese youngsters (odds ratios 1.55).

3. EFFECTS OF INSULIN RESISTANCE (HOMA-IR) ON THE PREVALENCE OF THE METABOLIC SYNDROME

We performed a multiple logistic regression analysis of risk factors associated with metabolic syndrome in childhood. Variables incorporated into the

Table 1. Metabolic characteristics of the cohort

	Lean $N = 20$	Overweight $N = 31$	Mod. obese $N = 244$	Sev. obese $N = 195$	*p* value Adjusted	Unadjusted
Fasting glucose (mg/dL)	87.4 (83.9–90.8)	86.8 (84.5–89.2)	90.5 (89.6–91.5)	90.2 (89.0–91.3)	$p = 0.04$	$p = 0.06$
Fasting insulin (μU/mL)	10.3 (8.0–13.2)	14.6 (11.8–18.2)	31.3 (29.2–33.3)	38.6 (34.8–42.4)	$p < 0.0001$	$p < 0.0001$
HOMA IR	2.20 (1.69–2.85)	3.12 (2.48–3.93)	7.05 (6.56–7.54)	8.69 (7.78–9.61)	$p < 0.0001$	$p < 0.0001$
Triglyceride (mg/dL)	48.4 (42.5–54.6)	83.1 (68.7–100.5)	104.6 (96.5–112.2)	96.5 (90.1–102.5)	$p < 0.0001$	$p < 0.0001$
HDL cholesterol (mg/dL)	58.5 (52.3–64.7)	46.7 (42.0–51.3)	41.1 (39.9–42.3)	39.9 (38.6–41.3)	$p < 0.0001$	$p < 0.0001$
Systolic blood pressure (mm Hg)	106 (102–110)	116 (112–121)	121 (119–123)	124 (122–126)	$p < 0.0001$	$p < 0.0001$
Percentage of impaired glucose tolerance	0 (0–20)	3.23 (0–17)	14.40 (10.3–19.60)	19.9 (15.5–24.5)	$p = 0.01$	$p = 0.01$
Adiponectin	9.6 (6.1–15.3)	8.0 (6.0–10.6)	6.7 (6.2–7.3)	5.8 (5.3–6.5)	$p = 0.001$	$p = 0.01$
hsCRP	0.014 (0.008–0.027)	0.05 (0.03–0.09)	0.13 (0.10–0.16)	0.33 (0.27–0.40)	$p < 0.001$	$p < 0.001$
IL-6	0.92 (0.32–2.58)	0.99 (0.64–1.53)	1.80 (1.58–2.05)	2.45 (2.05–2.94)	$p < 0.001$	$p < 0.001$

Data presented as mean (95% CI); *p* values are for trend across all weight groups (unadjusted and adjusted for gender, pubertal stage, and ethnicity). HOMA-IR, homeostatic model of assessment of insulin resistance; hsCRP, high-sensitivity C-reactive protein; IL-6, interleukin-6.

model were age, gender, BMI *z*-score, ethnicity, and HOMA-IR. Overall Each half-unit increase in the body mass index, converted to a *z*-score, was associated with an increase in the risk of the metabolic syndrome among overweight and obese subjects (odds ratio, 1.55; 95 percent confidence interval, 1.16 to 2.08), as was each unit of increase in insulin resistance as assessed with the homeostatic model (odds ratio, 1.12; 95% confidence interval, 1.07 to 1.18 for each additional unit of insulin resistance). Caucasians had a higher odds ratio to have the metabolic syndrome (OR = 1.10, CI 1.35–3.59); there was no significant difference in risk between Hispanic and black subjects. The prevalence of the metabolic syndrome increased significantly with increasing insulin

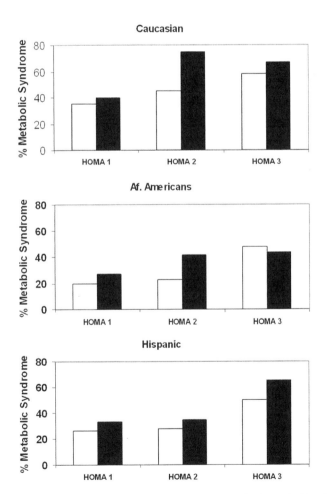

Figure 1. Prevalence of the metabolic syndrome by the degree obesity and of insulin resistance by ethnic background. HOMA-1, most sensitive; HOMA-3, most resistant; white bars, moderately obese; black bars, severely obese.

resistance after adjusting for ethnicity and degree of obesity as shown in Figure 1. CRP concentrations and IL-6 increased and adiponectin decreased with increasing obesity. This study showed that the prevalence of the metabolic syndrome is high among obese children and adolescents, and increases with worsening obesity. Biomarkers of increased risk of adverse cardiovascular outcomes are already present in youngsters. African Americans, Caucasians had a higher odds ratio for the metabolic syndrome (OR = 2.20, CI 1.35–3.59); there was no significant difference in risk between Hispanic and black subjects.

An intriguing finding in this study is that despite similar degrees of obesity and insulin resistance in African Americans and Caucasians, African-American children and adolescents were relatively protected from the metabolic syndrome, due primarily to a reduction in the prevalence of dyslipidemia. Of note, the threshold levels for triglycerides and HDL cholesterol in this study were ethnicity specific. As previously reported in adults, the lower prevalence of the metabolic syndrome in our African-American children was primarily related to more favorable lipid profiles. However, the lower prevalence of dyslipidemia in African-American children and adults seems to be in contrast with the high prevalence of cardiovascular disease in adult African Americans.

4. PROINFLAMMATORY AND ANTIINFLAMMATORY MARKERS AND INSULIN RESISTANCE

Recent accumulating evidence indicates that obesity is associated with subclinical chronic inflammation [21, 22]. The adipose tissue is not merely a simple reservoir of energy stored as triglycerides, but also serves as an active secretory organ releasing many peptides and cytokines into the circulation [23]. In the presence of obesity, the balance between these numerous molecules is altered, such that enlarged adipocytes produces more proinflammatory cytokines (i.e., TNF-α, IL-6) and less antiinflammatory peptides such as adiponectin [24]. The dysregulated production of adipocytokines has been found to participate in the development of metabolic and vascular diseases related to obesity [25]. Evidence indicates that as the degree of obesity increases, the adipose tissue is infiltrated by macrophages [21]. Such macrophages may be the major source of proinflammatory cytokines initiating a proinflammatory status that predates the development of insulin resistance and endothelial dysfunction [26]. Indeed, inflammation may be the missing link between obesity and insulin resistance. We also examined the effects of childhood obesity on two biomarkers of adverse cardiovascular outcomes: CRP and adiponectin. CRP is a general biomarker of inflammation that has been associated with adverse cardiovascular outcomes [27, 28] and altered glucose metabolism [29]. CRP levels in our cohort tended to rise as BMI z-score and as insulin resistance increased. Although these levels are still within the normal accepted range, even "high normal" levels have been suspected to indicate significant adverse outcomes [30]. The strong impact of the BMI z-score on the CRP levels suggests that the degree of low-grade inflammation increases in these youngsters as they become more obese. The implications of this low-grade inflammation on atherosclerosis and glucose metabolism are yet to be determined. Adiponectin, apart from being a biomarker of insulin sensitivity, has been implicated to play an important role in reducing vascular inflammation [31]. In contrast to CRP, adiponectin levels tended to drop as BMI z-score and insulin resistance increased. Lower levels of this adipocytokine have been demonstrated to increase the risk of cardiovascular disease [32]. Both biomarkers demonstrated a reciprocal trend as the degree of obesity increased, implicating a potential significant impact of "super" adiposity on adverse cardiovascular outcomes.

5. PATHOPHYSIOLOGICAL STUDIES OF THE PREDIABETIC PHENOTYPE IN YOUTH

The unabated rise in the prevalence and severity of childhood obesity has been accompanied by the appearance of a new pediatric disease: *type 2 diabetes* [33]. One dire prediction from the CDC estimated that, if current obesity rates continue, one in three babies born in 2000 will eventually develop T2DM [34]. African-American and Hispanic children are at greatest risk for both obesity and diabetes [35, 36].

In adults, type 2 diabetes develops over a long period [37]. Most, if not all, patients initially have IGT, which is an intermediate stage in the natural history of type 2 diabetes [38] and is highly predictive of diabetes and cardiovascular disease. With appropriate changes in lifestyle and/or pharmacologic interventions, progression from IGT to frank diabetes can be delayed or prevented [39, 40]. Thus, great emphasis has recently been placed on the early detection of IGT in adults. Before our project, little was known about this condition in pediatrics. Although severe obesity has a prominent role in the pathogenesis of type 2 diabetes in children and adolescents, it was unknown whether it is a risk factor for IGT. We determined the prevalence of IGT in a multiethnic clinic-based population of 55 obese children and 112 obese adolescents. Irrespective of ethnicity, IGT was detected in 25% of the obese children and 21% of the obese adolescents, and silent type 2 diabetes was identified in 4% of the obese adolescents [41]. Higher prevalence rates of IGT have been also reported in obese children from Thailand [42] and the Philippines [43] and in Latino children living in the United States [44], while lower prevalence rates of 15% were found in obese children in France [45].

6.   RELATIONSHIP BETWEEN INSULIN RESISTANCE AND TISSUE LIPID PARTITIONING

Insulin resistance is an important risk factor for the development of T2DM, but the decline in the acute insulin response to intravenous glucose determines disease progression in adults [46]. To address these issues, we studied differences in insulin sensitivity and secretion in obese adolescents with normal glucose tolerance (NGT) and IGT. These studies revealed profound insulin resistance in the obese adolescents with IGT compared with those with NGT [47]. Insulin resistance was mainly accounted for by a reduction in nonoxidative glucose disposal (storage). The lipid composition of skeletal muscle tissue, where most (70%) of the whole glucose disposal occurs, has attracted much attention recently as a major player in the development of muscle insulin resistance [48, 49]. This area of investigation has been greatly advanced by the recent development and validation of ^{1}H-nuclear magnetic resonance (^{1}H-NMR) for the noninvasive quantitation of fat stored inside the myocytes, the intramyocellular fat content (IMCL) [50, 51]. We used ^{1}H-NMR to measure IMCL in our obese children. These studies demonstrated excessive accumulation of IMCL in the soleus muscle of obese adolescents with IGT compared to age and adiposity matched obese adolescents with NGT (Figure 2). Abdominal MRI showed that subcutaneous fat in IGT subjects was significantly lower compared with NGT subjects while visceral fat tended to be higher in the IGT than in the NGT group (Figure 3). Our data are consistent with results obtained in both human and animal models of lipodystrophy, in which there is an absence of subcutaneous adipose tissue, leading to increased accumula-

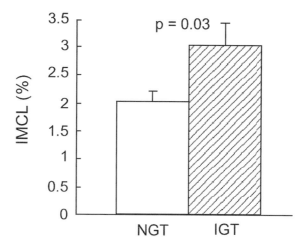

Figure 2. Intramyocellular lipid (IMCL) in obese subjects with normal and impaired glucose tolerance.

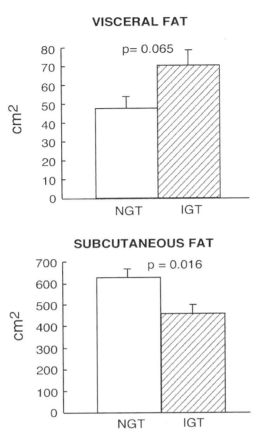

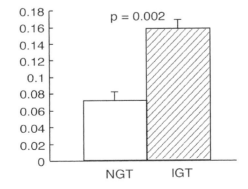

Figure 3. Visceral, subcutaneous, and the visceral to subcutaneous fat ratio in obese subjects with normal and impaired glucose tolerance.

tion of lipids in both myocytes and the visceral depot [52, 53]. It appears that the ability of peripheral subcutaneous fat tissue to vary its storage capacity is critical for regulating insulin sensitivity and ultimately protecting against diabetes. Consistent with this hypothesis is the evidence derived from the use of thiazolidinediones, which improve insulin sensitivity while increasing subcutaneous abdominal fat, and shunting lipid out of the visceral and liver fat depots [54].

These studies offer a novel insight into the pathogenesis of IGT in obese youth, namely that changes in glucose homeostasis are closely linked with altered partitioning of fat in both skeletal muscle and adipose tissues. Based on these studies, there is a strong rationale for changing the balance between visceral and subcutaneous fat and muscle lipid content in a more favorable pattern in order to improve insulin sensitivity.

7.   EARLY REDUCTION OF β-CELL SENSITIVITY TO GLUCOSE IN OBESE YOUTH WITH IMPAIRED GLUCOSE TOLERANCE

Studies in adults that evaluated alterations in insulin secretion in subjects with IGT have given inconsistent results [55]. The reason may be that many of these studies based their conclusions on variations in circulating plasma insulin concentrations rather than on more detailed assessments of insulin secretory rates. An important artifact in some of these studies is the analysis of β-cell function without considering the ambient insulin resistance and thus ignoring the intricate relationship between insulin sensitivity and secretion [56]. In collaboration with Dr. R. Bonadonna, we performed a detailed quantitative analysis of the components of β-cell function and their relationships with insulin resistance in obese youngsters across the entire spectrum of glucose tolerance [57].

We studied 62 obese youth: 29 with normal glucose tolerance (NGT), 24 with impaired glucose tolerance (IGT), and 9 with type 2 diabetes (T2DM). We assessed β-cell sensitivity to glucose via the hyperglycemic clamp, with applied modeling of c-peptide secretion to analyze several components of the β-cell response to a standardized glucose stimulus, including the sensitivity of the β cell for secretion during first and second phase. As shown in Figure 4, the model-derived first phase sensitivity of the β cell for c-peptide secretion was significantly reduced in the IGT group compared to the NGT group ($p < 0.008$). A further reduction was seen in the diabetic groups ($p < 0.0001$). In contrast, β-cell sensitivity for the second-phase c-peptide secretion was similar between NGT and IGT subjects yet decreased in the diabetic group ($p < 0.008$). Obese youngsters with prediabetes (IGT) thus have a reduced

Sensitivity of First Phase

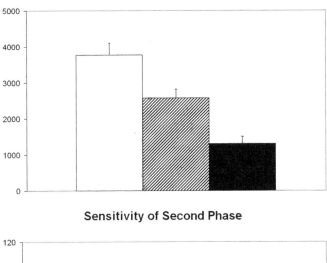

Sensitivity of Second Phase

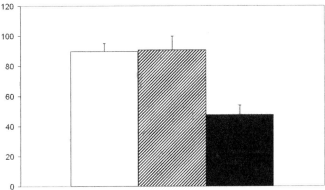

Figure 4. Sensitivity of the β-cell to first- and second-phase secretion in obese subjects with NGT (white), IGT (hatched), and T2DM (black).

sensitivity of the β-cell for first phase secretion compared to NGT subjects matched for age and percent body fat. Of note, these differences were not apparent when using conventional measures of insulin concentrations during the corresponding time points of the hyperglycemic clamp, yet they emerged through the analysis of c-peptide secretion using the minimal model modified by Bonadonna et al. [58]. Our study clearly demonstrates deterioration in the glucose sensitivity of β-cell secretion across the spectrum of glucose tolerance in obese youngsters.

8.   LONGITUDINAL STUDY OF CHANGES IN GLUCOSE TOLERANCE STATUS IN OBESE YOUTH

Cross-sectional studies demonstrated that IGT in obese youth is associated with severe insulin resistance, β-cell dysfunction and altered abdominal and muscle fat partitioning. Because of their design, these studies did not examine potential metabolic predictors of changes in glucose tolerance in these obese youngsters.

Transition from IGT to diabetes in adults is usually a gradual phenomenon, occurring over 5 to 10 years [59, 60], depending on the population studied. The early presentation of type 2 diabetes in youth raises the possibility of an accelerated process in these youngsters, compared to adults, thus shortening the transition time between IGT and diabetes. In contrast to the vast literature about metabolic predictors of deterioration of glucose tolerance in adults, little is known about this process in children and adolescents. Thus, our aim was to follow obese children and adolescents at risk for diabetes longitudinally and identify baseline metabolic and anthropometric parameters associated with later deterioration of glucose metabolism [61]. One hundred and seventeen obese children and adolescents were studied by performing an oral glucose tolerance test at baseline and after approximately 2 years. In the interim, participants received nutritional guidance and recommendations for increased physical activity, without any pharmacological intervention. Data from both glucose tolerance tests and changes in weight were examined to identify the youngsters at highest risk for developing diabetes and the factors that have the strongest impact on glucose tolerance.

Eighty four subjects had NGT and 33 had IGT at baseline. Eight subjects, all of which were IGT at baseline, developed T2DM while 15 subjects with IGT reverted to NGT. Severe obesity, impaired glucose tolerance, and African-American background emerged in this cohort as the best predictors of developing T2DM while fasting glucose, insulin, and c-peptide were nonpredictive. Changes in insulin sensitivity, strongly related to weight change, had a significant impact on the 2-hour glucose level on the follow-up study. Our study also clearly shows that glucose tolerance status in obese children is highly dynamic and can deteriorate fairly rapidly. Over a relatively short follow-up, roughly 10% of subjects initially classified as NGT developed IGT and 24% of subjects initially classified as IGT developed overt T2DM. These data suggest that the tempo of deterioration of β-cell function in children may be faster compared to that in adults [62, 63]. It should be noted, however, that our data also indicate that obese children with IGT can revert to NGT on follow-up testing. Such improvements in glucose tolerance do not appear to be artifacts of repeat testing, since these youngsters had lower BMI z-scores at baseline and maintained their weight without further weight gain by the time of the follow-up compared to youngsters who developed T2DM. These observations suggest that a focused and intensive intervention, similar to the one used in the Diabetes Prevention Program [64], may be useful in managing the severely obese child with IGT.

We conclude that severely obese children (BMI z-score > 2.5) with IGT, specifically of ethnic minority background, require the most intensive intervention and careful observation for prevention of development of T2DM. Cessation of weight gain and not necessarily weight loss may suffice to prevent further deterioration in glucose tolerance. As the risk in these patients seems very high and window of opportunity is narrow, pharmacological intervention, alongside lifestyle changes, should not be ruled out.

ACKNOWLEDGMENTS

This work was supported by grants RO1-HD40787, RO1-HD28016, and K24-HD01464 (to Dr. Caprio), MO1-RR00125 and MO1-RR06022 from the National Institutes of Health, and the Stephen I. Morse Pediatric Diabetes Research Fund (Dr. Weiss).

REFERENCES

[1] Ogden CL, Flegal KM, Carroll MD, Johnson CL. Prevalence and trends in overweight among US children and adolescents, 1999–2000. JAMA 2002;288:1728–1732.

[2] National Center of Health Statistics: NHANES III Reference Manuals and Reports. Hyattsville, MD: US Department of Health and Human Services, Public Health Service, Centers for Disease Control, 1996.

[3] Center for Disease Control and Prevention. Prevalence of overweight among adolescents, 1988–1991. MMWR 1994;43:818–821.

[4] Wang G, Dietz WH. Economic burden of obesity in youth aged 6–17 years: 1979–1999. Pediatrics 2002;109:E81–E82.

[5] Sinha R, Fisch G, Teague B, et al. Prevalence of impaired glucose tolerance among children and adolescents with marked obesity. N Engl J Med 2002;346(11):802–810.

[6] Weiss R, Dziura J, Burgert TS, et al. Obesity and the metabolic syndrome in children and adolescents. N Engl J Med 2004;350(23):2362–2374.

[7] Dietz WH. Health consequences of obesity in youth: Childhood predictors of adulthood disease. Pediatrics 1998;101(Suppl 3):518–525.

[8] Berenson GS, Srinivasan SR, Bao W, Newman WP III, Tracy RE, Wattigney WA. Association between multiple cardiovascular risk factors and atherosclerosis in children and young adults. N Engl J Med 1998;338:1650–1656.

[9] Reaven GM. Banting lecture 1988: Role of insulin resistance in human disease. Diabetes 1988;37(12):1595–1607.

[10] Isomaa B, Almgren P, Tuomi T, et al. Cardiovascular morbidity and mortality associated with the metabolic syndrome. Diabetes Care 2001;24(4):683–689.

[11] Levitt NS, Lambert EV. The foetal origins of the metabolic syndrome—a South African perspective. Cardiovasc J S Afr 2002;13(4):179–180.

[12] Ozanne SE, Hales CN. Early programming of glucose-insulin metabolism. Trends Endocrinol Metab 2002;13(9):368–373.

[13] Alberti KG, Zimmet PZ. Definition, diagnosis and classification of diabetes mellitus and its complications. Part 1: Diagnosis and classification of diabetes mellitus provisional report of a WHO consultation. Diabet Med 1998;15:539–553.

[14] National Institutes of Health. Third Report of the National Cholesterol Education Program Expert Panel on Detection, Evaluation, and Treatment of High Blood Cholesterol in Adults (Adult Treatment Panel III). NIH Publication 01-3670. Bethesda, MD: National Institutes of Health, 2001.

[15] Ford ES, Giles WH, Dietz WH. Prevalence of the metabolic syndrome among US adults: Findings from the Third National Health and Nutrition Examination survey. JAMA 2002;287:356–359.

[16] Ford ES, Giles WH, Mokdad AH. Increasing prevalence of the metabolic syndrome among U.S. Adults. Diabetes Care 2004;27(10):2444–2449.

[17] Rosenbloom AL, Joe JR, Young RS, Winter WE. Emerging epidemic of type 2 diabetes in youth. Diabetes Care 1999;22:345–354.

[18] Steinberger J, Daniels SR. Obesity, insulin resistance, diabetes, and cardiovascular risk in children. An American Heart Association Scientific Statement from the Atherosclerosis, Hypertension, and Obesity in the Young Committee (Council on Cardiovascular Disease in the Young) and the Diabetes Committee (Council on Nutrition, Physical Activity, and Metabolism). Circulation 2003;107:1448.

[19] Cook S, Weitzman M, Auinger P, Nguyen M, Dietz WH. Prevalence of a metabolic syndrome phenotype in adolescents: Findings from the third National Health and Nutrition Examination Survey, 1988–1994. Arch Pediatr Adolesc Med 2003;157(8):821–827.

[20] Cruz ML, Weigensberg MJ, Huang TT, Ball G, Shaibi GQ, Goran MI. The metabolic syndrome in overweight Hispanic youth and the role of insulin sensitivity. J Clin Endocrinol Metab 2004;89(1):108–113.

[21] Weisberg SP, McCann D, Desai M, et al. Obesity is associated with macrophage accumulation in adipose tissue. J Clin Invest 2003;112:1673–1808.

[22] Wellen KE, Hotamisligil GS. Obesity-induced inflammatory changes in adipose tissue. J Clin Invest 2003;112:1785–1788.

[23] Rajala MW, Scherer PE. The adipocyte at the crossroads of energy homeostasis, inflammation and atherosclerosis. Endocrinology 2003:3765–3773.

[24] Matsuzawa Y, Funahashi T, Nakamura T. Molecular mechanism of metabolic syndrome X: Contribution of adipocytokines adipocyte-derived bioactive substances. Ann NY Acad Sci 2000;146–154.

[25] Yudkin JS, Kumari M, Humphries SE, et al. Inflammation, obesity, stress and coronary heart disease: Is interleukin-6 the link? Atherosclerosis 2000;148;209–214.

[26] Pickup JC, Crook MA. Is type 2 diabetes mellitus a disease of the innate immune system? Diabetologia 1998;41:1241–1248.

[27] Koenig W, Sund M, Frohlich M, et al. C-reactive protein, a sensitive marker of inflammation, predicts future risk of coronary heart disease in initially healthy middle-aged men: Results from the MONICA (Monitoring Trends and Determinants in Cardiovascular Disease) Augsburg Cohort Study, 1984 to 1992. Circulation 1999;99(2):237–242.

[28] Ridker PM, Cushman M, Stampfer MJ, Tracy RP, Hennekens CH. Inflammation, aspirin, and the risk of cardiovascular disease in apparently healthy men. N Engl J Med 1997; 336(14):973–979.

[29] Tan KC, Wat NM, Tam SC, Janus ED, Lam TH, Lam KS. C-reactive protein predicts the deterioration of glycemia in Chinese subjects with impaired glucose tolerance. Diabetes Care 2003;26(8):2323–2328.

[30] Blake GJ, Rifai N, Buring JE, Ridker PM. Blood pressure, C-reactive protein, and risk of future cardiovascular events. Circulation 2003;108(24):2993–2999.

[31] Kumada M, Kihara S, Ouchi N, et al. Adiponectin specifically increased tissue inhibitor of metalloproteinase-1 through interleukin-10 expression in human macrophages. Circulation 2004;109(17):2046–2049.

[32] Maahs DM, Ogden LG, Kinney GL, et al. Low plasma adiponectin levels predict progression of coronary artery calcification. Circulation 2005;111(6):747–753.

[33] Rosenbloom AL, Joe JR, Young RS, Winter WE. Emerging epidemic of type 2 diabetes in youth. Diabetes Care 1999;22:345–354.

[34] Narayan KM, Boyle JP, Thompson TJ, Sorensen SW, Williamson DF. Lifetime risk for diabetes mellitus in the United States. JAMA 2003;290(14):1884–1890.

[35] Dabelea D, Pettitt DJ, Jones KL, Arslanian SA. Type 2 diabetes mellitus in minority children and adolescents. An emerging problem. Endocrinol Metab Clin North Am 1999; 28:709–729.

[36] Arslanian SA. Metabolic differences between Caucasian and African-American children and the relationship to type 2 diabetes mellitus. J Pediatr Endocrinol Metab 2002;15(Suppl 1):509–517.

[37] Polonsky KS, Sturis J, Bell GI. Seminars in Medicine of the Beth Israel Hospital, Boston. Non-insulin-dependent diabetes mellitus—a genetically programmed failure of the beta cell to compensate for insulin resistance. N Engl J Med 1996;334:777–783.

[38] Edelstein SL, Knowler WC, Bain RP, et al. Predictors of progression from impaired glucose tolerance to NIDDM: An analysis of six prospective studies. Diabetes 1997;46:701–710.

[39] Knowler WC, Barrett-Connor E, Fowler SE, et al. and Diabetes Prevention Program Research Group. Reduction in the incidence of type 2 diabetes with lifestyle intervention or metformin. N Engl J Med 2002;346(6):393–403.

[40] Tuomilehto J, Lindstrom J, Eriksson JG, and Finnish Diabetes Prevention Study Group. Prevention of type 2 diabetes mellitus by changes in lifestyle among subjects with impaired glucose tolerance. N Engl J Med 2001;344(18):1343–1350.

[41] Sinha R, Fisch G, Teague B, et al. Prevalence of impaired glucose tolerance among children and adolescents with marked obesity. N Engl J Med 2002;346(11):802–810.

[42] Keamseng C, Likitmaksul S, Kiattisakthavee P, et al. Risk of metabolic disturbance and diabetes development in Thai obese children, 29th Annual Meeting of the International Society for Pediatric and Adolescent Diabetes, Saint-Malo, France, September 3–6, 2003.

[43] Lee W, Tang J, Karim H, et al. Abnormalities of glucose tolerance in severely obese Singapore children, 29th Annual Meeting of the International Society for Pediatric and Adolescent Diabetes, Saint-Malo, France, September 3–6, 2003.

[44] Cruz ML, Weigensberg MJ, Huang TT, Ball G, Shaibi GQ, Goran MI. The metabolic syndrome in overweight Hispanic youth and the role of insulin sensitivity. J Clin Endocrinol Metab 2004;89(1):108–113.

[45] Tounian P, Aggoun Y, Dubern B, et al. Presence of increased stiffness of the common carotid artery and endothelial dysfunction in severely obese children: A prospective study. Lancet 2001;358:1400–1404.

[46] Weyer C, Bogardus C, Mott DM, Pratley RE. The natural history of insulin secretory dysfunction and insulin resistance in the pathogenesis of type 2 diabetes mellitus. J Clin Invest 1999;104(6):787–794.

[47] Weiss R, Dufour S, Taksali SE, et al. Prediabetes in obese youth: A syndrome of impaired glucose tolerance, severe insulin resistance, and altered myocellular and abdominal fat partitioning. Lancet 2003;362(9388):951–957.

[48] Kelley DE, Goodpaster BH, Storlien L. Muscle triglyceride and insulin resistance. Annu Rev Nutr 2002;22:325–346.

[49] Krssak M, Falk Petersen K, Dresner A, et al. Intramyocellular lipid concentrations are correlated with insulin sensitivity in humans: A 1H NMR spectroscopy study. Diabetologia 1999;42:113–116.

[50] Boesch C, Kreis R. Observation of intramyocellular lipids by [1]H-magnetic resonance spectroscopy. Ann NY Acad Sci 2000;904:25–31.

[51] Szczepaniak LS, Babcock EE, Schick F, et al. Measurement of intracellular triglyceride stores by H spectroscopy: Validation in vivo. Am J Physiol 1999;276(5 Pt 1):E977–E989.

[52] Petersen KF, Oral EA, Dufour S, et al. Leptin reverses insulin resistance and hepatic steatosis in patients with severe lipodystrophy. J Clin Invest 2002;109(10):1345–1350.

[53] Kim JK, Gavrilova O, Chen Y, Reitman ML, Shulman GI. Mechanism of insulin resistance in A-ZIP/F-1 fatless mice. J Biol Chem 2000;275:8456–8460.

[54] Bays H, Mandarino L, Defronzo R. Role of adipocyte, free fatty acids and ectopic fat in the pathogenesis of type 2 diabetes mellitus: Peroximal proliferator-activated receptor-agonists provide a rational therapeutic approach. J Clin Endocrinol Metab 2004,89(2):463–478.

[55] Kahn ES. The importance of beta cell failure in the development and progression of type 2 diabetes. J Clin Endocrinol Metab 2001;86(9):4047–4058.

[56] Ahren B, Pacini G. Importance of quantifying insulin secretion in relation to insulin sensitivity to accurately assess beta cell function in clinical studies. Eur J Endocrinol 2004; 150(2):97–104.

[57] Weiss R, Caprio S, Trombetta M, Taksali SE, Tamborlane WV, Bonadonna R. Beta cell function across the spectrum of glucose tolerance in obese youth. Diabetes (in press).

[58] Bonadonna RC, Stumvoll M, Fritsche A, et al. Altered homeostatic adaptation of first- and second-phase beta-cell secretion in the offspring of patients with type 2 diabetes: Studies with a minimal model to assess beta-cell function. Diabetes 2003;52(2):470–480.

[59] Edelstein SL, Knowler WC, Bain RP, et al. Predictors of progression from impaired glucose tolerance to NIDDM: An analysis of six prospective studies. Diabetes 1997;46:701–710.

[60] Saad MF, Knowler WC, Pettitt DJ, Nelson RG, Mott DM, Bennett PH. The natural history of impaired glucose tolerance in the Pima Indians. N Engl J Med 1988;319:1500–1506.

[61] Weiss R, Taksali SE, Tamborlane WV, Burgert TS, Savoye M, Caprio S. Predictors of changes in glucose tolerance status in obese youth. Diabetes Care 2005;28(4):902–909.

[62] Meigs JB, Muller DC, Nathan DM, Blake DR, Andres R; Baltimore Longitudinal Study of Aging. The natural history of progression from normal glucose tolerance to type 2 diabetes in the Baltimore Longitudinal Study of Aging. Diabetes 2003;52(6):1475–1484.

[63] Chou P, Li CL, Wu GS, Tsai ST. Progression to type 2 diabetes among high-risk groups in Kin-Chen, Kinmen. Exploring the natural history of type 2 diabetes. Diabetes Care 1998;21(7):1183–1187.

[64] Diabetes Prevention Program Research Group. Reduction in the incidence of type 2 diabetes with lifestyle intervention or metformin. N Engl J Med 2002;346:393–403.

Chapter 10

Evaluation of the Overweight and Obese Patient

George A. Bray and Donna H. Ryan

Pennington Biomedical Research Center, Baton Rouge, LA 70808, USA

1. INTRODUCTION

The increases in rates of overweight and obesity in the United States, which have become apparent in the last 30 years [1], prompt concern among medical personnel because of the health risks associated with excess adiposity. Of particular concern among public health officials is obesity's twin epidemic of type 2 diabetes [2]. However, the association of obesity as an independent risk factor for cardiovascular disease [3, 4] and as a contributor to risk for almost every type of cancer [5], are additional reasons for alarm. The societal and cultural values placed on slimness drive dieting patterns, even among those who are not at increased health risk for overweight. To help patients manage their health, physicians must be able to define the aspects of overweight that impose health risk. That indicates recognition of excess body fat, and in particular, excess central adiposity.

Overweight and obesity can be defined to inform health status from a population perspective and from an individual perspective. While the purpose of this chapter is to guide treating physicians, and thus our focus is on the individual, it is still informative to discuss overweight and obesity definitions from a population level. The current definition for the US population is to categorize overweight as body mass index (BMI) ≥ 25 to < 30 kg/m^2 and obesity as BMI ≥ 30 kg/m^2 [6]. Such a definition allows us to track population trends in overweight and obesity in the United States and around the world. Because BMI tracks well with total body fat on a population level [7], such a definition is acceptable from an epidemiologic standpoint. On an individual basis, these definitions do not always serve to identify those at health risk because of excess body fat. For those with increased muscle mass, such as body builders, BMI overestimates health risks because the total body fat may not be increased, and for the elderly, with a reduced lean mass, the BMI underestimates the health risk of fatness. Thus, because of the implications for health risks and increased demands on the health care system for advice and treatment, we need a set of ground rules that define overweight and obesity in terms of health risk to the individual and to guide a risk–benefit approach to selecting treatments. Health risks drive treatment options. Thus, information from waist circumference and the presence of comorbidities can be used in addition to BMI to determine an individual's risk status.

2.   DEFINITIONS

Obesity is an increase in body fat. In contrast, overweight is an increase in weight relative to some standard. Methods for determining body composition and the standards we use have improved over the past 25 years, greatly increasing the accuracy and ease of measuring body compartments in patients [8–11].

3.   ANTHROPOMETRIC MEASURES

3.1.   Height and Weight

Height and weight are best determined with a calibrated stadiometer and scales. It is best to standardize these procedures. In a research environment, these measures are made in a gown and without shoes according to a specific protocol. This approach can be adapted for the medical office, with attention to patient privacy, as is discussed later. In the office setting, it is only necessary to measure height once, but weight should be measured at each visit. These measures are used to determine BMI in kg/m^2. This index is in metric terms (weight in kilograms divided by the square of the height in meters), but it can also be calculated using pounds and inches if the appropriate correction factor is used. BMI = {weight (lbs)/[height (inches)]^2} × 703. Table 1 contains the BMI values for various heights and weights in lb/in and kg/m. In the office setting, BMI is determined from a chart like that in Table 1.

3.2.   Waist Circumference

The circumference of the waist is the second essential anthropometric measurement. There is no unified methodology for waist measurement. In a research setting, a tape measure device with a fixed tension is used to eliminate the effect of compression. One technique for positioning the tape measure is to mark a point midway between the highest point of the iliac crest and the lowest point of the costal margin in the mid-axillary line. The measure is then placed horizontally on this mark and the measure taken in a relaxed patient during expiration. In clinical practice, the most useful technique is to measure at the top of the iliac crest. In clinical practice, the value of the waist measurement is to identify persons with visceral adiposity. For BMI > 35 kg/m^2, the waist circumference is going to be increased and there is little to be gained by its

Table 1. Body mass index using either pounds and inches or kilograms and centimeters

													Body Mass Index (kg/m²)										
Inches	19	20	21	22	23	24	25	26	27	28	29	30	31	32	33	34	35	36	37	38	39	40	
58	*91*	*95*	*100*	*105*	*110*	*115*	*119*	*124*	*129*	*134*	*138*	*143*	*148*	*153*	*158*	*162*	*167*	*172*	*177*	*181*	*186*	*191*	Centimeters
	41	**43**	**45**	**48**	**50**	**52**	**54**	**56**	**58**	**61**	**63**	**65**	**67**	**69**	**71**	**73**	**76**	**78**	**80**	**82**	**84**	**86**	147
59	*94*	*99*	*104*	*109*	*114*	*119*	*124*	*128*	*133*	*138*	*143*	*148*	*153*	*158*	*163*	*168*	*173*	*178*	*183*	*188*	*193*	*198*	
	43	**45**	**47**	**50**	**52**	**54**	**56**	**59**	**61**	**63**	**65**	**68**	**70**	**72**	**74**	**77**	**79**	**81**	**83**	**86**	**88**	**90**	150
60	*97*	*102*	*107*	*112*	*118*	*123*	*128*	*133*	*138*	*143*	*148*	*153*	*158*	*164*	*169*	*174*	*179*	*184*	*189*	*194*	*199*	*204*	
	44	**46**	**49**	**51**	**53**	**55**	**58**	**60**	**62**	**65**	**67**	**69**	**72**	**74**	**76**	**79**	**81**	**83**	**85**	**88**	**90**	**92**	152
61	*100*	*106*	*111*	*116*	*121*	*127*	*132*	*137*	*143*	*148*	*153*	*158*	*164*	*169*	*174*	*180*	*185*	*190*	*195*	*201*	*206*	*211*	
	46	**48**	**50**	**53**	**55**	**58**	**60**	**62**	**65**	**67**	**70**	**72**	**74**	**77**	**79**	**82**	**84**	**86**	**89**	**91**	**94**	**96**	155
62	*104*	*109*	*115*	*120*	*125*	*131*	*136*	*142*	*147*	*153*	*158*	*164*	*169*	*175*	*180*	*186*	*191*	*196*	*202*	*207*	*213*	*218*	
	47	**50**	**52**	**55**	**57**	**60**	**62**	**65**	**67**	**70**	**72**	**75**	**77**	**80**	**82**	**85**	**87**	**90**	**92**	**95**	**97**	**100**	158
63	*107*	*113*	*118*	*124*	*130*	*135*	*141*	*146*	*152*	*158*	*163*	*169*	*175*	*180*	*186*	*192*	*197*	*203*	*208*	*214*	*220*	*225*	
	49	**51**	**54**	**56**	**59**	**61**	**64**	**67**	**69**	**72**	**74**	**77**	**79**	**82**	**84**	**87**	**90**	**92**	**95**	**97**	**100**	**102**	160
64	*110*	*116*	*122*	*128*	*134*	*140*	*145*	*151*	*157*	*163*	*169*	*174*	*180*	*186*	*192*	*198*	*203*	*209*	*215*	*221*	*227*	*233*	
	50	**52**	**55**	**58**	**60**	**63**	**66**	**68**	**71**	**73**	**76**	**79**	**81**	**84**	**87**	**89**	**92**	**94**	**97**	**100**	**102**	**105**	162
65	*114*	*120*	*126*	*132*	*138*	*144*	*150*	*156*	*162*	*168*	*174*	*180*	*186*	*192*	*198*	*204*	*210*	*216*	*222*	*228*	*234*	*240*	
	52	**54**	**57**	**60**	**63**	**65**	**68**	**71**	**74**	**76**	**79**	**82**	**84**	**87**	**90**	**93**	**95**	**98**	**101**	**103**	**106**	**109**	165
66	*117*	*124*	*130*	*136*	*142*	*148*	*155*	*161*	*167*	*173*	*179*	*185*	*192*	*198*	*204*	*210*	*216*	*223*	*229*	*235*	*241*	*247*	
	54	**56**	**59**	**62**	**65**	**68**	**71**	**73**	**76**	**79**	**82**	**85**	**87**	**90**	**93**	**96**	**99**	**102**	**104**	**107**	**110**	**113**	168
67	*121*	*127*	*134*	*140*	*147*	*153*	*159*	*166*	*172*	*178*	*185*	*191*	*198*	*204*	*210*	*217*	*223*	*229*	*236*	*242*	*248*	*255*	
	55	**58**	**61**	**64**	**66**	**69**	**72**	**75**	**78**	**81**	**84**	**87**	**90**	**92**	**95**	**98**	**101**	**104**	**107**	**110**	**113**	**116**	170
68	*125*	*131*	*138*	*144*	*151*	*158*	*164*	*171*	*177*	*184*	*190*	*197*	*203*	*210*	*217*	*223*	*230*	*236*	*243*	*249*	*256*	*263*	
	57	**60**	**63**	**66**	**69**	**72**	**75**	**78**	**81**	**84**	**87**	**90**	**93**	**96**	**99**	**102**	**105**	**108**	**111**	**114**	**117**	**120**	173
69	*128*	*135*	*142*	*149*	*155*	*162*	*169*	*176*	*182*	*189*	*196*	*203*	*209*	*216*	*223*	*230*	*237*	*243*	*250*	*257*	*264*	*270*	
	58	**61**	**64**	**67**	**70**	**74**	**77**	**80**	**83**	**86**	**89**	**92**	**95**	**98**	**101**	**104**	**107**	**110**	**113**	**116**	**119**	**123**	175
70	*132*	*139*	*146*	*153*	*160*	*167*	*174*	*181*	*188*	*195*	*202*	*209*	*216*	*223*	*230*	*236*	*243*	*250*	*257*	*264*	*271*	*278*	
	60	**63**	**67**	**70**	**73**	**76**	**79**	**82**	**86**	**89**	**92**	**95**	**98**	**101**	**105**	**108**	**111**	**114**	**117**	**120**	**124**	**127**	178
71	*136*	*143*	*150*	*157*	*165*	*172*	*179*	*186*	*193*	*200*	*207*	*215*	*222*	*229*	*236*	*243*	*250*	*258*	*265*	*272*	*279*	*286*	
	62	**65**	**68**	**71**	**75**	**78**	**81**	**84**	**87**	**91**	**94**	**97**	**100**	**104**	**107**	**110**	**113**	**117**	**120**	**123**	**126**	**130**	180
72	*140*	*147*	*155*	*162*	*169*	*177*	*184*	*191*	*199*	*206*	*213*	*221*	*228*	*235*	*243*	*250*	*258*	*265*	*272*	*280*	*287*	*294*	
	64	**67**	**70**	**74**	**77**	**80**	**84**	**87**	**90**	**94**	**97**	**100**	**104**	**107**	**111**	**114**	**117**	**121**	**124**	**127**	**131**	**134**	183
73	*144*	*151*	*159*	*166*	*174*	*182*	*189*	*197*	*204*	*212*	*219*	*227*	*234*	*242*	*250*	*257*	*265*	*272*	*280*	*287*	*295*	*303*	
	65	**68**	**72**	**75**	**79**	**82**	**86**	**89**	**92**	**96**	**99**	**103**	**106**	**110**	**113**	**116**	**120**	**123**	**127**	**130**	**133**	**137**	185
74	*148*	*155*	*163*	*171*	*179*	*187*	*194*	*202*	*210*	*218*	*225*	*233*	*241*	*249*	*256*	*264*	*272*	*280*	*288*	*295*	*303*	*311*	
	67	**71**	**74**	**78**	**81**	**85**	**88**	**92**	**95**	**99**	**102**	**106**	**110**	**113**	**117**	**120**	**124**	**127**	**131**	**134**	**138**	**141**	188
75	*152*	*160*	*168*	*176*	*184*	*192*	*200*	*208*	*216*	*224*	*232*	*240*	*247*	*255*	*263*	*271*	*279*	*287*	*295*	*303*	*311*	*319*	
	69	**72**	**76**	**79**	**83**	**87**	**90**	**94**	**97**	**101**	**105**	**108**	**112**	**116**	**119**	**123**	**126**	**130**	**134**	**137**	**141**	**144**	190
76	*156*	*164*	*172*	*180*	*189*	*197*	*205*	*213*	*221*	*230*	*238*	*246*	*254*	*262*	*271*	*279*	*287*	*295*	*303*	*312*	*320*	*328*	
	71	**74**	**78**	**82**	**86**	**89**	**93**	**97**	**101**	**104**	**108**	**112**	**115**	**119**	**123**	**127**	**130**	**134**	**138**	**142**	**145**	**149**	193
BMI	19	20	21	22	23	24	25	26	27	28	29	30	31	32	33	34	35	36	37	38	39	40	BMI

The Body Mass Index is shown as **Bold Underlined** numbers at the top and bottom
To determine your BMI, select your height in either inches or cm and move across
the row until you find your weight in pounds or inches. Your BMI can be read at the top or bottom.
The Italics are for pounds and inches ; **The bold is for kilograms and centimeters.**
Copyright 1999 George A. Bray

measurement. It is acceptable to omit waist measurement for class II obesity (BMI 35 to < 40) and class III obesity (BMI ≥ 40), in consideration of the sensitivity of the patient.

4.   INSTRUMENTAL METHODS FOR MEASURING BODY FAT

The number and precision of methods for measuring body composition have improved greatly over the past 25 years [9–12], but some of these methods are expensive, limiting their usefulness in clinical practice (Table 2).

Table 2. Methods for measuring body composition

	Cost	Ease of use	Can measure regional fat	External radiation
Anthropometric				
Height and weight	$	E	No	
Diameters	$	E	+	
Circumferences	$	E	+	
Skinfolds	$	M	+	
Instrumental				
Hydrodensitometry	$$	E[a]	No	
Air displacement (plethysmography)	$$$$	D[a]	No	
Dual x-ray absorptio-metry (DXA)	$$$	M[a]	+	Trace
Isotope dilution	$$	M[a]	No	
Impedance (BIA)	$$	E[a]	+	
Potassium counting	$$$$	D[a]	No	
Conductivity (TOBEC)	$$$	D[a]	±	
Computed tomography	$$$$	D[a]	++	Some
Magnetic resonance imaging	$$$$	D[a]	++	
Neutron activation	$$$$	D[a]	No	Larger
Ultrasound	$$	M[a]	+	

[a]Special equipment; E = easy; M = moderately difficult; D = difficult.

$ = inexpensive; $$ = more expensive; $$$ = expensive; $$$$ = very expensive.

+ = good; ++ = very good; ± = possibly.

4.1.   Dual X-ray Absorptiometry

Dual x-ray absorptiometry (DXA) instruments [9, 10] were developed to evaluate osteoporosis. DXA has replaced underwater weighing as the gold standard for determining body fat and lean body mass. In addition to accuracy, this method has the advantage of convenience and speed, as measurements can be done in about 10 minutes for individuals in a hospital gown.

4.2.   Density

By weighing an individual in air and under water it is possible to divide the body weight into fat and nonfat compartments, based on the fact that fat floats and the nonfat components sink [13]. Underwater weighing is a good method, but DXA is preferred, on the basis of both accuracy and convenience.

4.3. Isotope Dilution

Estimating body water by injecting a nonradioactive tracer of isotopic water (D_2O; $H_2{}^{18}O$; ^3H_2O) makes it possible to calculate body fat and thus partition body weight into lean body mass and body fat. This method, density, and DXA have comparable accuracy [15]; however, the method is expensive and time consuming.

4.4. Bioelectric Impedance

Measurement of the impedance of the body to an alternating current provides an easy and relatively inexpensive way to estimate body water [16]. However, most formulas for bioelectric impedance underestimate body fat in overweight patients [15], and, thus, bioelectric impedance analysis sacrifices accuracy to convenience.

5. IMAGING TECHNIQUES FOR BODY COMPOSITION

Regional body fat distribution can be reliably determined by either computed tomography (CT) or magnetic resonance imaging (MRI) [4, 5]. Because of their expense, these techniques should not be used for routine evaluation of visceral fat in the clinical setting. The waist circumference is the most useful clinical measure to assess visceral adiposity.

6. SUMMARY OF CLINICAL RECOMMENDATIONS FOR MEASUREMENT OF BODY COMPOSITION

Careful measurement of height, weight, and waist circumference are the essential measurements needed to begin evaluation of an overweight patient. If the clinician is concerned that lean body mass is increased, and thus the contribution of body fat to an elevated BMI being difficult to assess, DXA (also density or isotope dilution) may be considered to more accurately assess total body fat. Although impedance measurements are used in many clinical settings, they often underestimate fat.

7. BODY FAT THROUGH THE LIFE SPAN

Several factors modify the percentage of body fat, including gender, age, level of physical activity, and hormonal status [17]. The percentage of body fat steadily increases with age in both men and women, as illustrated in Figure 1. Women have a higher percentage of body fat than do men for a comparable

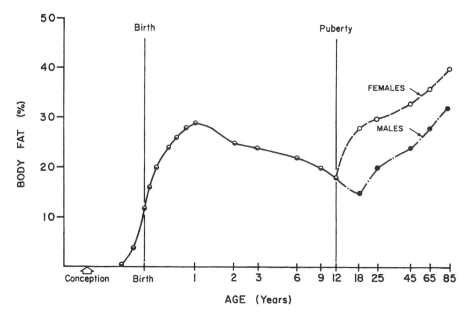

Figure 1. Changing body composition from gestation through adult life. There is a gradual increase in the proportion of body fat in adulthood. After puberty, females have greater proportion of body fat than do males. (From Friis-Hansen. In: Brozed J, ed, Human Body Composition. Oxford: Pergamon Press, 1965;191–209.)

height and weight at all ages after puberty. Visceral fat in women is lower during the reproductive years, but rises rapidly to nearly male levels in the postmenopausal years, when risk for cardiovascular and other diseases increase sharply. Indeed, when differences in body fat distribution are considered, almost all of the differences in excess mortality of men over women disappear, suggesting that the underlying factors leading to differences in fat distribution are significant in the risk of diabetes, heart disease, high blood pressure, and stroke in men.

8.   PREVALENCE OF OVERWEIGHT

BMI is a useful measure for comparing populations; it allows us to divide a population into groups, compare these groups across national boundaries, and examine time trends.

Using measurements of a representative sample of the US population, the percentage of overweight and obese Americans has been determined by NHANES (National Health and Nutrition Examination Survey), beginning in 1960 [18] (Figure 2). The percentage of obese men and women defined as a BMI $\geq$ 30 kg/m^2 increased slowly in each of the first three surveys, but there

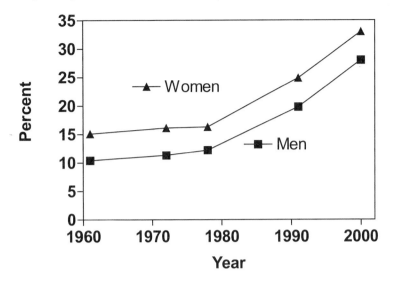

Figure 2. Prevalence of obesity (BMI $\geq$ 30 kg/m^2) in US adults as measured by NHANES surveys since 1963. There has been a dramatic increase in the prevalence of obesity, with doubling of rates in the last 25 years [18].

was a striking rise between 1980 and 1990. The increase in percentage of men with a BMI $\geq$ 30 kg/m^2 nearly doubled, and the percentage of women with a BMI $\geq$ 30 kg/m^2 rose by more than 50%. An even greater concern is the skewing of the population distribution. The problem is not just that the population distribution has shifted slightly to the right because of a small weight gain in the population. The problem is confounded by the rising prevalence of extreme obesity. The prevalence of class III obesity (BMI $\geq$ 40 kg/m^2) was 4.7% of the adult US population in the 1999–2000 NHANES survey, increased from 2.9% in the 1988–1994 survey [1]. Minorities are at particular risk. A larger percentage of Hispanics and African Americans are overweight and obese than whites. Of particular concern is the 15.1% prevalence of class III obesity among African-American females in the 1999–2000 NHANES survey, which compares to 4.9% for non-Hispanic whites [1]. Over all, females are more likely to be obese than men [1].

The prevalence of overweight in children is also rising, according to surveys conducted over the past 30 years [19] (Figure 3). For children, overweight is defined as BMI > 95th percentile for height. From 1963 to 1970, six to 11-year-olds had a prevalence of 4.3% and in 12- to 17-year-olds, it was 4.6%. From 1976 to 1980, according to the NHANES II survey, 7.5% of the six to 11-year-olds and the 12- to 17-year-olds were overweight. In the NHANES III survey from 1988 to 1991, the prevalence in the younger children rose to 13.5% and to 11.5% in the 12- to 17-year-olds [19].

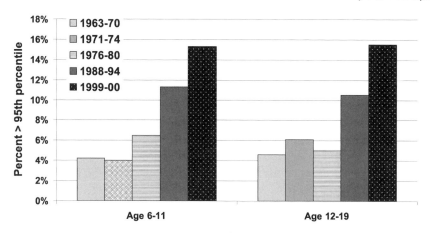

Figure 3. Prevalence of overweight in US children and adolescents as measured in NHANES surveys since 1963. There has been a dramatic increase, with tripling of rates for overweight in US children in the last 25 years [19].

9.   CLINICAL EVALUATION OF OVERWEIGHT PATIENTS

Evaluation of health risks from weight status is the first step in formulating a treatment plan. Thus, both clinical and laboratory information are needed to evaluate overweight patients. Several reports provide guidance for this evaluation (NHLBI [6, 20]; AOA [21]; WHO [22]).

9.1.   Body Mass Index

Overweight is usually assessed by measuring the BMI (see Table 1), and this step is the first in screening for obesity. BMI was originally proposed by Quetelet more than 150 years ago and correlates more closely with body fat content than do other anthropometric relationships of height and weight. Its advantages are ease of determination and the accuracy with which both height (stature) and weight can be measured. Its chief limitation is that, particularly in the normal BMI range (18.5 to 24.9 kg/m^2), the correlation with actual body fat content is sufficiently low that it is a poor guide to individual fat level. For BMI values above 25 kg/m^2 and especially above 30 kg/m^2, it is a much better guide to the degrees of excess fat and risk to health.

Table 3 lists BMI ranges and the relative risk associated with each as modified by taking waist circumference into account. This table is derived from the National Institutes of Health guidance on prevention and treatment of obesity [6, 20]. As is discussed later, health risk may also be elevated for any given BMI level, based on a history of comorbid condition, sedentary lifestyle, or of history of weight gain, among other factors.

Table 3. Classification of overweight and obesity by BMI, waist circumference and associated disease risk

| | BMI (kg/m²) | Obesity class | Disease risk[a] relative to normal weight and waist circumference | |
			Men ≤ 102 cm (≤ 40 in) Women ≤ 88 cm (≤ 35 in)	> 102 cm (> 40 in) > 88 cm (> 35 in)
Underweight	18.5		–	–
Normal[b]	18.5–24.9		–	–
Overweight	25.0–29.9		Increased	High
Obesity	30.0–34.9	I	High	Very high
	35.0–39.9	II	Very high	Very high
Extreme obesity	≥ 40	III	Extremely high	Extremely high

[a]Disease risk for type 2 diabetes, hypertension, and CVD.

[b]Increased waist circumference can also be a marker for increased risk even in persons of normal weight [6].

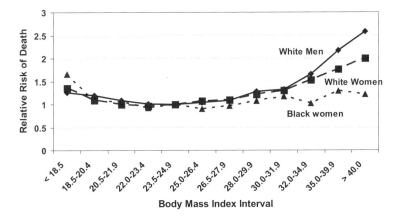

Figure 4. Relationship of BMI to risk for mortality in the US Physicians and Nurses Health Studies [23].

BMI shows a curvilinear relationship to risk for mortality [23], and although many longitudinal population studies demonstrate this, we choose to illustrate the relationship with data from the Nurses and Physicians Health Study cohorts (Figure 4). Several points can be made from these data. They illustrate the recently popular focus on the relatively small increase for mortality that is evident in this population in the overweight category, BMI $25 < 30$ kg/m². They take a very large study, and long periods of follow-up, to demonstrate the increased mortality risk for those in the overweight category, while the increased risk for obese among American whites is readily demonstrated as

BMI exceeds 30. Other measures besides BMI, such as waist circumference and other risk factors, can serve to identify those with high risk in the BMI 25 to < 30 category. The cut points to define overweight and obese are derived from data collected on Caucasians. It is now clear that different ethnic groups have different percentages of body fat for the same BMI. For a given BMI, Asians tend to have more fat and African Americans the same or less fat. For the black American women in Figure 4, the risk for mortality with elevations in BMI is less prominent than for whites.

9.2. Waist Circumference

Estimation of body fat distribution can aid in assessing health risk. This is particularly true for those with BMI < 35 kg/m^2, and we do not endorse the routine ascertainment of waist circumference for BMI $\geq$ 35 kg/m^2, because the waist circumference is almost certainly elevated. Visceral fat and central fatness can be evaluated by several methods, but for practical purposes, the waist circumference is recommended. In the clinic, waist circumference can be measured with a flexible tape placed horizontally at the level of the natural waistline or narrowest part of the torso as seen anteriorly [24]. Measuring the change in waist circumference is a good tool for following the progress of weight loss. It is particularly valuable when patients become more physically active. Physical activity may slow loss of muscle mass, and thus slow weight loss while fat continues to be mobilized. Waist circumference can help in making this distinction. As with BMI, the relationship of central fat to risk factors for health varies among populations as well as within them. Japanese Americans and Indians from South Asia have relatively more visceral fat, and are thus at higher risk for a given BMI or total body fat than are Caucasians. Even though the BMI may be below 25 kg/m^2, central fat may be increased and, thus, adjustment of BMI for central adiposity is important, particularly with BMI between 22 and 29 kg/m^2.

9.3. Weight Gain

Patients with a weight gain of more than 1 kg/year or more than 10 kg overall have an increased risk to health [25].

9.4. Sedentary Lifestyle

A sedentary lifestyle also increases the risk of early death. Individuals with no regular physical activity are at higher risk than individuals with modest levels of physical activity [26].

9.5. Laboratory and Other Measures

The relationship between obesity and increasing blood pressure is well known, and careful assessment of blood pressure should be part of the evaluation. Laboratory measurements should include, as a minimum, lipids (total cholesterol, low-density lipoprotein [LDL] cholesterol, high-density lipoprotein [HDL] cholesterol, and triglycerides), glucose, and uric acid. Sleep apnea and osteoarthritis should be assessed by a careful history.

10. THE METABOLIC SYNDROME

Identification of a constellation of risk factors that imposes higher risk for the development of type 2 diabetes and for cardiovascular disease is a key part of health risk appraisal in the office. In the United States, the National Cholesterol Education Program (NCEP) Adult Treatment Panel III has promoted a working diagnosis for metabolic syndrome that relies on the presence of three or more of the risk factors illustrated in Figure 5 [27]. The NCEP's goal in promoting recognition of metabolic syndrome was to encourage physicians to prescribe lifestyle approaches as a way to prevent cardiovascular disease. The NCEP's recommendation is that weight reduction, healthy diet, and physical activity be incorporated into the lifestyle of all individuals with the metabolic syndrome.

Recently, the International Diabetes Federation (IDF) has promoted another definition of metabolic syndrome [28] (Figure 6). The IDF definition relies on waist circumference as its central criteria and is easily applied in the clinical setting. The waist circumference cited by the IDF is lower than that used in the NCEP criteria, but the IDF states, "In the USA, the ATP III values (102 cm

Risk Factor	Defining Level
• **Abdominal Adiposity**	
(Waist Circumference)	
– **Men**	**>102 cm (> 40 in)**
– **Women**	**> 88 cm (> 35 in)**
• **HDL-Cholesterol**	
– **Men**	**< 40 mg/dL**
– **Women**	**< 50 mg/dL**
• **Triglycerides**	**≥150 mg/dL**
• **Blood Pressure**	**≥130/≥85 mm Hg**
• **Fasting Glucose**	**≥ 110-125 mg/dL**

Figure 5. Criteria for the metabolic syndrome, NCEO Adult Treatment Panel III, 2001, criteria. At least three of the conditions must be met for the diagnosis of metabolic syndrome under this classification [27].

Required Criterion:
•Central obesity (defined as waist circumference $\geq$94 cm for Europid men and $\geq$80 cm for Europid women, with ethnicity specific values for other groups)

Plus any two of the following four factors:
• raised TG level: $\geq$150 mg/dL, or specific treatment for this lipid abnormality
• reduced HDL cholesterol: <40 mg/dL in males and <50 mg/dL in females, or specific treatment for this lipid abnormality
• raised blood pressure: systolic BP $\geq$130 or diastolic BP $\geq$85 mm Hg, or treatment of previously diagnosed hypertension
• raised fasting plasma glucose (FPG) $\geq$100 mg/dL, or previously diagnosed type 2 diabetes

Figure 6. Criteria for the metabolic syndrome, IDF criteria, 2005. To meet the criteria for metabolic syndrome in this classification, the waist circumference must be elevated and two other conditions must be met [28].

male; 88 cm female) are likely to continue to be used for clinical purposes." It is the hope of the International Diabetes Federation that their consensus definition of the metabolic syndrome will be adopted world-wide. The waist circumference criteria are listed for Europid ethnic groups, but specific cutpoints are provided for other ethnicities.

11. ETIOLOGIC FACTORS UNDERLYING OBESITY

As part of the evaluation of overweight and obese patients in the clinical setting, etiologic factors causing obesity should be identified, if possible [29, 30].

- *Genetic diseases and genetic predisposition.* There are several extremely rare single-gene causes of obesity, but the usual genetic basis is to enhance susceptibility to environmental factors.
- *Hypothalamic obesity.* Hypothalamic obesity is rare in humans [31], but can be regularly produced in animals by injuring the ventromedial or paraventricular region of the hypothalamus or the amygdala. Hypothalamic obesity can follow surgical intervention in the hypothalamic-pituitary area or result from hypothalamic disease or trauma.
- *Cushing's syndrome.* Obesity is one of the cardinal features of Cushing's syndrome, and the differential diagnosis of obesity from Cushing's syndrome and pseudo-Cushing's syndrome is clinically important for therapeutic decisions [32, 33]. If Cushing's syndrome cannot be excluded, an endocrine consultation would be appropriate.

Table 4. Drugs that produce weight gain and alternatives to their use

Category	Drugs that cause weight gain	Possible alternatives
Neuroleptics	Thioridazine; olanzaepine; quetiapine; riesperidone; clozapine	Molindone; haloperidol; ziprasiodone
Antidepressants		
Tricyclics	Amitriptyline; nortriptyline	Protriptyline; bupropion;
Monoamine oxidase inhibitors	Imipramine mitrazapine	nefazoadone
Selective serotonin reuptake inhibitors	Paroxetine	
Anticonvulsants	Valproate; carbamazepine; gabapentin	Fluoxetine, sertraline; topiramate; lamotrigine; zonisamide
Antidiabetic drugs	Insulin; sulfonylureas; thiazolidinediones	Acarbose; miglitol; metformin; exenatide; pramlintide; orlistat; sibutramine
Antiserotonin	Pizotifen	
Antihistamines	Cyproheptidine	Inhalers; decongestants
-Adrenergic blockers	Propranolol	ACE inhibitors; calcium
-Adrenergic blockers	Terazosin	channel blockers
Steroid hormones	Contraceptives; gluco-corticoids; proges-tational steroids	Barrier methods; non-steroidal antiinflam-matory agents

- *Hypothyroidism.* Women with hypothyroidism frequently gain weight because of a generalized slowing of metabolic rate. Some of this gain is fat. However, the weight gain is usually modest, and marked obesity is uncommon. In the United States, hypothyroidism is common, particularly in older women, where measurement of thyroid-stimulating hormone (TSH) is a valuable diagnostic test.
- *Polycystic ovary syndrome.* More than 50% of women with PCOS are obese [34]. The cardinal features of this syndrome are oligomenorrhea with infertility, hirsutism, and polycystic ovaries.
- *Drug-induced weight gain.* Several drugs can cause weight gain, including a variety of psychoactive agents [35] and hormones (Table 4). The degree of weight gain can be severe with some high-dose corticosteroids, psychoactive drugs, or with valproate.
- *Cessation of smoking.* Weight gain is very common when individuals stop smoking and is at least partly mediated by nicotine withdrawal. Weight gain

of 1 to 2 kg in the first few weeks is often followed by an additional 2- to 3-kg weight gain over the next 4 to 6 months. Average weight gain is 4 to 5 kg, but can be much greater.

- *Sedentary lifestyle*. A sedentary lifestyle lowers energy expenditure and promotes weight gain in both animals and humans.
- *Dietary factors*. The amount of energy intake relative to energy expenditure is the central reason for the development of obesity. However, diet composition may also be important in the pathogenesis. Dietary factors become important in a variety of settings.

  (a) *Breast feeding*. Failure to breast feed or breast feeding for less than 3 months is associated with increased risk of weight gain when children enter school [36].
  (b) *Maternal smoking*. Offspring of children whose mother smoked during pregnancy have a significantly increased risk of overweight later in life [37].
  (c) *Overeating*. Voluntary overeating (repeated ingestion of energy exceeding daily energy needs) can increase body weight in normal-weight men and women. When these subjects stop overeating, they invariably lose most or all of the excess weight. The use of overeating protocols to study the consequences of food ingestion has shown the importance of genetic factors in the pattern of weight gain [38]. Progressive hyperphagic obesity is one clinical form of overeating where individuals gain 5 kg/year or more year after year [31]. Japanese sumo wrestlers who eat large quantities of food twice a day for many years are another obvious example.
  (d) *Dietary fat intake*. Epidemiologic data suggest that a high-fat diet is associated with obesity. The relative weight in several populations, for example, is directly related to the percentage of dietary fat in the diet [39]. A high-fat diet introduces palatable, often high-fat foods into the diet, with a corresponding increase in energy density (i.e., lesser weight of food for the same number of calories). This makes overconsumption more likely. Increased portion sizes are another component of environmental food presentation that contributes to obesity.
  (e) *Dietary carbohydrate and fiber*. Dietary fiber is inversely related to body weight in population studies [40]. The consumption of sugar-sweetened beverages in children may enhance the risk of more rapid weight gain. Both the baseline consumption and the change in consumption over two years were positively related to the increase in BMI over two years [41].
  (f) *Dietary calcium*. A negative relationship between body mass index and dietary calcium intake has been noted in several studies [42].

12.   INTRODUCTION TO TREATMENT: RISK–BENEFIT ASSESSMENT

Once the workup for etiologic and complicating factors is complete, health risk can be refined beyond the BMI assessment, according to the algorithm shown in Figure 7 [12, 21–23], which is only one of many. Because health risk determines the treatment choices, it is important to individualize assessments based on more than just BMI.

Individuals with a BMI below 25 kg/m^2 are at very low health risk, but nonetheless, nearly half of those in this category at ages 20 to 25 will become overweight by age 60 to 69. Thus, a large group of pre-overweight individuals need preventive strategies. Risk rises with a BMI above 25 kg/m^2 (Figure 6). The presence of complicating factors further increases this risk. Thus, an attempt at a quantitative estimate of these complicating factors is important.

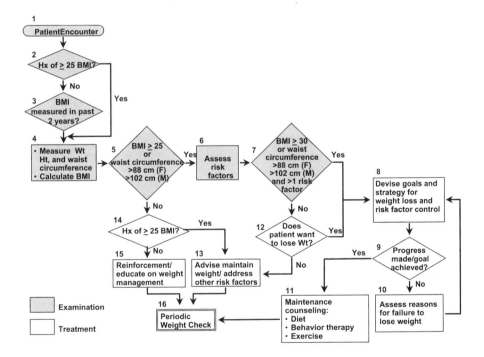

Figure 7. Treatment algorithm for evaluation of overweight and obesity [20].

13.   CONCLUSION

Determining body mass index and waist circumference are the first steps in evaluating the risk to an individual patient. This can be complemented by more sophisticated methods and supplemented with laboratory data. If no specific etiologies are identified as contributory, and which could be ameliorated, then treatment can be designed, taking into considerations the patients needs and the realities of obesity. It is the role of the physician to evaluate individual patients and to estimate their health risk from obesity and aberrant fat deposition. As treatment approaches become more sophisticated and more effective, a proactive approach to risk assessment is an imperative.

REFERENCES

[1] Flegal KM, Carroll MD, Ogden CL, et al. Prevalence and trends in obesity among US adults, 1999–2000. JAMA 2002;288:1723–1727.

[2] Bray GA. Obesity—a time bomb to be defused. Lancet. 1998;352:160–161.

[3] Manson JE, Willett WC, Stampfer MJ, et al. Body weight and mortality among women. N Engl J Med 1995;333:677–685.

[4] Garrison RJ, Castelli WP. Weight and 30-year mortality of men in the Framingham Study. Ann Intern Med 1985;103:1006–1009.

[5] Calle EE, Rodriguez C, Walker-Thurmond K, et al. Overweight, obesity, and mortality from cancer in a prospectively studied cohort of US adults. N Engl J Med 2003;348:1625–1638.

[6] NHLBI Obesity Education Initiative Expert Panel on the Identification, Evaluation, and Treatment of Overweight and Obesity in Adults. Clinical guidelines on the identification, evaluation, and treatment of overweight and obesity in adults—the evidence report. Obes Res 1998;6:51S–63S.

[7] Gallagher D, Visser M, Sepulveda D, et al. How useful is body mass index for comparison of body fitness across age, sex and ethnic groups? Am J Epidemiol 1996;143:228–239.

[8] Bioelectrical Impedance Analysis in Body Composition Measurement. Proceedings of a National Institutes of Health Technology Assessment Conference. Bethesda, MD, December 12–14, 1994. Am J Clin Nutr 1996;64:387S–532S.

[9] Heymsfield SB, Allison DB, Wang ZM. Evaluation of total and regional body composition. In: Bray GA, Bouchard C, James WP, eds. Handbook of Obesity. New York: Marcel Dekker, 1997;41–77.

[10] Lohman TG. Advances in Body Composition Assessment. Champaign, IL: Human Kinetics, 1992.

[11] Seidell JC, Rissanen AM. Time trends in worldwide prevalence of obesity. In: Bray GA, Bouchard C, James WP, eds. Handbook of Obesity. New York: Marcel Dekker, 1997;79–91.

[12] Sjostrom L, Kvist H, Cederblad A, et al. Determination of total adipose tissue and body fat in women by computed tomography, ^{40}K, and tritium. Am J Physiol 1986;250:E736–E745.

[13] Heymsfield SB, Wang ZM. Measurement of total-body fat by underwater weighing: New insights and uses for old method. Nutrition 1993;9(5):472–473.

[14] Westerterp KR. Body composition, water turnover and energy turnover assessment with labelled water. Proc Nutr Soc 1999;58(4):945–951.

[15] Bray GA. Predicting obesity in adults from childhood and adolescent weight. Am J Clin Nutr 2002;76:497–498.

[16] Foster KR, Lukaski HC. Whole-body impedance—what does it measure? Am J Clin Nutr 1996:(Suppl 3):388S–396S.

[17] Kotani KK, Tokunaga K, Fujioka S, et al. Sexual dimorphism of age-related changes in whole-body fat distribution in the obese. Int J Obes Relat Metab Disord 1994;18:207–212.

[18] Flegal KM, Carroll MD, Kuczmarski RJ, et al. Overweight and obesity in the United States: Prevalence and trends. Int J Obes 1998;22:39–47.

[19] Troiano RP, Flegal KM. Overweight children and adolescents: Description, epidemiology, and demographics. Pediatrics 1998;101:497–504.

[20] The Practical Guide: Identification, Evaluation and Treatment of Overweight and Obesity in Adults vs Department of Health and Human Services, Public Health Service, National Institutes of Health, National Heart, Lung and Blood Institute: NIH Publication No. 00-4084, October 2000.

[21] American Obesity Association and Shape Up America! Guidance for Treatment of Adult Obesity. Available at: http://www.shapeup.org/sua/bmi/guidance/.

[22] World Health Organization. Obesity: Preventing and Managing the Global Epidemic. Geneva: World Health Organization, 1999.

[23] Calle EE, Thun MJ, Petrelli JM, et al. Body mass index and mortality in a prospective cohort of U.S. adults. N Engl J Med 1999;341(15):1097–1105.

[24] Roche A, Heymsfield SB, Lohman T. Human Body Composition. Champaign, IL: Human Kinetics, 1996.

[25] Manson JE, Willett WC, Stampfer MJ, et al. Body weight and mortality among women. N Engl J Med 1995;333:677–685.

[26] Blair SN, Khol HW, Poffenburger RS, et al. Physical fitness and all-cause mortality: A prospective study of healthy men and women. JAMA 1989;262:2392–2401.

[27] Expert Panel on Detection, Evaluation and Treatment of High Blood Cholesterol in Adults. Executive Summary of the Third Report of the National Cholesterol Education Program (NCEP) Expert Panel on the Detection, Evaluation and Treatment of High Blood Cholesterol in Adults (Adult Treatment Panel III). JAMA 2001;285:2486–2497.

[28] http://www.idf.org/webdata/docs/IPF_Metasyndrome_definition.pdf

[29] Bray GA. Definition, measurement and classification of the syndromes of obesity. Int J Obes 1978;2:99–112.

[30] Bray GA, Gray DS. Obesity. Part II—Treatment. West J Med 1988;149:555–571.

[31] Bray GA. Contemporary Diagnosis and Management of Obesity and the Metabolic Syndrome. Newtown, PA: Handbooks in Healthcare, 2002.

[32] Orth DN. Cushing's syndrome. N Engl J Med 1995;332(12):791–803.

[33] Wajchenberg BL, Bosco A, Marone MM, et al. Estimation of body fat and lean tissue distribution by dual energy X-ray absorptiometry and abdominal body fat evaluation by computed tomography in Cushing's disease. J Clin Endocrinol Metab 1995;80(9):2791–2794.

[34] Kiddy DS, Sharp PS, White DM, et al. Differences in clinical and endocrine features between obese and non-obese subjects with polycystic ovary syndrome: An analysis of 263 consecutive cases. Clin Endocrinol (Oxf) 1990;332:213–220.

[35] Allison DB, Mentore JL, Heo M, et al. Antipsychotic-induced weight gain: A comprehensive research synthesis. Am J Psychiatry 1999;156:1686–1696.

[36] Von Kries R, Koletzko B, Sauerwald T, et al. Breast feeding and obesity: Cross sectional study. BMJ 1999;319(7203):147–150.

[37] Toschke AM, Montgomery SM, Pfeiffer U, et al. Early intrauterine exposure to tobacco-inhaled products and obesity. Am J Epidemiol 2003;158(11):1068–1074.

[38] Rankinen T, Perusse L, Weisnagel SJ, et al. The human obesity gene map: The 2001 update. Obes Res 2002;10:196–243.

[39] Bray GA, Popkin BM. Dietary fat intake does affect obesity! Am J Clin Nutr 1998;68:1157–1173.

[40] Kromhout D, Bloemberg B, Seidell JC, et al. Physical activity and dietary fiber determine population body fat levels: The Seven Countries Study. Int J Obes Relat Metab Disord 2001;25(3):301–306.

[41] Ludwig DS, Peterson KE, Gortmaker SL. Relation between consumption of sugar-sweetened drinks and childhood obesity: A prospective, observational analysis. Lancet 2001;357:505–508.

[42] Zemel MB, Shi H, Greer B, et al. Regulation of adiposity by dietary calcium. FASEB J 2000;14(9):1132–1138.

Chapter 11

Dietary Approaches to Obesity and the Metabolic Syndrome

Angela P. Makris and Gary D. Foster

Temple University, School of Medicine, Philadelphia, PA 19140, USA

1. INTRODUCTION

According to the National Health and Nutrition Examination Survey (NHANES), rates of the metabolic syndrome (MetS) have risen in conjunction with increasing rates of obesity, affecting approximately 27% of adults in the United States [1, 2]. Certain dietary patterns have been associated with MetS, particularly, those high in fat (i.e., 37.9% of total energy) and sugar and low in vegetables and fiber [3].

Weight management through dietary modification (i.e., reducing saturated fat and cholesterol and increasing fiber intake) has been identified by the National Cholesterol Education Program's Adult Treatment Panel III (NCEP ATP-III) as an important strategy to prevent and reverse MetS and decrease the risk of associated adverse health conditions such as cardiovascular disease and diabetes [1]. Currently, the best dietary approach to weight loss is a matter of debate among professionals and the public alike. Likewise, the optimal dietary intervention for MetS has not been identified. However, strategies that improve any one of the metabolic disturbances associated with MetS (i.e., abdominal obesity, dyslipidemia, hypertension, and insulin resistance) may be effective in treating the condition.

During the last 20 years, the focus has been on decreasing fat intake [4, 5]. This recommendation is guided by the high energy density of dietary fat and the link between increased risk of chronic disease and saturated fat [6–8]. Although low-calorie, low-fat approaches are effective in reducing weight, improving blood pressure, decreasing cardiovascular risk, and improving insulin sensitivity in the short term, they have not proven to be sustainable for many living in an environment in which palatable, inexpensive, and high-fat foods are easily accessible [9]. Recently, researchers have begun to explore other means of reducing energy intake (e.g., manipulating the amount and/or type of carbohydrate and protein in the diet) and have evaluated the effects of these diets on weight and various metabolic parameters.

This chapter reviews dietary approaches to the treatment of obesity and the conditions associated with MetS, with an emphasis on the relative roles of fat, carbohydrate, and protein. Each section begins with a description of various diets (i.e., low-, very low-, and moderate-fat diets, low-carbohydrate diets, low glycemic index diets, or high-protein diets) and concludes with a review of their efficacy for the treatment of obesity, dyslipidemia, insulin resistance, and/or hypertension.

2.   LOW-FAT DIETS

The *Dietary Guidelines for Americans 2005* (associated with MyPyramid) provides one example of a low-fat eating plan [10]. The guidelines are based on the premise that a low-fat (20% to 35%), high-carbohydrate (45% to 65%) diet results in optimal health [10]. By consuming a variety of foods and the recommended number of servings from each food group, individuals will meet their protein requirements, as well as their RDA for vitamins and minerals, and consume adequate amounts of fiber. In addition, healthy limits on total fat, saturated fat, cholesterol, and sodium are encouraged. Other examples of a low-fat diet are the DASH diet and those recommended by the American Diabetes Association [11], American Heart Association [12], and American Cancer Society [13], as well as commercial programs such as Weight Watchers.

2.1.   Efficacy of Low-fat Diets on Weight Loss, Hypertension, and Diabetes

Low-fat diets are the best studied of all approaches to weight loss. Three large, multicenter, randomized studies (i.e., the PREMIER trial, Diabetes Prevention Program, and the Finnish Diabetes Prevention study) have demonstrated that low-fat, low calorie diets in combination with intensive group therapy, individual counseling, and 150 to 180 minutes of moderate intensity physical activity per week are effective in reducing body weight by approximately 5% to 10% of initial weight during the first 6 months of treatment [14–17]. Improvements in blood pressure and cardiovascular complications, as well as reductions in the incidence of type 2 diabetes, have been observed. Findings from these studies are summarized in Table 1.

The PREMIER trial investigated the effects of the DASH diet (i.e., Dietary Approaches to Stop Hypertension), a diet high in fruits and vegetables, fiber and mineral content (such as calcium, magnesium, and potassium) and low in total and saturated fat and cholesterol and refined sugar. This diet was combined with recommendations known to individually lower blood pressure (i.e., sodium and alcohol restriction, exercise, and weight loss) and evaluated for reduction in weight loss and hypertension [14]. Eight hundred and ten obese,

Table 1. Summary of findings from low- and moderate-fat studies

	Premier (6-month data)	DPP (6-month data)	Finnish Prevention (12-month data)	McManus (18-month data)
Sample size (*n*)	810	3234	522	101
Control	273	1082	257	51
Intervention 1	268	1079	265	50
Intervention 2	269	1073	N/A	N/A
Sex				
Male	310	1,043	172	10
Female	500	2,191	350	91
Age (years)				
Control	49.5	50.3	55	44
Intervention 1	50.2	50.9	55	44
Intervention 2	50.2	50.6	N/A	N/A
Baseline BMI (kg/m^2)				
Control	32.9	34.2	31.0	33
Intervention 1	33.0	33.9	31.3	34
Intervention 2	33.3	33.9	N/A	N/A
Weight loss (kg)				
Control	−1.1	−0.1	−0.8	2.9
Intervention 1	−4.9	−5.6	−4.2	−4.1
Intervention 2	−5.8	−2.1	N/A	N/A

Premier: Intervention 1 = established intervention; Intervention 2 = established intervention plus DASH; Control = advice only.

DPP: Intervention 1 = intensive lifestyle group; Intervention 2 = metformin; Control = placebo.

Finnish PP: Intervention 1 = detailed diet and exercise instruction in 7 sessions during year 1; Control = diet and exercise information at baseline and annual visit.

McManus: Intervention 1 = moderate-fat; Control = low-fat.

nonhypertensive, and hypertensive participants were randomly assigned to either a control group (single advice-giving session for consuming a DASH diet) or one of two intervention groups. One intervention group instructed participants to reduce calories through the DASH diet (Established Intervention plus DASH) and exercise. The other encouraged calorie restriction and exercise (Established Intervention) alone. Both intervention groups included behavior modification instruction.

There were significant differences in dietary intake, weight loss, and blood pressure between the control and intervention groups at 6 months. The Established Intervention plus DASH group consumed more fruits and vegetables and dairy products than the other two groups. Significantly greater weight losses were observed in the Established Intervention and the Established Intervention plus DASH groups compared to the control group at 6 months (see Table 1). There were no significant differences in weight loss between the Established

Intervention and Established Intervention plus DASH groups. Although blood pressure decreased in all three groups at 6 months, the greatest reduction was observed in the Established Intervention plus DASH group. Seventy-seven percent of stage 1 hypertensive participants in the Established Intervention plus DASH group and 66% stage 1 hypertensive participants in the Established group had systolic and diastolic blood pressure less than 140 mm Hg and 90 mm Hg, respectively, at 6 months [18]. Even greater decreases in blood pressure have been observed in previous DASH studies [19, 20], in which fruits and vegetables were provided and intake of these foods was higher (7.8 servings in Premier study vs. 9.6 servings in DASH study).

The Diabetes Prevention Program was a 27-center randomized clinical trial that evaluated the effects of lifestyle intervention and pharmacotherapy on the incidence of type 2 diabetes in individuals with impaired glucose tolerance [15]. In this study 3,234 overweight participants were randomly assigned to one of three groups: (1) placebo plus standard lifestyle recommendations, (2) metformin plus standard lifestyle recommendations, and (3) intensive lifestyle intervention. Participants in the medication and placebo group were provided written information on the Food Guide Pyramid and the National Cholesterol Education Program Step 1 diet and were seen annually in individual sessions. Participants in the lifestyle intervention group were prescribed fat and calorie goals and were asked to monitor their intake daily. Calorie levels were based on initial body weight and were designed to produce a weight loss of 0.5 to 1.0 kg/week.

Participants in the intensive lifestyle group lost significantly more weight than those in the metformin and placebo groups (see Table 1). The intensive lifestyle group also had a significantly lower incidence of type 2 diabetes than the placebo or metformin groups at one year (see Table 1). Compared to the placebo group, the incidence of diabetes was reduced by 58% and 31% in the intensive lifestyle and metformin groups, respectively [15].

Similar to the Diabetes Prevention Program, the Finnish Diabetes Prevention study investigated the ability of lifestyle intervention to prevent or delay the onset of type 2 diabetes in 522 overweight participants with impaired glucose tolerance [16]. Participants were randomly assigned to either a control group, which received verbal and written diet and exercise information at baseline and at annual visits, or to an intervention group, which was provided detailed dietary and exercise instructions in seven sessions with a nutritionist during the first year and every 3 months after the first year. These latter participants were instructed to consume less than 30% of energy from fat (i.e., consuming low-fat dairy and meat products), less than 10% from saturated fat (i.e., increase consumption of vegetable oils rich in monounsaturated fat), 15 g/1000 kcal of fiber from whole grain products, vegetables, and berries and other fruits. They were also told to engage in moderate activity for 30 minutes or more per day.

Results showed that there was a significantly greater reduction in the incidence of type 2 diabetes and greater weight loss in the intervention group. Greater reductions in mean body weight were observed in the intervention group compared to the control group in the first year and remained significantly greater in the intervention group than after 2 years (see Table 1).

Taken together these findings suggest that consumption of a low-fat, low-calorie diet, in the context of intensive group and/or individual counseling emphasizing moderate intensity physical activity, is an effective strategy for weight management, hypertension, and diabetes. A major limitation of these studies is that the control and intervention groups did not receive the same number of treatment visits. Participant–clinician contact and instruction was greater in the intervention groups. It can also be argued that these studies do not simulate treatment in the "real" world because of their high intensity and frequency. While not effectiveness studies, these well-designed efficacy studies show that low-calorie, low-fat, high-fiber diets have positive effects on weight control and, more importantly, on the comorbid conditions associated with MetS.

3.   VERY-LOW-FAT DIETS

Some argue that a reduction in fat greater than 20% to 35% of calories is necessary for optimal health [21]. Diets that provide < 10% fat are defined as very-low-fat [22]. Pritikin and Ornish diets are examples of very-low-fat diets. The Ornish diet is a plant-based diet and therefore encourages consumption of high-complex-carbohydrate, high- fiber foods (e.g., fruits, vegetables, whole grains); beans; soy; and moderate amounts of reduced fat dairy, eggs, and limited amounts of sugar and white flour [22]. The Pritikin diet is similar. However, limited quantities of lean meats and fish are also allowed. The major difference between low- and very-low-fat diets is that the latter are more restrictive in terms of the types of foods permitted. Unlike low-fat plans that incorporate all foods, the very-low-fat diets strongly discourage consumption of foods containing high amounts of refined carbohydrate and/or fat such as sugar, high-fructose corn syrup, white flour, and rice.

3.1.   Efficacy of Very-low-fat Diets on Weight Loss and Cardiovascular Disease

Few randomized studies have evaluated the effects of very-low-fat diets on weight loss and none have systematically examined the efficacy of these diets on the conditions associated with MetS; however, the Lifestyle Heart Trial was a long-term randomized trial on 48 patients with coronary atherosclerosis that evaluated the effects of a very-low-fat diet and intensive lifestyle modification on the progression of this disease [23]. Twenty participants were randomly assigned to an intervention group and 28 to a control group. The intervention group consumed a very-low-fat vegetarian diet and was prescribed a behavior modification program that included moderate aerobic activity, stress management, and smoking cessation. Those in the control group followed recommendations consistent with conventional guidelines for a healthy lifestyle (provided by their primary care physician).

Participants in the intervention group reduced their fat intake from 29.7% to 6.22% at 1 year. The decrease in the control group (e.g., from 30.5% to 28.8%) was less dramatic. Participants in the intervention and control groups lost 10.8 kg and 1.5 kg respectively, at 1 year. Furthermore, there were significant differences in coronary artery outcomes. The average coronary artery percent diameter stenosis in the intervention group decreased (i.e., 1.75 absolute percentage points) at 1 year, while it increased (i.e., 2.3 absolute percentage points) in the control group. These data suggest that a very-low-fat diet, in combination with lifestyle change, can result in regression of coronary atherosclerosis. However, when part of a multicomponent lifestyle intervention program (i.e., diet, exercise, stress management, smoking cessation), it is hard to separate the impact of dietary treatment from other factors. Further, adherence to these dietary and lifestyle recommendations outside of clinical trials is unknown.

4.   MODERATE-FAT DIETS

While many argue that intake of 35% fat or less is the most favorable approach for treating obesity and preventing chronic disease, others note that many European countries with relatively high percentages of fat intake (e.g., France, Italy) have a low prevalence of obesity [24] and lower rates of cardiovascular disease [25, 26] and mortality [27–29]. Moreover, there is some evidence to suggest that individuals who follow a diet higher in fat may be better able to sustain weight losses over the long term compared to those who adhere to a diet lower in fat [30].

Mediterranean diets are considered moderate fat diets because they may contain over 40% of total calories from fat [31, 32]. Mediterranean diets differ depending upon the region of the Mediterranean from which they originate. The percentage of fat can range from 26% to 42% of total calories from fat. Despite differences in the total percentage of fat, Mediterranean diets generally contain a higher proportion of monounsaturated fat and omega 3 fatty acids than western diets. A traditional Mediterranean diet is rich in natural whole foods and relies heavily on foods from plant sources such as fruits, vegetables (including wild types such as purslane), legumes, breads and grains, and nuts and seeds. These plant foods along with olive oil and low to moderate amounts of cheese, yogurt, and wine are consumed daily [33]. Rather than red meat, fish, chicken, and eggs are consumed on a weekly basis. The diet is low in saturated and trans-fats because of limited intakes of butter, red meat and processed foods. Fresh or dried fruit with nuts (e.g., figs stuffed with walnuts) is viewed as a typical daily dessert rather than commercially baked foods.

4.1. Efficacy of Moderate-fat Diets on Weight Loss, Cardiovascular Disease, and Diabetes

McManus et al. examined the effects of a moderate-fat diet (35% of total energy) and a lower-fat control diet (e.g., 20% of total energy) in 101 overweight men and women [30]. Women were instructed to consume 1200 kcal per day while men were asked to consume 1500 kcal per day in both groups. All subjects participated in weekly behavior modification sessions. There were no differences between the moderate-fat and low-fat groups in weight loss at 6 and 12 months. However, at 18 months they were significantly different because participants in the moderate-fat group maintained their weight loss while the low-fat group regained weight (see Table 1). Further, there were greater reductions in percent body fat and waist circumference in the moderate-fat group.

Although some studies evaluating diets with characteristics similar to the Mediterranean diet (i.e., moderate-fat diets or diets rich in fiber and grains) have reported beneficial effects on weight [30, 34, 35], few studies have directly investigated the effects of Mediterranean diets on weight management [36, 37]. Schroder et al. reported that adherence to a traditional Mediterranean diet (i.e., greater intake of olive oil, fruits, vegetables, legumes, nuts and seeds, fish, and poultry and a lower percentage of saturated fat) is associated with a lower prevalence of obesity [36]. Similarly, Goulet et al. showed that women who adapt a Mediterranean pattern of eating consume fewer calories and have modest reductions in body weight and waist circumference after 12 weeks [37]. Effects varied as a function of baseline waist circumference and age in this study. Reductions in waist circumference, low-density lipoprotein (LDL)-cholesterol and apo-B concentrations were more pronounced in women with the highest baseline waist circumferences. Unlike younger women who had significant reductions in both weight and waist circumference, significant reductions in waist circumference were observed only in older women. Older women also had more pronounced reductions in LDL-cholesterol.

A number of studies have examined the effects of Mediterranean diets on chronic disease; however, diets in these studies are relatively low in fat (i.e., approximately 30% energy from fat). The Lyon Diet Heart Study was a randomized trial comparing the effects of a Mediterranean-type diet (i.e., consumption of more root and green vegetables, fruit, fish, wine in moderation, margarine with a fatty acid profile similar to olive oil instead of butter, and less red meat) and a prudent diet (i.e., basic dietary advice from the hospital dietitian or attending physician) on the prevention of coronary events in 605 overweight patients surviving a first myocardial infarction [38–40]. Compared to those consuming the control (prudent) diet, participants consuming a Mediterranean-type diet consumed fewer total calories from fat (30% vs. 34%), less saturated fat (8% vs. 12%) and cholesterol (203 mg/day vs. 312 mg/day), more monounsaturated fat (13% vs. 11%), and more fiber (19 g/day vs. 16 g/day). After 46 months on a Mediterranean-type diet, participants decreased their risk for cardiac death, nonfatal heart attacks, unstable angina, heart failure, and pulmonary or peripheral embolism by 50% to 70%.

Proinflammatory cytokines such as interleukin-6 (IL-6) and interleukin-18 (IL-18) have been associated with thrombotic cardiovascular events and endothelial dysfunction. In addition, it is thought that increased production of IL-6 and low adiponectin may be associated with insulin resistance; therefore, beneficial changes in proinflammatory cytokine concentration may reduce risk for the development of cardiovascular disease and type 2 diabetes. Esposito et al. used a Mediterranean-type diet to examine the effect of weight loss on markers of vascular inflammation, blood pressure, and insulin sensitivity (via homeostasis model assessment [HOMA]) in 120 obese women without diabetes, hypertension, or hyperlipidemia [41]. Participants randomized to the Mediterranean-type diet group met with a dietitian monthly and received instruction for following a hypocaloric (i.e., 1300 kcal/day at year 1, 1500 kcal/day at year 2) Mediterranean-type diet (i.e., high in fruits, vegetables, grains, less saturated fat and more monounsaturated fat) while participants in the control group were given general information about healthy eating and exercise over a 2-year period. Although decreases in blood pressure, glucose, insulin, triglycerides, cytokines, and weight were observed in both groups after 2 years, greater decreases were observed in participants consuming a Mediterranean-type diet. Participants in the Mediterranean-type diet group lost 14 kg compared to 3 kg in the control group. Adiponectin levels were greater and HOMA scores were lower in the intervention group compared to the control group. Findings from this study suggest that weight loss can reduce risk for cardiovascular disease and type 2 diabetes by decreasing markers of vascular inflammation and improving insulin sensitivity.

In a similar study, Esposito et al. [42] examined the effects of a Mediterranean-type diet on markers of vascular inflammation and endothelial function in 180 overweight patients with metabolic syndrome. Individuals ($n = 90$) randomized to the Mediterranean-type diet were instructed to follow an American Heart Association Step 1 diet, eat specific amounts of fruit, vegetables, walnuts, and whole grains, and increase their intake of olive oil. Participants randomized to the control group were given general information about following a low-fat, high-carbohydrate diet. Group meetings, led by a dietitian, were held monthly for the first year and bi-monthly for the second year. In general, participants in the Mediterranean-type diet group consumed more complex carbohydrates, fiber, and monounsaturated fat and less saturated fat than the control group. Those in the Mediterranean-type diet group lost significantly more weight than the control group, 4.0 versus 1.2 kg, respectively, at the end of 2 years. In addition, decreases in HOMA scores, blood pressure, total cholesterol, triglycerides, and serum concentrations of IL-6, IL-7, IL-18, and C-reactive protein were greater in participants following a Mediterranean-type diet. While no change in endothelial function was observed in the control group, scores improved in the Mediterranean-type diet group. Results were adjusted for changes in body weight. After 2 years, a greater number of participants were still classified as having MetS in the control group compared to the Mediterranean-type diet group (i.e., 78 participants vs. 40 participants). Taken together, these findings suggest that adherence to a hypocaloric, 30% fat Mediterranean diet can result in beneficial changes in body composition and improvements in vascular parameters, blood pressure, and insulin sensitivity.

In summary, many studies have assessed the effects of fat intake on weight loss and disease risk. Compared to very-low-fat and moderate-fat diets, low-fat diets are the best studied. These diets have been shown to be effective in treating obesity and reducing blood pressure and the incidence of type 2 diabetes. Although the low-fat diet is an effective weight loss strategy, there are questions concerning long-term adherence. Moderate-fat and relatively low-fat Mediterranean diets are less studied for weight loss but have impressive risk reducing effects on cardiovascular disease (i.e., decreasing markers of vascular inflammation and lipids) and type 2 diabetes (i.e., improving insulin sensitivity) and have been shown to decrease mortality from cardiovascular disease, coronary heart disease, and cancer [28]. Shifting the focus from low-fat to healthy fat (e.g., eating more nuts, fish, and unsaturated oils) and focusing on portion control may be a more enjoyable and sustainable approach to weight management for some people. Additional studies comparing the effects of low-fat and moderate-fat diets on weight loss, satiety, and adherence would help clarify the amount of fat that is most effective for long-term weight control and health.

5. HIGH-PROTEIN DIETS

There is no standard definition of a "high-protein diet"; however, intakes greater than 25% total energy or 1.6 g/kg per day can be considered high [43].

The Zone diet (30% protein, 40% carbohydrate, and 30% fat) is an example of a high-protein diet. The most prominent difference between a high-protein diet such as the Zone and a low-carbohydrate diet like the Atkins diet is that a high-protein diet is typically low in fat.

5.1.   Efficacy of High-protein Diets on Weight Loss

No studies have examined the effects of a high-protein diet in individuals with MetS. One 12-month study evaluated the effects of a high-protein diet on body composition in obese adults [44, 45] and a limited number of short-term studies (< 6 months) have investigated the effects of high-protein diets on weight loss and body composition in obese individuals with hyperinsulinemia or type 2 diabetes [46–48]. In a recent investigation, 50 overweight and obese (body mass index [BMI] of 25 to 35 kg/m^2) individuals were randomly assigned to an *ad libitum* low-protein diet (12% protein, 30% fat, 58% carbohydrate) or high-protein regimen (25% protein, 30% fat, 45% carbohydrate) [44, 45]. During the first 6 months of the study, foods were provided to ensure that the prescribed diet was consumed. Between months 6 and 12, foods were no longer provided but participants were asked to maintain their dietary prescription and attend biweekly group behavior therapy sessions.

The high-protein group lost significantly more weight than the low-protein group after 6 months (-9.4 kg vs. -5.9 kg). Not surprisingly, the high-protein group had a greater decrease than the low-protein group in waist circumference, waist-to-hip ratio, and intraabdominal adipose tissue (assessed by dual-energy x-ray absorptiometry). At the 24-month assessment, the high-protein group continued to have a greater weight loss than the low protein group (-6.4 kg vs. -3.2 kg) but this difference was not significant because a large number of participants were lost to follow-up.

These findings suggest that although participants in the high-protein group regained weight after 6 months, there was a trend toward better weight maintenance in these individuals. In addition to weight loss, there was a greater reduction in waist circumference, waist-to-hip ratio, and intraabdominal adipose tissue, even after weight was regained. The effect on intraabdominal adipose tissue remained after adjustments were made for weight loss, which is important because this measure is highly correlated with MetS and certain chronic conditions such as type 2 diabetes and cardiovascular disease. Reductions in abdominal adipose tissue have been associated with improvements in insulin sensitivity, glycemic control, and dyslipidemia in insulin resistant subjects [49–51].

Short-term studies have also suggested that high-protein diets are superior to high-carbohydrate diets in either reducing body weight [46], preserving lean body mass [47], or promoting fat loss [48]. In one study 13 obese, hyperinsulinemic men were randomized to either a hypocaloric (i.e., 80% resting energy expenditure) high-protein (45% protein, 25% carbohydrate, 30% fat) or high-carbohydrate (12% protein, 58% carbohydrate, 30% fat) diet for 4 weeks [46]. To enhance compliance to the diet, food was provided and participants attended weekly counseling sessions. In addition to anthropometric measurements, fasting insulin, glucose, and plasma lipid concentrations were measured. Although weight loss was observed in both groups, participants in the high-protein group lost significantly more weight than those in the high-carbohydrate group (−8.3 kg vs. −6.0 kg) as well as more body water (−1.0 kg vs. −0.3 kg). Insulin levels decreased in both groups but only those in the high-protein group were within normal limits. Blood lipids improved but no differences were observed between groups with the exception of high-density lipoprotein (HDL)-cholesterol. A significant decrease in HDL-cholesterol was observed in the high-protein group.

Beneficial effects of high-protein diets on body composition were observed in a 16-week (i.e., 12-week weight loss phase and 4-week weight maintenance phase) study comparing the effects of hypocaloric (i.e., 1500 kcal) high-protein (30% protein, 40% carbohydrate, 30% fat) and standard protein (15% protein, 55% carbohydrate, 30% fat) diets on body composition, fasting glucose and insulin, lipid levels, and blood pressure in 66 overweight and obese, hyperinsulinemic adults over [47]. Like the previous study, participants were provided with fixed menu plans and a significant amount of food to enhance compliance.

Despite similarities in weight and total and abdominal fat loss in both groups, women in the high protein group lost significantly less lean body mass than those in the standard protein group. The researchers point out that the high-protein diet provided women approximately 1.4 g protein/kg of ideal body weight, a level sufficient to suppress proteolysis in women but not in men, as it only provided approximately 1.1 g protein/kg of ideal body weight for men. Intakes of 1.5 g protein/kg ideal body weight have also been shown to prevent loss of lean body mass [52, 53].

With the exception of greater decreases in fasting triglyceride concentrations in the high-protein group, the high-protein diet was no more efficacious than the standard protein diet in decreasing total and LDL cholesterol, increasing HDL, reducing blood pressure, or improving insulin resistance in this study. In another study conducted by this group, a high-protein diet did not confer any additional benefits on glycemic control, blood pressure, or HDL concentrations over a 12-week period in individuals with type 2 diabetes; however, total and LDL cholesterol decreased more in individuals following the high-protein diet [48]. There were no significant differences in weight loss between the two dietary groups; however, women on a high-protein diet lost significantly more total and abdominal fat than women on a low-protein diet.

The change in fat mass did not appear to alter insulin sensitivity in this subset of participants. Less lean body mass was lost in those following a high-protein diet but the differences between groups were not statistically significant.

Based on these findings, it does not appear that hypocaloric high-protein diets are more advantageous than low-protein diets in stabilizing glycemic response or improving blood lipids; however, there is some evidence from short-term studies to suggest that high-protein diets confer an advantage in promoting weight loss and reductions in abdominal adipose tissue independent of weight loss. Mechanisms regarding the greater changes in body composition in the high-protein group are unknown but may be due to the satiating effect of protein resulting in a lower intake of calories [45]. Some speculate that high-protein diets may lead to smaller reductions in resting energy expenditure resting (REE) or to greater diet-induced thermogenesis; however, it appears that both high- and low-protein diets produce similar effects on REE and diet induced thermogenesis in individuals with type 2 diabetes [54] and hyperinsulinemia [55]. Limitations of these studies include small sample sizes and short duration of treatment.

6.   LOW-CARBOHYDRATE DIETS

Although it gained some recognition in the 70's [56] and 90's [57], the popularity of the low carbohydrate diet remained dormant until 2002 [58] when it reemerged as an alternative to conventional low-fat diets. diet exist (i.e., Atkins diet, South Beach diet), each with a unique interpretation of optimal low-carbohydrate eating. Unlike low-fat diets, the FDA has not established a clear definition for "low-carbohydrate." Much attention has focused on the high fat and protein content of the diet. However, the focus of low-carbohydrate diets, as the name implies, is on carbohydrate, not fat or protein. Low-carbohydrate approaches encourage consumption of controlled amounts of nutrient-dense carbohydrate-containing foods (i.e., low glycemic index [low-GI] vegetables, fruits, and whole grain products) and eliminate intake of carbohydrate-containing foods based on refined carbohydrate (i.e., white bread, rice, pasta, cookies, and chips). Although consumption of foods that do not contain carbohydrate (i.e., meats, poultry, fish, as well as butter and oil) is not restricted, the emphasis is on moderation and quality rather than quantity.

6.1.   Efficacy of Low-carbohydrate Diets on Weight Loss, Insulin Sensitivity, and Lipids

Five randomized studies have now compared the short-term (≤ 12 months) effects of a low-carbohydrate diet and a calorie-controlled, low-fat diet on weight, body composition, and cardiovascular risk factors in obese adults [59–64]. Only one of these studies has evaluated the effects of low-carbohydrate diets in individuals with diabetes or metabolic syndrome [61, 62]. (Note that the Samaha and Stern papers refer to the same study but report 6 month and 12 month data, respectively). With the exception of one study which prescribed nutritional supplements including vitamins, minerals, essential oils, and chromium picolinate to the low-carbohydrate group but not the low-fat group [63], diet prescriptions in these studies were comparable (e.g., a low-carbohydrate diet containing less than 60 grams of carbohydrate). BMIs and ages ranged from 33–43 kg/m^2 and 43–54 years, respectively, in all four studies. While there were many similarities in diet prescriptions and participant characteristics, a few differences emerged. The majority of the studies were predominately of females [59, 60, 63, 64] except for one [61, 62]. Comorbidities and amount of clinician contact also differed slightly between these studies. Two of the investigations evaluated effects in healthy adults [59, 60], three examined effects in adults with significant comorbidities such as diabetes, MetS [61, 62], hyperlipidemia [63], and other cardiovascular risk factors [64]. Treatment occurred primarily in a self-help setting in one study [59] and in individual and/or group treatment in the others [60–64]. Only three studies evaluated these effects at one year [59, 62, 64]. Findings of these studies are summarized in Table 2.

Participants who followed a low-carbohydrate diet lost significantly more weight than those who adhered to a low-fat diet during the first 6 months of treatment [59–63]. However, differences in weight loss did not persist at 1 year [59, 62, 64] (Table 2). Two studies [59, 64] observed weight regain in both groups after 6 months with a greater regain in the low-carbohydrate group. While participants in the low-carbohydrate group did not regain weight in the Stern et al. study, those in the low-fat group continued to lose weight after 6 months, resulting in similar weight losses at one year [62].

In studies that compared low-carbohydydrate and low-fat diets over the course of 6–12 months there were no differences in total cholesterol or low density lipoprotein (LDL) cholesterol concentration between groups [59–63, 65]. One study reported that low-carbohydrate diet was less effective than the low-fat diet in reducing total cholesterol and LDL cholesterol at one year [64]. Only one study reported a small, transient increase in total cholesterol and LDL cholesterol during the third month of a 1 year treatment [59]. Furthermore, compared with the conventional group, those in the low-carbohydrate group experienced greater improvements in high density lipoprotein (HDL) cholesterol [59, 63] and triglycerides [59–61, 63]. Only one study reported decreases in HDL cholesterol in participants following a low-carbohydrate diet but the decrease was less than the decrease in the low-fat group [62]. Findings of these studies are summarized in Table 2. It is worth noting that in the

Table 2. Summary of findings from low-carbohydrate studies

	Brehm (6-month data)	Yancy (6-month data)	Stern (12-month data)	Foster (12-month data)	Dansinger (12-month data)
Sample size (*n*)	53	119	132	63	80
LC	26	59	64	33	40
C	27	60	68	30	40
Sex					
Male	N/A	28 (15 LC/ 13 C)	109 (51 LC/ 58 C)	20 (12 LC/ 8 C)	36 (19 LC/ 17 C)
Female	53 (26 LC/ 27 C)	91 (44 LC/ 47C)	23 (13 LC/ 10 C)	43 (21 LC/ 22 C)	44 (21 LC/ 23 C)
Age (years)					
LC	44.2	44.2	53.0	44.0	47
C	43.1	45.6	54.0	44.2	49
Baseline BMI (kg/m^2)					
LC	33.2	34.6	42.9	33.9	35.0
C	34.0	34.0	42.9	34.4	35.0
Weight loss (% change)					
LC	−9.3	−12.9	−3.9	−7.3	−3.9
C	−4.2	−6.7	−2.3	−4.5	−4.8
			Percent change		
Triglycerides					
LC	−23.4	−47.2	−28.6	−28.1	N/A
C	1.6	−14.4	2.7	1.4	
Total cholesterol					
LC	−0.4	−3.3	3.4	0.2	−3.8
C	−0.9	−5.6	−4.2	−5.5	−5.7
LDL					
LC	−0.7	1.0	6.2	0.5	−9.9
C	−5.3	−5.0	−3.2	−5.8	−10.0
HDL					
LC	13.4	9.8	−2.8	18.2	13.3
C	8.4	−2.9	−12.3	3.1	11.1

C, conventional diet; LC, low-carbohydrate diet.

Yancy et al. study, 2 subjects in the low carbohydrate withdrew due to high LDL levels while none did in the low calorie group. These small numbers are difficult to interpret, but they suggest that mean values may obscure important individual differences. A meta-analysis of these data suggests that while the low-carbohydrate diet produced more favorable changes in triglycerides and HDL cholesterol concentrations, the low-fat diet produced more favorable changes in total cholesterol and LDL cholesterol concentrations [66]. As such, further research is needed to understand whether the improvements in triglycerides and HDL concentrations outweigh the relatively smaller effects low-carbohydrate diets have on total and LDL cholesterol as compared to low-fat diets. No significant differences in blood pressure were observed between groups in any of the studies.

There is some evidence to suggest that a low-carbohydrate diet may be more efficacious in improving insulin sensitivity in nondiabetic individuals than a low-fat diet in the short term (i.e., after 6 months) but not in the long term (i.e., at 1 year) [61, 62]. Although the effects of low-carbohydrate diets on insulin sensitivity in diabetic participants were not measured in this study, the effects of low-carbohydrate diets on glycosylated hemoglobin in diabetic participants were examined [61, 62]. Greater decreases in glycosylated hemoglobin values were observed, independent of weight loss, in diabetic participants consuming a low-carbohydrate diet after 6 and 12 months [61, 62]. The significance of glycosylated hemoglobin was not maintained when the analysis included individuals who only completed the study or when baseline values were carried forward.

These data suggest that although participants in the low-carbohydrate group were not instructed to limit their energy intake, as were individuals in the conventional group, those in the low-carbohydrate group consumed fewer calories [60, 63]. It is interesting to note that at 6 months, across all four studies, subjects who were instructed to count carbohydrate consumed fewer calories than those who were instructed to count calories. The reason for this is unknown but may include greater satiety on a higher protein, low-GI diet. Greater weight loss may also be the result of the increased structure (i.e., clear boundaries about what foods are allowed). Structured approaches, including meal replacements and food provision, have been shown to increase the magnitude of weight loss [67–74].

Although few in number, it is interesting to note that findings are remarkably consistent despite differences across studies (e.g., gender, comorbid conditions, and clinician contact). These initial results are encouraging but very preliminary and do not signal a call for revised dietary guidelines. Limitations of these studies include small sample sizes, high attrition, and short duration of treatment and assessments limited to glycemic control and lipids. These preliminary data need to be replicated in larger and longer trials that include more comprehensive assessment of safety including measures of bone health and kidney function.

7.   LOW GLYCEMIC INDEX DIET

As consumption of carbohydrate has increased, more attention has been focused on the impact of high- and low-GI foods on food intake and obesity. The low-GI diet is an example of a unique blend of low-fat, low-carbohydrate, and low energy density concepts. Recommendations for this dietary approach are based not only on the GI values of foods but also on the overall nutritional content of the diet [75]. Like the low-fat diet, a low-GI diet should consist of a variety of foods that are low in saturated fat and sodium and high in fiber, vitamins, and minerals. The main focus, however, is increased consumption of low-GI foods such as whole grains, legumes, vegetables, and fruit. Refined and highly processed grains should be replaced with whole grain versions. Unlike the low-carbohydrate diet, this approach allows foods that may be relatively high on the GI scale as long as they are nutrient dense. Individuals following this dietary plan are also encouraged to consume foods low in energy density (e.g., number of calories in a given weight of food) and to recognize that "low-fat" does not necessarily mean that a food is healthy. By making wise GI choices, individuals should feel satisfied without having to overly restrict food intake, which should make adherence to this weight loss approach easier [75].

7.1.   Effects of Low Glycemic Index Diets on Hunger and Weight Loss and Insulin Sensitivity

There is considerable discussion regarding whether clinicians should recommend low-GI diets to overweight and obese patients [76–78]. Some suggest that low-GI diets produce greater decreases in weight and fat [79–82], and better preservation of lean body mass [83]. Others argue that these findings are not consistently observed and that there is insufficient evidence to conclude that low-GI diets are more effective than high-GI, low-fat diets in reducing food intake and producing weight loss [77]. The effects of low-GI diets on weight loss have not been extensively studied. Two studies have examined outcomes in obese but otherwise healthy children [80] and adolescents [81]. Three small crossover studies have compared the effects of low- and high-GI diets in obese hyperinsulinemic women [79], patients with non-insulin-dependent diabetes [83], and overweight but healthy nondiabetic men [82]. One large multicenter randomized trial evaluated the effects of diets consisting of simple versus complex carbohydrates on body weight in obese adults [84]. Although all studies evaluated the effects of increased intake of low-GI foods, these studies differed in study duration and dietary instruction and macronutrient composition, making it difficult to compare studies.

In a nonrandomized study, Speith et al. compared the effects of an *ad libitum* low-GI diet (45% to 50% carbohydrate, 20% to 25% protein, 30% to 35% fat) low-fat diet (55% to 60% carbohydrate, 15% to 20% protein, 25% to 30% fat) in 107 children (mean age 10 years) attending an outpatient obesity program [80]. Participants in the low-GI group were instructed to follow the Low-GI Pyramid and focus on food selection rather than energy restriction while those in the low-fat group were prescribed a calorie-controlled diet based on the Food Guide Pyramid. Children who consumed a low-GI diet had a significantly larger decrease in BMI (-1.53 kg/m^2) compared to children who followed a low-fat diet (-0.06 kg/m^2).

Ebbeling et al. found similar effects on weight in a study comparing an *ad libitum* reduced glycemic load diet with an energy-restricted low-fat diet in 16 obese adolescents (ages 13 to 21 years) [81]. Macronutrient distributions were the same as those in the Speith study. Participants also received behavior therapy during treatment. The study consisted of a 6-month intervention phase and 6-month follow up. Significantly greater reductions in BMI (-1.3 kg/m^2 vs. 0.7 kg/m^2) and fat mass (-3.0 kg vs. 1.8 kg) were observed in the low-GI group at 12 months. In addition, while insulin resistance, measured by HOMA, increased in the low fat-group, no changes were observed in the low glycemic load diet.

Taken together, these studies suggest that children who follow an *ad libitum* low-GI diet are more successful in losing weight than those who adhere to a standard low-fat diet. However, it is unclear whether these effects are due to differences between diets in GI or macronutrient composition. A blunted increase in insulin resistance in participants consuming a low-GI load diet suggests that this diet may reduce the risk for diabetes; however, the sample size in this study is too small on which to base conclusions.

Slabber et al. compared the effects of low- and high-GI energy restricted diets on weight loss and plasma insulin concentrations in 42 obese, hyperinsulinemic women during a 12-week period. Both diets were similar in macronutrient composition (50% carbohydrate, 20% protein, and 30% fat) and differed primarily in the types of carbohydrate-containing foods permitted (i.e., high-GI foods were excluded from the low-GI food plan) [79]. The Exchange List for Meal Planning was used in both groups to aid in meal selection. Participants in the low-GI group lost 9.3 kg while those in the high-GI group lost 7.4 kg after 12 weeks of treatment. Despite similar weight loss, fasting insulin concentrations dropped significantly more in the low-GI group than the high-GI group.

Similarly, Bouche et al. examined whether differences in glucose and lipid metabolism, as well as in total fat mass, would be observed in nondiabetic men who adhere to low-GI diets or a high-GI diet for 5 weeks [82]. With the exception of the type of carbohydrate prescribed, total energy and macronutrient intakes of the experimental diets were similar to those of the regular diet for each participant. Participants in the low-GI group were instructed to consume foods with a GI $< 45\%$ while those in the high-GI group were asked to consume foods with a GI > 60%. Each participant was provided a substitution list allowing exchanges within food groups and a list of commonly consumed foods. No significant changes in body weight were observed during the 5 weeks in either group. However, participants who consumed a low-GI diet had lower postprandial plasma glucose and insulin profiles, as well as lower postprandial cholesterol and triglycerides compared to those in the high-GI group. In another small 6-week study that compared low-GI and high-GI diets, overall blood glucose and lipid control were improved in patients with non-insulin-dependent diabetes mellitus following a low-GI diet. Similar amounts of weight were lost on both diets (i.e., −1.8 kg on the low-GI diet and −2.5 kg on the high-GI diet) [83].

Using a 2 × 2 design McMillan-Price et al. [85] evaluated the effects of low and high GI diets, varying in carbohydrate and protein, on weight loss and cardiovascular risk in 129 overweight or obese young adults. Participants consumed one of four reduced fat, high fiber diets for 12 weeks: (1) high Gl, high carbohydrate (55% of total energy), (2) high GI, high protein (25% of total energy), (3) low GI, high carbohydrate, or (4) low GI, high protein. Mean weight loss was similar across all 4 groups; however, a significantly greater proportion of participants consuming low GI, high carbohydrate (i.e., 56%) or high GI, high protein (i.e., 66%) diets lost at least 5% of body weight than participants consuming low GI, high protein (i.e., 33%) or high GI, high carbohydrate diets (i.e., 31%). Reductions in LDL cholesterol were observed in participants consuming the low GI, high carbohydrate diet but not in the high GI, high protein diet. These findings suggest that the effects of GI on weight loss and lipids may be dependent on the overall macronutrient composition of the diet. Although findings from this study suggest that the low GI, high carbohydrate diet was most efficacious in reducing both weight and LDL cholesterol, additional research is needed to determine which Gl-macronutrient combination is optimal for reducing weight, improving lipid profiles, and insulin and glucose concentrations. Saris et al. found that simply substituting simple carbohydrate for complex carbohydrate in the context of a low-fat diet does not result in significant differences in weight after 6 months of treatment [84].

Findings from the studies in children and adolescents suggest that *ad libitum* low-GI diets that provide slightly higher percentages of protein and fat may be more efficacious in reducing weight than standard energy-restricted diets. However, based on these limited findings in adults, there appear to be no advantages in terms of weight loss when GI is altered and energy and macronutrient composition are held constant. Findings in adults do suggest, however, that low-GI diets that are rich in fiber may play an important role in improving fasting insulin concentrations as well as postprandial glucose, insulin, cholesterol, and triglyceride concentrations. Many studies have shown that foods high in fiber, and particularly soluble fiber, improve blood lipid profiles and reduce the risk for cardiovascular disease [86–88].

8. CLINICAL IMPLICATIONS AND FUTURE DIRECTIONS FOR RESEARCH

Popular dietary approaches for weight loss have generated widespread interest and considerable debate. Despite the publicity surrounding the myriad of dietary approaches, very little is known about their efficacy in treating MetS or their comparative short- and long-term effects. It appears that in our results-oriented society more attention has been devoted to the potential for "success" of various weight loss approaches, traditionally measured by the general public in terms of pounds of lost, rather than their potential health effects and long-term sustainability. As such, overweight and obese individuals often find themselves in a vicious cycle of weight loss and regain looking for the next "best" diet.

More effective weight loss options are needed to support healthy and sustainable eating behaviors. Energy balance remains the cornerstone of weight control (i.e., calories still count). Randomized control weight loss trials have been designed to assess which diet is best but perhaps researchers have been asking the wrong question. The "winner take all" mentality does not serve the field or patients well. Rather than asking which is the best diet, investigators should be asking for which type of patients (i.e., individuals with diabetes, cardiovascular disease, hypertension, or MetS) do certain diets work best. Future research might focus more on how macronutrients or more specific characteristics or components of food such as GI or fiber affect the metabolic abnormalities that define MetS. Given the importance of weight maintenance for the management of MetS, more research is needed to better understand cravings, satiety, hunger, and other behavioral factors that often undermine dieters in the long-term. These studies will require large samples that will allow for examination of various behavioral and metabolic subtypes.

REFERENCES

[1] Executive Summary of The Third Report of The National Cholesterol Education Program (NCEP) Expert Panel on Detection, Evaluation, and Treatment of High Blood Cholesterol in Adults (Adult Treatment Panel III). Expert Panel on Detection, Evaluation, and Treatment of High Blood Cholesterol in Adults. JAMA 2001;285:2486–2497.

[2] Ford ES, Giles WH, Mokdad AH. Increasing prevalence of the metabolic syndrome among U.S. adults. Diabetes Care 2004;27:2444–2449.

[3] Sonnenberg L, Pencina M, Kimokoti R, Quatromoni P, Nam BH, D'Agostino R, Meigs JB, Ordovas J, Cobain M, Millen B. Dietary patterns and the metabolic syndrome in obese and non-obese Framingham women. Obes Res 2005;13:153–162.

[4] National Institute of Health/National Heart Lung and Blood Institute. Clinical Guidelines on the Identification, Evaluation, and Treatment of Overweight and Obesity in Adults. The Evidence Report, National Institutes of Health, September 1998;1–228.

[5] Lauber RP, Sheard NF; American Heart Association. The American Heart Association Dietary Guidelines for 2000: A summary report. Nutr Rev 2001;59:298–306.

[6] Tanasescu M, Cho E, Manson JE, Hu FB. Dietary fat and cholesterol and the risk of cardio-vascular disease among women with type 2 diabetes. Am J Clin Nutr 2004;79:999–1005.

[7] Wolfram G. Dietary fatty acids and coronary heart disease. Eur J Med Res 2003;8:321–324.

[8] Minehira K, Tappy L. Dietary and lifestyle interventions in the management of the metabolic syndrome: Present status and future perspective. Eur J Clin Nutr 2002;56:7 1262–1267.

[9] Wadden TA, Brownell KD, Foster GD. Obesity: Responding to the global epidemic. J Consult Clin Psychol 2002;70(3):510–525.

[10] US Department of Agriculture and the US Department of Health and Human Services. Dietary Guidelines for Americans, 6th edn. Washington, DC: US Government Printing Office, 2005.

[11] Irwin T. New dietary guidelines from the American Diabetes Association. Diabetes Care 2002;25:1262–1263.

[12] Kinsella A. American Heart Association issues new dietary guidelines. Home Health Nurse 2002;20:86–88.

[13] Byers T, Nestle M, McTiernan A, Doyle C, Currie-Williams A, Gansler T, Thun M; American Cancer Society 2001 Nutrition and Physical Activity Guidelines Advisory Committee. American Cancer Society guidelines on nutrition and physical activity for cancer prevention: Reducing the risk of cancer with healthy food choices and physical activity. CA Cancer J Clin 2002;52:92–119.

[14] Svetkey LP, Harsha DW, Vollmer WM, Stevens VJ, Obarzanek E, Elmer PJ, Lin PH, Champagne C, Simons-Morton DG, Aickin M, Proschan MA, Appel LJ. Premier: A clinical trial of comprehensive lifestyle modification for blood pressure control: Rationale, design and baseline characteristics. Ann Epidemiol 2003;13(6):462–471.

[15] Knowler WC, Barrett-Connor E, Fowler SE, Hamman RF, Lachin JM, Walker EA, Nathan DM. Diabetes Prevention Program Research Group. Reduction in the incidence of type 2 diabetes with lifestyle intervention or metformin. N Engl J Med 2002;346(6):393–403.

[16] Lindstrom J, Eriksson JG, Valle TT, Aunola S, Cepaitis Z, Hakumaki M, Ilanne-Parikka P, Keinanen-Kiukaanniem S, Laakso M, Louheranta A, Mannelin M, Martikkala V, Moltchanov V, Rastas M, Salminen V, Sundvall J, Uusitupa M, Tuomilehto J. Prevention of diabetes mellitus in subjects with impaired glucose tolerance in the Finnish Diabetes Prevention Study: Results from a randomized clinical trial. J Am Soc Nephrol 2003;14(7):S108–113.

[17] Wadden TA, Butryn ML, Byrne KJ. Efficacy of lifestyle modification for long-term weight control. Obes Res 2004;12(Suppl):151S–162S.

[18] Appel LJ, Champagne CM, Harsha DW, Cooper LS, Obarzanek E, Elmer PJ, Stevens VJ, Vollmer WM, Lin PH, Svetkey LP, Stedman SW, Young DR. Effects of comprehensive lifestyle modification on blood pressure control: Main results of the PREMIER clinical trial. JAMA 2003;289:2083–2093.

[19] Appel LJ, Moore TJ, Obarzanek E, Vollmer WM, Svetkey LP, Sacks FM, Bray GA, Vogt TM, Cutler JA, Windhauser MM, Lin PH, Karanja N. A clinical trial of the effects of dietary patterns on blood pressure. DASH Collaborative Research Group. N Engl J Med 1997;336:1117–1124.

[20] Sacks FM, Svetkey LP, Vollmer WM, Appel LJ, Bray GA, Harsha D, Obarzanek E, Conlin PR, Miller ER 3rd, Simons-Morton DG, Karanja N, Lin PH. Effects on blood pressure of reduced dietary sodium and the Dietary Approaches to Stop Hypertension (DASH) diet. DASH-Sodium Collaborative Research Group. N Engl J Med 2001;344(1):3–10.

[21] Ornish D. Low-fat diets. N Engl J Med 1998;338:127;128–129.

[22] Freedman MR, King J, Kennedy E. Popular diets: A scientific review. Obes Res 2001; 9(1):1S–40S.

[23] Ornish D, Scherwitz LW, Billings JH, Brown SE, Gould KL, Merritt TA, Sparler S, Armstrong WT, Ports TA, Kirkeeide RL, Hogeboom C, Brand RJ. Intensive lifestyle changes for reversal of coronary heart disease. JAMA 1998;280:2001–2007.

[24] Marques-Vidal P, Ruidavets JB, Cambou JP, Ferrieres J. Trends in overweight and obesity in middle-aged subjects from southwestern France, 1985–1997. Int J Obes Relat Metab Disord 2002;26(5):732–734.

[25] Willett WC, Sacks F, Trichopoulou A, Drescher G, Ferro-Luzzi A, Helsing E, Trichopoulos D. Mediterranean diet pyramid: A cultural model for healthy eating. Am J Clin Nutr 1995;61(Suppl 6):1402S–1406S.

[26] Kok FJ, Kromhout D. Atherosclerosis—epidemiological studies on the health effects of a Mediterranean diet. Eur J Nutr 2004;43(Suppl 1):I2–I5.

[27] Trichopoulou A, Costacou T, Bamia C, Trichopoulos D. Adherence to a Mediterranean diet and survival in a Greek population. N Engl J Med 2003;348(26):2599–2608.

[28] Knoops KT, de Groot LC, Kromhout D, Perrin AE, Moreiras-Varela O, Menotti A, van Staveren WA. Mediterranean diet, lifestyle factors, and 10-year mortality in elderly European men and women: The HALE project. JAMA 2004;292:1433–1439.

[29] Esposito K, Marfella R, Ciotola M, Di Palo C, Giugliano F, Giugliano G, D'Armiento M, D'Andrea F, Giugliano D. Effect of a mediterranean-style diet on endothelial dysfunction and markers of vascular inflammation in the metabolic syndrome: A randomized trial. JAMA 2004;292:1440–1446.

[30] McManus K, Antinoro L, Sacks F. A randomized controlled trial of a moderate-fat, low-energy diet compared with a low-fat, low-energy diet for weight loss in overweight adults. Int J Obes Relat Metab Disord. 2001;25(10):1503–1511.

[31] Karamanos B, Thanopoulou A, Angelico F, Assaad-Khalil S, Barbato A, Del Ben M, Dimitrijevic-Sreckovic V, Djordjevic P, Gallotti C, Katsilambros N, Migdalis I, Mrabet M, Petkova M, Roussi D, Tenconi MT. Nutritional habits in the Mediterranean Basin. The macronutrient composition of diet and its relation with the traditional Mediterranean diet. Multi-centre study of the Mediterranean Group for the Study of Diabetes (MGSD). Eur J Clin Nutr 2002;56(10):983–991.

[32] Trichopoulou A, Katsouyanni K, Gnardellis C. The traditional Greek diet. Eur J Clin Nutr 1993;47(Suppl 1):S76–S81.

[33] Simopoulos AP. The Mediterranean diets: What is so special about the diet of Greece? The scientific evidence. J Nutr 2001;131(Suppl 11):3065S–3073S.

[34] Liu S, Willett WC, Manson JE, Hu FB, Rosner B, Colditz G. Relation between changes in intakes of dietary fiber and grain products and changes in weight and development of obesity among middle-aged women. Am J Clin Nutr 2003;78(5):920–927.

[35] Koh-Banerjee P, Franz M, Sampson L, Liu S, Jacobs DR Jr, Spiegelman D, Willett W, Rimm E. Changes in whole-grain, bran, and cereal fiber consumption in relation to 8-y weight gain among men. Am J Clin Nutr 2004;80(5):1237–1245.

[36] Schroder H, Marrugat J, Vila J, Covas MI, Elosua R. Adherence to the traditional mediterranean diet is inversely associated with body mass index and obesity in a Spanish population. J Nutr 2004;134(12):3355–3561.

[37] Goulet J, Lamarche B, Nadeau G, Lemieux S. Effect of a nutritional intervention promoting the Mediterranean food pattern on plasma lipids, lipoproteins and body weight in healthy French-Canadian women. Atherosclerosis 2003;170(1):115–124.

[38] Kris-Etherton P, Eckel RH, Howard BV, St Jeor S, Bazzarre TL; Nutrition Committee, Population Science Committee and Clinical Science Committee of the American Heart Association. AHA Science Advisory: Lyon Diet Heart Study. Benefits of a Mediterranean-style, National Cholesterol Education Program/American Heart Association Step I Dietary Pattern on Cardiovascular Disease. Circulation 2001;103(13):1823–1825.

[39] de Lorgeril M, Salen P, Martin JL, Monjaud I, Delaye J, Mamelle N. Mediterranean diet, traditional risk factors, and the rate of cardiovascular complications after myocardial infarction: Final report of the Lyon Diet Heart Study. Circulation 1999;99(6):779–785.

[40] de Lorgeril M, Renaud S, Mamelle N, Salen P, Martin JL, Monjaud I, Guidollet J, Touboul P, Delaye, J. Mediterranean alpha-linolenic acid-rich diet in secondary prevention of coronary heart disease. Lancet 1994;343:1454–1459.

[41] Esposito K, Pontillo A, Di Palo C, Giugliano G, Masella M, Marfella R, Giugliano D. Effect of weight loss and lifestyle changes on vascular inflammatory markers in obese women: A randomized trial. JAMA 2003;289(14):1799–1804.

[42] Esposito K, Marfella R, Ciotola M, Di Palo C, Giugliano F, Giugliano G, D'Armiento M, D'Andrea F, Giugliano D. Effect of a mediterranean-style diet on endothelial dysfunction and markers of vascular inflammation in the metabolic syndrome: A randomized trial. JAMA 2004;292(12):1440–1446.

[43] Eisenstein J, Roberts SB, Dallal G, Saltzman E. High-protein weight-loss diets: Are they safe and do they work? A review of the experimental and epidemiologic data. Nutr Rev 2002;1:189–200.

[44] Skov AR, Toubro S, Ronn B, Holm L, Astrup A. Randomized trial on protein vs carbohydrate in ad libitum fat reduced diet for the treatment of obesity. Int J Obes Relat Metab Disord 1999;23:528–536.

[45] Due A, Toubro S, Skov AR, Astrup A. Effect of normal-fat diets, either medium or high in protein, on body weight in overweight subjects: A randomised 1-year trial. Int J Obes Relat Metab Disord 2004;28:1283–1290.

[46] Baba NH, Sawaya S, Torbay N, Habbal Z, Azar S, Hashim SA. High protein vs high carbohydrate hypoenergetic diet for the treatment of obese hyperinsulinemic subjects. Int J Obes Relat Metab Disord 1999;23(11):1202–1206.

[47] Farnsworth E, Luscombe ND, Noakes M, Wittert G, Argyiou E, Clifton PM. Effect of a high-protein, energy-restricted diet on body composition, glycemic control, and lipid concentrations in overweight and obese hyperinsulinemic men and women. Am J Clin Nutr 2003;78(1):31–39.

[48] Parker B, Noakes M, Luscombe N, Clifton P. Effect of a high-protein, high-mono-unsaturated fat weight loss diet on glycemic control and lipid levels in type 2 diabetes. Diabetes Care 2002;25(3):425–430.

[49] Stewart KJ, Bacher AC, Turner K, Lim JG, Hees PS, Shapiro EP, Tayback M, Ouyang P. Exercise and risk factors associated with metabolic syndrome in older adults. Am J Prev Med 2005;28:9–18.

[50] Laaksonen DE, Kainulainen S, Rissanen A, Niskanen L. Relationships between changes in abdominal fat distribution and insulin sensitivity during a very low calorie diet in abdominally obese men and women. Nutr Metab Cardiovasc Dis 2003;13(6):349–356.

[51] Janssen I, Fortier A, Hudson R, Ross R. Effects of an energy-restrictive diet with or without exercise on abdominal fat, intermuscular fat, and metabolic risk factors in obese women. Diabetes Care 2002;25:431–438.

[52] Piatti PM, Monti F, Fermo I, Baruffaldi L, Nasser R, Santambrogio G, Librenti MC, Galli-Kienle M, Pontiroli AE, Pozza G. Hypocaloric high-protein diet improves glucose oxidation and spares lean body mass: Comparison to hypocaloric high-carbohydrate diet. Metabolism 1994;43(12):1481–487.

[53] Hoffer LJ, Bistrian BR, Young VR, Blackburn GL, Matthews DE. Metabolic effects of very low calorie weight reduction diets. J Clin Invest 1984;73(3):750–758.

[54] Luscombe ND, Clifton PM, Noakes M, Parker B, Wittert G. Effects of energy-restricted diets containing increased protein on weight loss, resting energy expenditure, and the thermic effect of feeding in type 2 diabetes. Diabetes Care 2002;25(4):652-657.

[55] Luscombe ND, Clifton PM, Noakes M, Farnsworth E, Wittert G. Effect of a high-protein, energy-restricted diet on weight loss and energy expenditure after weight stabilization in hyperinsulinemic subjects. Int J Obes Relat Metab Disord 2003;27(5):582–590.

[56] Atkins RC. Dr. Atkins' Diet Revolution. New York: David McKay Inc. Publishers, 1972.

[57] Atkins RC. Dr. Atkins' New Diet Revolution. New York: Avon Books, Inc., 1992.

[58] Atkins RC. Dr. Atkins' New Diet Revolution. New York: Avon Books, Inc., 2002.

[59] Foster GD, Wyatt HR, Hill JO, McGuckin BG, Brill C, Mohammed S, Szapary PO, Rader DJ, Edman JS, Klein S. A randomized trial of a low-carbohydrate diet for obesity. N Engl J Med 2003;348:2082–2090.

[60] Brehm BJ, Seeley RJ, Daniels SR, D'Allesio DA. A randomized trial comparing a very low-carbohydrate diet and a calorie-restricted low-fat diet on body weight and cardiovascular risk factors in healthy women. J Clin Endocrinol Metab 2003;88:1617–1623.

[61] Samaha FF, Iqbal N, Seshadri P, Chicano KL, Daily DA, McGrory J, Williams T, Williams M, Gracely EJ, Stern L. A low-carbohydrate as compared with a low-fat diet in severe obesity. N Engl J Med 2003;348:2074–2081.

[62] Stern L, Iqbal N, Seshadri P, Chicano KL, Daily DA, McGrory J, Williams M, Gracely EJ, Samaha FF. The effects of low-carbohydrate versus conventional weight loss diets in severely obese adults: One-year follow-up of a randomized trial. Ann Intern Med 2004;140:778–785.

[63] Yancy WS, Olsen MK, Guyton JR, Bakst RP, Westman EC. A low-carbohydrate, ketogenic diet versus a low-fat diet to treat obesity and hyperlipidemia. Ann Intern Med 2004;140:769–777.

[64] Dansinger ML, Gleason JA, Griffith JL, Selker HP, Schaefer EJ. Comparison of the Atkins, Ornish, Weight Watchers, and Zone diets for weight loss and heart disease risk reduction: A randomized trial. JAMA 2005;293:43–53.

[65] Lean ME, Han TS, Prvan T, Richmond PR, Avenell A. Weight loss with high and low carbohydrate 1200 kcal diets in free living women. Eur J Clin Nutr 1997;51:243–248.

[66] Nordmann AJ, Nordmann A, Briel M, Keller U, Yancy WS Jr, Brehm BJ, Bucher HC. Effects of low-carbohydrate vs low-fat diets on weight loss and cardiovascular risk factors: A meta-analysis of randomized controlled trials. Arch Intern Med 2006;166:285–293.

[67] Jeffery RW, Wing RR, Thorson C, et al. Strengthening behavioral interventions for weight loss: A randomized trial of food provision and monetary incentives. J Consult Clin Psychol 1993;6:1038–1045.

[68] Wing RR, Jeffery RW, Burton LR, Thorson C, Nissinoff KS, Baxter JE. Food provision vs structured meal plans in the behavioral treatment of obesity. Int J Obes Relat Metab Disord 1996;20:56–62.

[69] Ditschuneit HH, Flechtner-Mors M. Value of structured meals for weight management: Risk factors and long-term weight maintenance. Obes Res 2001;9(Suppl 4):284S–289S.

[70] Ditschuneit HH, Flechtner-Mors M, Johnson TD, Adler G. Metabolic and weight loss effects of a long-term dietary intervention in obese patients. Am J Clin Nutr 1999; 69:198–204.

[71] Rothacker DQ, Staniszewski BA, Ellis PK. Liquid meal replacement vs traditional food: A potential model for women who cannot maintain eating habit change. J Am Diet Assoc 2001;101(3):345–347.

[72] Ashley JM, St Jeor ST, Perumean-Chaney S, Schrage J, Bovee V. Meal replacements in weight intervention. Obes Res 2001;9:312S–320S.

[73] Hannum SM, Carson, L, Evans EM, et al. Use of portion-controlled entrees enhances weight loss in women. Obes Res 2004;12:538–546.

[74] Metz JA, Stern JS, Kris-Etherton P, et al. A randomized trial of improved weight loss with a prepared meal plan in overweight and obese patients. Arch Intern Med 2000; 160:2150–2158.

[75] Brand-Miller J, Wolever TMS, Foster-Powell K, Colagiuri S. The New Glucose Revolution. New York: Marlowe & Co., 1996;71–94, 173–195.

[76] Pawlak DB, Ebbeling CB, Ludwig DS. Should obese patients be counseled to follow a low-glycaemic index diet? Yes. Obes Rev 2002;3:235–243.

[77] Raben A. Should obese patients be counseled to follow a low-glycaemic index diet? No. Obes Rev 2002;3:245–256.

[78] Pi-Sunyer FX. Glycemic index and disease. Am J Clin Nutr 2002;76:290S–298S.

[79] Slabber M, Barnard HC, Kuyl JM, Dannhauser A, Schall R. Effects of a low-insulin-response, energy-restricted diet on weight loss and plasma insulin concentrations in hyperinsulinemic obese females. Am J Clin Nutr 1994;60:48–53.

[80] Speith LE, Harnish JD, Lenders CM, Raezer LB, Pereira MA, Hangen J, Ludwig DS. A low-glycemic index diet in the treatment of pediatric obesity. Arch Pediatr Adolesc Med 2000;154:947–951.

[81] Ebbling CB, Leidig MM, Sinclair KB, Hangen JP, Ludwig DS. A reduced-glycemic load diet in the treatment of adolescent obesity. Arch Pediatr Adolesc Med 2003;157:773–779.

[82] Bouche C, Rizkalla SW, Luo J, Vidal H, Veronese A, Pacher N, Fouquet C, Lang V, Slama G. Five-week, low-glycemic index diet decreases total fat mass and improves plasma lipid profile in moderately overweight nondiabetic men. Diabetes Care 2002;25:822–828.

[83] Wolever TM, Jenkins DJ, Vuksan V, Jenkins AL, Wong GS, Josse RG. Beneficial effect of low-glycemic index diet in overweight NIDDM subjects. Diabetes Care 1992;15:562–564.

[84] Saris WH, Astrup A, Prentice AM, Zunft HJ, Formiguera X, Verboeket-van de Venne WP, Raben A, Poppitt SD, Seppelt B, Johnston S, Vasilaras TH, Keogh GF. Randomized controlled trial of changes in dietary carbohydrate/fat ratio and simple vs complex carbohydrates on body weight and blood lipids: The CARMEN study. The Carbohydrate Ratio Management in European national diets. Int J Obes Relat Metab Disord 2000;24(10):1310–1318.

[85] McMillan-Price J, Petocz P, Atkinson F, O'neill K, Samman S, Steinbeck K, Caterson I, Brand-Miller J. Comparison of 4 diets of varying glycemic load on weight loss and cardiovascular risk reduction in overweight and obese young adults: A randomized controlled trial. Arch Intern Med 2006; 166:1466–1475.

[86] Anderson JW, Spencer DB, Hamilton CC, Smith SF, Tietyen J, Bryant CA, Oeltgen P. Oat-bran cereal lowers serum total and LDL cholesterol in hypercholesterolemic men. Am J Clin Nutr 1990;52(3):495–499.

[87] Anderson JW, Zeigler JA, Deakins DA, Floore TL, Dillon DW, Wood CL, Oeltgen PR, Whitley RJ. Metabolic effects of high-carbohydrate, high-fiber diets for insulin-dependent diabetic individuals. Am J Clin Nutr 1991;54(5):936–943.

[88] Marckmann P, Sandstrom B, Jespersen J. Low-fat, high-fiber diet favorably affects several independent risk markers of ischemic heart disease: Observations on blood lipids, coagulation, and fibrinolysis from a trial of middle-aged Danes. Am J Clin Nutr 1994;59(4):935–939.

Chapter 12

Exercise as an Approach to Obesity and the Metabolic Syndrome

John M. Jakicic and Amy D. Otto

Department of Health and Physical Activity, Physical Activity and Weight Management Research Center, University of Pittsburgh, 140 Trees Hall, Pittsburgh, PA 15261, USA

1. INTRODUCTION

More than 65% of adults in the United States are classified as either overweight (body mass index ≥ 25.0 kg/m^2) or obesity (body mass index ≥ 30 kg/m^2). These prevalence rates are of significant public health concern because of the link with numerous chronic health-related conditions such as heart disease, diabetes, and various forms of cancer [1]. Thus, examining strategies to effectively reduce body, prevent weight gain, and impact the health-related conditions associated with excess body weight are of significant public health importance.

While overweight and obesity can be linked to a variety of factors including behavior, metabolism, and genetics, ultimately body weight is affected by energy balance. Therefore, to reduce body weight or to prevent weight gain, energy intake must not exceed energy expenditure, with manipulation of either of these parameters influencing body weight control and related health risks. The most variable component of energy expenditure is exercise and other forms of physical activity, which suggests that this component of energy balance may be an appropriate target for interventions related to weight control. More importantly, exercise has been shown to independently impact health-related factors that appear to be common in overweight and obese individuals. Therefore, the purpose of this review is to summarize the effect of exercise on body weight control and associated health risks.

2. EFFECT OF EXERCISE ON HEALTH-RELATED PARAMETERS

Based on a growing body of scientific literature, it is widely accepted that increased energy expenditure through exercise and physical activity can positively influence health [2]. Data from the Harvard Alumni Study have repeated demonstrated the inverse association between leisure-time physical activity and mortality from all-causes for men [3, 4]. For example, it has been demonstrated that individuals reporting ≥ 2000 kcal/week of leisure-time physical activity have a 28% reduction in all-cause mortality compared to those individuals reporting < 2000 kcal/week of leisure-time physical activity [3]. Lee et al. [5] have reported that vigorous exercise and physical activity (≥ 6 METS) show a significant reduction in risk of mortality compared to nonvigorous forms of exercise and physical activity (< 6 METS). However, maintaining activity levels of at least 4.5 METS over an 11- to 15-year period was shown to reduce the relative risk of all-cause mortality by 29% when compared to those maintaining activity patterns of < 4.5 METS [4]. Moreover, individuals increasing from < 4.5 METS to ≥ 4.5 METS over this same period showed a reduction in relative risk of all-causes mortality of 23% when compared to those reporting < 4.5 METS over this same period of time [4].

The effect of higher levels of energy expenditure on health-related outcomes have also been demonstrated for women [6–8]. Manson et al. [8] reported that women who exercised at least once per week had an age-adjusted relative of 0.67 for developing type 2 diabetes mellitus. Helmrich et al. [9] reported that for every 500-kcal increase in energy expenditure there is a 6% reduction in age-adjusted risk for type 2 diabetes. It has also been reported that ≥ 1 hour of walking per week reduces the risk of coronary heart disease by approximately 50% in women [6]. Moreover, data from the Nurses' Health Study indicate that regular exercise that is ≥ 6 METS is associated with a 30 to 40 reduction in coronary heart disease in women [7], which is similar to the results reported by Hu et al. [10]. Thus, the positive effects of physical activity on health-related outcomes are not limited to men, but are also observed in women.

The impact of exercise and physical activity on improving health-related outcomes and reducing both morbidity and mortality may operate through improvements in cardiorespiratory fitness, with numerous studies reporting an inverse association between cardiorespiratory fitness and mortality. Blair et al. have reported that the relative risk of all-cause mortality is 3.44 in men and 4.65 in women with the lowest levels of fitness when compared to those with the highest levels of fitness [11]. When comparing individuals grouped as having the lowest 20% of fitness to those with higher levels of fitness, low fitness resulted in a relative risk of 2.03 and 2.23 for all-cause mortality in men and women, respectively [12]. Moreover, it has been shown that an increase in cardiorespiratory fitness results in a reduction in risk of death, whereas a decrease in cardiorespiratory fitness is associated with an increase in the risk of death [13]. When viewed in combination with the data available on the relationship between energy expenditure and health risk, it appears that energy expenditure that results in improvements in fitness may have the most influence on the reduction in health risk. This may have implications for interventions that focus on improving health-related outcomes.

The link between both exercise and fitness with mortality and morbidity may be partially explained through the effect on specific risk factors such as the metabolic syndrome. For example, Rennie et al. [14] reported that the odds ratio for developing metabolic syndrome was 0.78 and 0.52 for individuals engaging in moderate or vigorous activity, respectively. With regard to fitness, individuals with low to moderate levels of cardiorespiratory fitness have been shown to have a higher relative risk of metabolic syndrome when compared to those individuals with high levels of cardiorespiratory fitness [15]. Moreover, data from the HERITAGE Study demonstrated that after 20 weeks of exercise training, the prevalence of metabolic syndrome was reduced by approximately 30% [16].

These findings may have particular implications for the overweight and obese adult. While excess body weight is associated with increased health risk from numerous chronic health conditions [1], a number of studies have demonstrated that the health improvements associated with higher levels of cardiorespiratory fitness and energy expenditure appear to be present even in adults classified as overweight or class I or II obesity [17–19]. Moreover, the odds ratio for metabolic syndrome is increased in overweight and obese individuals [20]. Thus, because of the observed beneficial influence of higher levels of exercise and fitness on factors associated with the metabolic syndrome, it would be advantageous for overweight and obese adults to engage in efforts to modify exercise patterns and improve fitness. Moreover, it appears that there is sufficient scientific evidence to recommend that overweight and obese adults increase energy expenditure through exercise and other forms of physical activity, even in the absence of weight reduction, to improve health-related outcomes.

3.   IMPACT OF EXERCISE ON WEIGHT LOSS

Because of the association between excess body weight and health risk, it is important to understand how increases in energy expenditure resulting from exercise and other forms of physical activity can impact body weight control. Interventions of ≤ 6 months have consistently demonstrated that exercise alone results in significantly less weight loss when compare to diet alone or the combination of diet plus exercise [1, 21]. For example, Wing et al. [22] reported weight losses of 2.1 kg, 9.1 kg, and 10.3 kg in the exercise, diet, and diet plus exercise groups, respectively. This pattern of weight loss is similar to the results of a 12-week study by Hagan et al. [23] that reported reductions in body weight of 11.4%, 8.4%, and 0.3% in men and 7.5%, 5.5%, and 0.6% for women in response to diet plus exercise, diet alone, or exercise alone, respectively. In contrast, Ross et al. [24] have reported similar reductions in body weight when a similar energy deficit was elicited with either diet (reduction in energy intake) or exercise (increase in energy expenditure). However, to achieve the typically recommended 1 to 2 pounds of weight loss per week [25], a 90.7-kg (200 lb) individual would need to engage in approximately 82.7 min/day (1 hour 23 minutes/day) to 165.4 minutes/day (2 hour 45 minutes/day) of brisk walking (4 METS), which may not be practical. Thus, the most effective short-term interventions for weight loss do not appear to be limited to exercise alone to increase energy expenditure, but rather include a diet component to also reduce energy intake, and this is consistent with the clinical guidelines developed by the National Heart, Lung and Blood Institute [1].

The importance of exercise and other forms of physical activity may be most important for long-term weight loss outcomes. It has been demonstrated that higher levels of exercise are associated with improved weight loss and the prevention of weight regain. For example, Jakicic et al. [26, 27] reported improved weight loss outcomes with increased levels of exercise across 12- to 18-month interventions in women. Moreover, both Weinsier et al. [28] and McGuire et al. [29] have reported lower levels of physical activity energy expenditure are associated with weight gain or regain. However, the existing scientific evidence appear to indicated that the need to continue to observe appropriate dietary practices in combination with exercise to enhance weight loss maintenance. Jakicic et al. [30] demonstrated that the greatest magnitude of weight loss was achieved through the combination of increased energy expenditure through exercise and the reduction in energy intake. Moreover, data from the National Weight Control Registry demonstrate that individuals who successfully maintain significant weight loss long-term report engaging in both high levels of leisure-time physical activity and consume a moderate energy intake [31], with the ability to maintain significant body weight loss influenced by both components of energy balance [29]. Therefore, similar to short-term findings, it appears that the combination of adequate levels of exercise along with the maintenance of appropriate levels of energy intake are most important for maximizing long-term weight control outcomes in overweight and obese adults.

4.   EXERCISE PRESCRIPTION CONSIDERATIONS FOR LONG-TERM WEIGHT CONTROL

The importance of exercise and physical activity in management of body weight and risk associated with chronic diseases has been highlighted in the recent US Dietary Guidelines [32]. However, it is important to understand that the recommended level of exercise varies based on the health outcome that is desired. For example, 30 minutes/day of moderate intensity activity is recommended to reduce the risk associated with the onset of various chronic diseases, and this is consistent with earlier recommendations [2, 33]. Moreover, this level of activity is consistent with the recommendation to accumulate at least 10,000 steps per day, which has been shown to be associated with improvements in health-related outcomes [34]. However, 60 minutes/day of moderate intensity activity is recommended to prevent weight gain, with 60 to 90 minutes/day recommended to prevent weight regain after significant weight loss [32], which is similar to previously recommended levels of exercise to control body weight [25–27, 31, 35–37]. Therefore, based on the existing data, clinicians should initially target at least 30 minutes/day of moderate intensity activity to reduce the risk of chronic diseases, with activity progressively increasing to 60 to 90 minutes/day for individuals to maximize long-term weight loss and to prevent weight regain after weight loss.

The current recommendations indicate that activity should be performed at a moderate level of intensity. However, there has been some debate regarding the appropriate intensity of exercise required for weight loss, with current research suggesting that energy expenditure rather than exercise intensity is the most important factor for controlling body weight [27, 38]. Both Duncan et al. [38] and Jakicic et al. [27] reported similar changes in body weight between moderate and vigorous intensity exercise when total energy expenditure did not differ between the conditions. These data appear to suggest overweight and obese adults do not need to participate in vigorous intensity exercise, but rather moderate intensity exercise is sufficient provided that overall energy expenditure is adequate to impact body weight.

The majority of research related to the effect of exercise on weight control and associated risk factors has focused primarily on aerobic forms of exercise. However, there may be interest in examining alternative forms of exercise such as resistance exercise. A relatively recent review of the literature concludes that resistance exercise offers little to no improvement for weight loss when compared to other forms of exercise [39]. For example, Kraemer et al. [40] reported weight losses of 6.2 kg, 6.8 kg, and 7.0 kg in response to 12 weeks of diet alone, diet plus endurance exercise, and diet plus both endurance and resistance exercise, respectively. Moreover, the reduction in body fatness was not improved with the addition of resistance exercise. The review by Donnelly et al. [39] also revealed that few long-term studies have been conducted to examine the effect of resistance exercise on long-term weight loss outcomes, which indicates that there is a research need in this area. Despite the minimal impact of resistance on weight loss outcomes in the majority of studies published to date, there may be additional benefits of including resistance exercise in interventions for overweight and obese adults. For example, resistance exercise has been demonstrated to improve muscular strength [40, 41], and this may lead to functional improvements in overweight and obese adults [34]. Moreover, Jurca et al. [42] have reported that after controlling for cardiorespiratory fitness, higher levels of muscular strength are associated with a 20% reduction in the relative risk for all-cause mortality, with this reduction being 30% to 40% for individuals classified with high levels or muscular strength and cardiorespiratory fitness.

5. SUMMARY

Increases in energy expenditure resulting from exercise and other forms of physical activity appear to be important for weight loss and to impact risk factors associated with excess body weight. They may be an important component of effective interventions to enhance initial weight loss and the prevention of weight regain. While 30 minutes/day of exercise appears to have the desired impact on risk factors for numerous chronic diseases, to maximize weight loss and prevention weight regain it appears that overweight and obese adults may need to progress to as much as 60 to 90 minutes/day of exercise, which is consistent with current recommendations [32]. Therefore, it is important to have interventions target these levels of physical activity to improve health-related outcomes and to facilitate long-term weight control, and to develop effective interventions to progress overweight and obese individuals to levels of exercise conducive with successful long-term weight loss.

ACKNOWLEDGMENTS

The efforts of Dr. Jakicic and Dr. Otto in the development of this manuscript are supported by research grants provided by the National Institutes of Health (HL070257, HL67826, and DK066150).

REFERENCES

[1] National Institutes of Health. Clinical Guidelines on the Identification, Evaluation, and Treatment of Overweight and Obesity in Adults—The Evidence Report. Obes Res 1998;6(Suppl 2).

[2] US Department of Health and Human Services. Physical Activity and Health: A Report of the Surgeon General. Atlanta, GA: US Department of Health and Human Services, Centers for Disease Control and Prevention, National Center for Chronic Disease Prevention and Health Promotion, 1996.

[3] Paffenbarger RS, Hyde RT, Wing AL, Hsieh CC. Physical activity, all-cause mortality, and longevity of college alumni. N Engl J Med 1986;314:605–613.

[4] Paffenbarger RS, Hyde RT, Wing AL, Lee I-M, Jung DL, Kampert JB. The association of changes in physical-activity level among other lifestyle characteristics with mortality among men. N Engl J Med 1993;328:538–545.

[5] Lee I-M, Hsieh CC, Paffenbarger RS. Exercise intensity and longevity in men. The Harvard Alumni Study. JAMA 1995;273:1179–1184.

[6] Lee I-M, Rexrode KM, Cook NR, Manson JE, Buring JE. Physical activity and coronary heart disease in women. JAMA 2001;285(11):1447–1454.

[7] Manson JE, Hu FB, Rich-Edwards JW, Colditz GA, Stampfer MJ, Willett WC. A prospective study of walking as compared with vigorous exercise in the prevention of coronary heart disease in women. N Engl J Med 1999;341:650–658.

[8] Manson JE, Rimm EB, Stampfer MJ, et al. Physical activity and incidence of non-insulin-dependent diabetes mellitus in women. Lancet 1991;338:774–778.

[9] Helmrich SP, Ragland DR, Leung RW, Paffenbarger RS. Physical activity and reduced occurence of non-insulin-dependent diabetes mellitus. N Engl J Med 1991;325:147–152.

[10] Hu FB, Sigal RJ, Rich-Edwards JW, et al. Walking compared with vigorous physical activity and risk of type 2 diabetes in women. A prospective study. JAMA 1999;282:1433–1439.

[11] Blair SN, Kohl III H, Paffenbarger RS, Clark DG, Cooper KH, Gibbons LW. Physical fitness and all-cause mortality. A prospective study of healthy men and women. JAMA 1989;262(17):2395–2401.

[12] Blair SN, Kampert JB, Kohl III H, et al. Influence of cardiorespiratory fitness and other precursors on cardiovascular disease and all-cause mortality in men and women. JAMA 1996;276:205–210.

[13] Blair SN, Kohl III H, Barlow CE, Paffenbarger RS, Gibbons LW, Macera CA. Changes in physical fitness and all-cause mortality: A prospective study of healthy and unhealthy men. JAMA 1995;273:1093–1098.

[14] Rennie KL, McCarthy N, Yazdgerdi S, Marmot M, Brunner E. Association of the metabolic syndrome with both vigorous and moderate physical activity. Int J Epidemiol 2003;32:600–606.

[15] Lee S, Kuk JI, Katzmarzyk PT, Blair SN, Church TS, Ross R. Cardiorespiratory fitness attenuates metabolic risk independent of subcutaneous and visceral fat in men. Diabetes Care 2005;28:895–901.

[16] Katzmarzyk PT, Leon AS, Wilmore JH, et al. Targeting the metabolic syndrome with exercise: Evidence from the HERITAGE Family Study. Med Sci Sports Exerc 2003;35(10):1703–1709.

[17] Wei M, Kampert J, Barlow CE, et al. Relationship between low cardiorespiratory fitness and mortality in normal-weight, overweight, and obese men. JAMA 1999;282(16):1547–1553.

[18] Barlow CE, Gibbons LW, Blair SN. Physical activity, mortality, and obesity. Int J Obes 1995;19:S41–S44.

[19] Farrell SW, Braun L, Barlow CE, Cheng YJ, Blair SN. The relation of body mass index, cardiorespiratory fitness, and all-cause mortality in women. Obes Res 2002;10(6):417–423.

[20] Katzmarzyk PT, Church TS, Janssen I, Ross R, Blair SN. Metabolic syndrome, obesity, and mortality. Diabetes Care 2005;28(2):391–397.

[21] Wing RR. Physical activity in the treatment of adulthood overweight and obesity: Current evidence and research issues. Med Sci Sports Exerc 1999;31(Suppl 11):S547–S552.

[22] Wing RR, Venditti EM, Jakicic JM, Polley BA, Lang W. Lifestyle intervention in overweight individuals with a family history of diabetes. Diabetes Care 1998;21(3):350–359.

[23] Hagan RD, Upton SJ, Wong L, Whittam J. The effects of aerobic conditioning and/or calorie restriction in overweight men and women. Med Sci Sports Exerc 1986;18(1):87–94.

[24] Ross R, Dagnone D, Jones PJH, et al. Reduction in obesity and related comorbid conditions after diet-induced weight loss or exercise-induced weight loss in men. Ann Intern Med 2000;133:92–103.

[25] Jakicic JM, Clark K, Coleman E, et al. American College of Sports Medicine position stand: Appropriate intervention strategies for weight loss and prevention of weight regain for adults. Med Sci Sports Exerc 2001;33(12):2145–2156.

[26] Jakicic JM, Winters C, Lang W, Wing RR. Effects of intermittent exercise and use of home exercise equipment on adherence, weight loss, and fitness in overweight women: A randomized trial. JAMA 1999;282(16):1554–1560.

[27] Jakicic JM, Marcus BH, Gallagher KI, Napolitano M, Lang W. Effect of exercise duration and intensity on weight loss in overweight, sedentary women. A randomized trial. JAMA 2003;290:1323–1330.

[28] Weinsier RL, Hunter GR, Desmond RA, Byrne NM, Zuckerman PA, Darnell BE. Free-living activity energy expenditure in women successful and unsuccessful at maintaining a normal body weight. Am J Clin Nutr 2002;75:499–504.

[29] McGuire MT, Wing RR, Klem ML, Lang W, Hill JO. What predicts weight regain in a group of successful weight losers? J Consult Clin Psychol 1999;67(2):177–185.

[30] Jakicic JM, Wing RR, Winters-Hart C. Relationship of physical activity to eating behaviors and weight loss in women. Med Sci Sports Exerc 2002;34(10):1653–1659.

[31] Klem ML, Wing RR, McGuire MT, Seagle HM, Hill JO. A descriptive study of individuals successful at long-term maintenance of substantial weight loss. Am J Clin Nutr 1997;66:239–246.

[32] Department of Health and Human Services, and US Department of Agriculture. Dietary Guidelines for Americans: http://www.healthierus.gov/dietaryguidelines; 2005.

[33] Pate RR, Pratt M, Blair SN, et al. Physical activity and public health: A recommendation from the Centers for Disease and Prevention and the American College of Sports Medicine. JAMA 1995;273(5):402–407.

[34] Jakicic JM. Physical activity considerations for the treatment and prevention of obesity. Am J Clin Nutr 2005;82(Suppl 1):226S–229S.

[35] Saris WHM, Blair SN, van Baak MA, et al. How much physical activity is enough to prevent unhealthy weight gain? Outcome of the IASO 1st Stock Conference and consensus statement. Obes Rev 2003;4:101–114.

[36] Institute of Medicine. Dietary Reference Intakes for Energy, Carbohydrates, Fiber, Fat, Protein and Amino Acids (Macronutrients). Washington, DC: The National Academies Press, 2002.

[37] Schoeller DA, Shay K, Kushner RF. How much physical activity is needed to minimize weight gain in previously obese women. Am J Clin Nutr 1997;66:551–556.

[38] Duncan JJ, Gordon NF, Scott CB. Women walking for health and fitness: How much is enough? JAMA 1991;266(23):3295–3299.

[39] Donnelly JE, Jakicic JM, Pronk NP, et al. Is resistance exercise effective for weight management? Evidence Based Prevent Med 2004;1(1):21–29.

[40] Kraemer WJ, Volek JS, Clark KL, et al. Physiological adaptations to a weight-loss dietary regimen and exercise programs in women. J Appl Physiol 1997;83(1):270–279.

[41] Kraemer WJ, Volek JS, Clark KL, et al. Influence of exercise training on physiological and performance changes with weight loss in men. Med Sci Sports Exerc 1999;31:1320–1329.

[42] Jurca R, LaMonte MJ, Church TS, et al. Association of muscle strength and aerobic fitness with metabolic syndrome in men. Med Sci Sports Exerc 2004;36(8):1301–1307.

Chapter 13

Behavioral Strategies for Controlling Obesity

Donald A. Williamson, Corby K. Martin and Tiffany M. Stewart

Pennington Biomedical Research Center, Baton Rouge, LA 70810, USA

1.   INTRODUCTION

Obesity occurs when the energy consumed exceeds the amount of energy expended, and the long-term result is excess body weight caused by storage of "extra" energy in body fat stores [1]. The prevalence of overweight and obesity is considered a serious public health issue in the United States [2]. Over the past few decades, overweight and obesity prevalence rates among children, adolescents, and adults have increased markedly across all racial/ethnic groups and men and women [3–5]. Overweight and obesity have been shown to be associated with chronic and life threatening disorders, such as diabetes, hypertension, and hyperlipidemia [6]. However, it has recently been suggested that comorbid symptoms (e.g., cardiovascular disease) and mortality rates associated with obesity are improving (lower than previous estimates) [7]. This finding is of interest because it contradicts prior conclusions [8, 9] concerning the costs and health outcomes associated with the current epidemic of obesity. Nevertheless, there is no evidence to suggest that obesity rates are decreasing [10]. Further, for severe underweight and obesity, particularly higher levels of obesity (body mass index [BMI] $\geq$ 30), mortality rates relative to normal weight individuals continue to be a concern [7].Thus, despite recent evidence that comorbid symptoms of obesity have improved, obesity remains to be a significant public health problem for which effective treatment strategies are needed.

Behavioral approaches for weight management have been extensively studied as one strategy for addressing this health problem. Modest weight loss (5% to 10% of total body weight) through lifestyle intervention approaches has been found to have a beneficial effect on comorbid conditions, particularly hypertension and type 2 diabetes. Recent lifestyle intervention research also suggests that moderate weight loss may delay or prevent the onset of type 2 diabetes [11]. In 2003, the Diabetes Prevention Program [11] reported that a lifestyle intervention for obesity reduced the risk of diabetes by 58%. This study found that lifestyle intervention was more effective than metformin, and was effective in individuals of every gender, age and BMI group. These results suggest that there is great promise for the application of lifestyle behavioral interventions for the reduction of obesity and the risk for comorbid health conditions [12].

Effective behavioral treatment of obesity involves modification of eating and physical activity behavior patterns to yield negative energy balance. This chapter describes the behavioral approach for weight management and summarizes research findings. These studies have found that interventions that combine a low-calorie diet, increased physical activity, and behavior therapy are most effective for weight loss and maintenance. Further, extended length of treatment contact, weight loss satisfaction, and social support may promote positive long-term outcomes in obese adults, adolescents, and children. Given the success of lifestyle intervention for the induction of moderate weight loss, behavioral treatment for obesity is a logical initial treatment option for people who are overweight, moderately obese, or desire to adopt a healthier lifestyle.

2.   HISTORY OF BEHAVIORAL STRATEGIES FOR CONTROLLING OBESITY

The origins of behavioral treatment for obesity date back to the late 1960s. Since the 1970s, behavioral treatment programs for obesity have been intensified in terms of length and aggressiveness, yielding average weight losses ranging from 7% to 10% of initial body weight. On average, most people reach their maximum point of weight loss about 6 months after the initiation of treatment. However, it is important to note that these weight losses usually occur in the short term and are not maintained in the long-term, after treatment ends. Thus, maintenance of weight loss is an important focus of treatment outcome research.

2.1.   Philosophy of Treatment

A general principle underlying the theory of behavior therapy for obesity (based on Social Learning Theory) is that obese individuals have learned eating and exercise patterns that are contributing to weight gain and/or maintenance of obesity. These behaviors can be modified to produce weight loss. Learning principles from both classical and operant conditioning are applied in training new behaviors. Behavioral treatment of obesity seeks to alter the environment, since some environmental reinforcement contingencies shape eating behavior and physical activity.

3. BEHAVIORAL TREATMENT FOR ADULTS

3.1. Approach and Outcomes

Behavioral studies of weight management have focused on changing physical activity, eating behavior, and motivational strategies to improve weight loss. Behavioral treatment is best coordinated by the collaboration of a multidisciplinary team of professionals, including medical doctors, psychologists, dietitians, and exercise physiologists. The two phases of the behavioral treatment approach are (1) weight loss induction and (2) weight maintenance. To induce weight loss, specific calorie goals for food intake and specific goals for physical activity are prescribed for each individual. These goals are designed to yield a 1- to 2-pound weight loss per week. Physical activity and exercise goals are gradually increased until individuals engage in a minimum of 150 minutes (30 to 45 minutes, 5 days per week) of moderate intensity activity (e.g., brisk walking) per week [13]. Treatment typically involves attendance to weekly outpatient treatment groups during the 6 months of the weight loss induction phase and is reduced to biweekly or monthly meetings thereafter. Generally, longer duration of treatment (at least 6 months) and the combination of diet and exercise have been shown to yield greater success in weight loss and weight maintenance over time [14].

3.2. Duration of Treatment

In an effort to make weight loss therapies more effective, treatment length has been increased over time from an average of 8 weeks in 1974 to an average of 21 weeks by the 1990s. Comparable increases in weight loss have occurred with increases in treatment duration. In 1974, the average weight loss associated with the 8-week treatment protocol was 3.8 kg, and in 1990, the average weight loss associated with a 21-week treatment protocol was 8.5 kg. In 2000, Jeffery et al. [15] estimated that average weight losses in behavioral treatment studies have increased by approximately 75% between 1974 and 1994. In 1989, Perri et al. [16] reported that treating participants for 40 weeks as opposed to 20 weeks was associated with more weight loss. In a review of this research in 1998, Perri [17] concluded that extended contact with participants yielded better weight loss. Therefore, longer duration of treatment has been consistently associated with greater weight loss.

3.3. Targets and Tools

The targets for the behavioral treatment of obesity include the individuals' eating and physical activity as well as ways in which they interact with the environment. The primary goal of treatment is to create negative energy balance, i.e., caloric expenditure exceeds caloric intake. Accomplishment of this goal requires many behavior and lifestyle alterations. In recent years, there has been a growing trend toward individually tailoring treatment. To accomplish individualized treatment plans, the weight management therapist needs many therapeutic "tools." These tools include self-monitoring, stimulus control, goal setting, behavioral contracting and reinforcement, nutrition education, meal planning, portion-controlled foods (e.g., meal replacements), modification of physical activity, social support, cognitive restructuring, and problem-solving. Each of these primary tools for change are described in Table 1; however, further description and research outcome related to the use of some of these tools is described below.

3.3.1. Meal planning. Prescribed meal plans are typically based on dietary exchange programs, utilization of portion controlled foods, or meal replacements, and/or structured meal planning. Use of structured meal plans with food provision (actually providing the persons with the appropriate food) can increase initial weight loss, but is no more effective in the long term than provision of a calorie goal such as 1000 to 1500 kcal/day. The most important component of structured meal plans is the provision of structure for foods that are to be consumed and the provision of grocery shopping lists. Therefore, it is not the provision of food per se that is important. Structured meal plans appear to be useful because they provide assistance for selecting healthy foods, and by creating a regular meal pattern (i.e., breakfast, lunch, dinner, snacks).

3.3.2. Portion control. Utilization of meal replacement plans (e.g., Slim Fast®) has also been studied. These studies prescribed meal plans for consuming 1200 to 1500 kcal per day by eating two or three meal replacements and one healthy meal, usually at dinner in the evening. This approach has yielded weight losses of 7 kg over the first 3 months of treatment, and 10.2 kg at 24-month follow-up for those who continued on meal replacements [18]. A meta-analysis of studies that included partial meal replacements and reduced calorie diets indicated that meal replacements were associated with greater weight loss and less attrition at 1 year compared to reduced calorie diets [19]. These studies suggest that meal replacements or portion-controlled foods facilitate adherence to the meal plan and the prescribed calorie level.

3.3.3. Modification of physical activity and exercise. Physical activity alone does not reliably produce significant weight loss, but physical activity is a predictor of long-term weight loss maintenance. A number of studies have investigated different aspects of physical activity and weight loss, including: (1) lifestyle activity vs. structured exercise, (2) long bout vs. short bout of exercise, and (3) home-based vs. group-based exercise. In long-term weight loss (1 year or longer follow-up), Wing [20] concluded that there was greater

Table 1. Behavioral strategies that can be used to promote weight loss and weight maintenance

Self-monitoring	Self-monitoring of food intake and physical activity helps people become aware of their eating and exercise habits. Self-monitoring also allows the counselor to monitor behaviors and note changes that occur over time.
Stimulus control	Stimulus control involves altering the environmental antecedents that affect eating and exercise behaviors. The environment is changed to provide cues for healthy behavior, such as eating healthy and exercising.
Goal setting/shaping	Setting small attainable goals helps foster motivation for behavior change and create feelings of accomplishment when they are achieved. As treatment progresses, the goals gradually become more challenging.
Behavioral contracting/ reinforcement	Rewarding oneself for attaining a goal helps maintain motivation for behavior change and give the person a sense of accomplishment.
Nutrition education	Patients are educated on the nutritional aspects of weight loss and weight maintenance.
Meal planning	Patients are encouraged to plan the type and amount of foods that are to be eaten for their meals. Meals should also be regularly scheduled.
Portion-controlled foods	Portion-controlled foods, including nutrition shakes and bars, and microwavable entrees, are an easy way for patients to eat healthy. These foods are affordable and easy to prepare and eat while away from home.
Modification of physical activity	Decreasing sedentary behavior and increasing physical activity are important for weight loss maintenance.
Social support	Social support may be derived from a spouse, family member, or friends. Family and friends are encouraged to support the patient in making lifestyle changes.
Cognitive restructuring	Cognitive restructuring helps patients identify and the negative consequences of dysfunctional thoughts, which might be associated with repeated dieting attempts, depressed mood, or body image dissatisfaction. Negative dysfunction thoughts can contribute to depressed mood and eating behavior. Patients are taught how to combat these thoughts and replace them with more adaptive ones.
Problem-solving	Problem-solving training teaches patients to systematically overcome problematic situations.

long-term weight loss for groups receiving diet plus exercise treatment, though the effects of the combined treatment were often only marginally better than those achieved by diet alone. It has been suggested that the limited long-term impact of exercise programs may be due to the inability of most people to maintain physical activity regimens over a long duration of time. With regard to improvement of exercise adherence, studies of supervised group exercise versus home-based approaches to physical activity have reported that home-based programs may have a long-term advantage, because they promote greater adherence. In addition, short-bout exercise prescription was shown to yield higher maintenance of physical activity in the long term (12 to 18 months) as well as overall better weight loss than long-bout exercise programs [14, 20].

The amount of exercise has been shown to be an important variable in the success in weight loss and weight maintenance over time. Typical exercise prescriptions recommended in behavioral weight loss programs consist of at least 150 minutes of moderate intensity physical activity per week. Nevertheless, it appears that the duration of physical activity is associated with long-term weight loss. Reports from the National Weight Control Registry (adults who have lost significant weight and maintained it for at least one year) have indicated that successful weight loss maintenance was achieved by an average of 2800 kcal per week of physical activity [21]. Thus, higher levels of exercise than are typically prescribed in behavioral programs may be necessary for long-term weight maintenance.

3.3.4.   Social support.   Enhancement of social support has been studied as a means for improving long-term weight loss [22]. The most common way to enhance social support has been to include spouses, family members, or close friends in the treatment process. These studies have reported that there are both short-term and long-term weight loss benefits for inclusion of strong family support [22].

3.3.5.   Satisfaction with weight loss.   Obese adults often have difficulty establishing reasonable weight loss goals. Setting unreasonable weight loss goals in the behavioral treatment of obesity often leads to disappointing outcomes and little motivation to continue adherence to treatment programs. A recent study [23] investigated whether informing obese persons of the expectation of a weight loss of 5% to 15% would influence them to adopt more realistic expectation for weight loss. This study found that simply providing information promoting an expectation of moderate weight loss (5% to 15%) had no significant impact on weight loss expectations. Therefore, if weight loss expectations are to be modified, it appears that a more intensive effort will be required.

3.4.   Weight Maintenance Strategies

The primary strategy used to facilitate weight maintenance is to extend the length of treatment and maintain longer therapeutic support and/or booster treatment as needed. The increased length of contact should result in continuous use of weight loss strategies, and thus, weight maintenance. Perri [17] concluded that the addition of therapist contact via the telephone and mail, significantly enhanced maintenance of weight loss for a group that received behavior therapy plus relapse prevention training. Similar results have been obtained with the use of booster sessions to enhance maintenance of weight loss [24].

3.4.1.   Internet approaches.   Also, in recent years, the Internet has been employed as a means of increasing therapist contact to improve long-term weight maintenance, and preliminary results of this approach are encouraging [25]. Overall, four studies have investigated the use of the internet for the purpose of delivering a weight management program in adults. The research designs of two of the studies [26, 27] compared the efficacy of interactive Internet-based interventions to health education Web sites. Both studies found a 2.5-kg difference between the two treatments at the end of 6 to 12 months. A third study [28] tested the efficacy of an Internet-based intervention as a weight maintenance strategy for adults who had lost weight using a face-to-face behavioral counseling approach. The study reported negative results in that the Internet-based intervention did not yield good weight maintenance in comparison to face-to-face contact. A recent study [29] reported no differences in weight maintenance results between face-to-face contact and Internet support. Thus, mixed evidence has been found for the efficacy of utilizing the Internet as a means for yielding long-term weight maintenance.

3.4.2.   Relapse prevention and problem solving.   There is a general consensus [24] that development of skills to respond immediately to overeating, periods of inactivity, or to small weight gains, is useful for long-term management of obesity. Relapse prevention is based on the idea that individuals will encounter "high-risk" situations that threaten behavior change. Relapse prevention training, which develops plans to cope with situations that place the person at risk for returning to previous unhealthy patterns of behaviors, is incorporated into many treatments for weight loss. An alternative approach for long-term weight maintenance is called problem-solving therapy, which has been found to be superior to relapse-prevention training for promoting long-term weight loss maintenance [30]. Problem-solving therapy advocates that patients require professional guidance and advice to effectively cope with situations that put their weight loss maintenance at risk. This model, therefore, involves continued contact with a professional.

3.5.   Special Considerations

3.5.1.   Cultural considerations.   Cultural issues may influence one's motivation and ability to succeed in weight loss. For example, the stigma of obesity varies across cultures, genders, and races. Women, more than men, are likely to attempt weight loss for appearance reasons. Men are more likely to enter into obesity treatment programs when they believe that their overweight status has negative health consequences or when they have been prompted by a health care professional. Generally, African Americans are less likely to experience social pressures to lose weight and may therefore be less motivated to seek treatment. For some individuals, it may be useful to emphasize health-related benefits of weight loss rather than appearance-based reasons for weight loss.

3.5.2.   Health considerations.   An individual's physical health must be considered when prescribing caloric restriction and/or a physical activity regimen. A physician should evaluate the safety of caloric restriction and increased exercise on an individual basis. A dietitian or nutritionist should be consulted to formulate dietary recommendations. Individuals with type 2 diabetes or cardiovascular disease may require special diets and medical monitoring throughout the course of any weight loss program. Further, overweight individuals may experience knee or other joint problems; in such cases, physical activity may be limited.

3.5.3.   Psychosocial consequences.   It is also important to consider the psychological sequelae of obesity. In American culture, there is a stigma associated with obesity. The "obesity stereotype" is that people who are overweight tend to be less socially competent, lazier, and less intelligent than normal weight individuals. In addition, most obese people have experienced various forms of discrimination and teasing about their weight. As a result, obese people often suffer from low self-esteem and may be very concerned about their body size and shape. In addition, many individuals may have attempted unsuccessfully to lose weight in the past, or they may have lost weight only to regain it later. A pattern of unsuccessful weight loss attempts frequently leads to frustration and lowered self-esteem. It is important that clinicians remain sensitive to these issues when treating obesity.

3.5.4.   Eating disorders.   Finally, it is important to identify individuals with eating disorders. The most common type of eating disorder associated with obesity is binge eating disorder (BED). BED is characterized by recurrent episodes of binge eating in which the individual consumes large amounts of food and perceives a loss of control over eating. Unlike the pattern of behavior observed in bulimia nervosa (BN), binge eating episodes in BED do not occur with compensatory behaviors to prevent weight gain (e.g., fasting, purging, excessive exercise). BED occurs in fewer than 2% of obese people, though binge-eating as a behavioral symptom is much more common. When such problems are identified, the treatment strategy should incorporate a component to reduce the frequency of binge episodes.

4.   BEHAVIORAL TREATMENT FOR CHILDREN AND ADOLESCENTS

4.1.   Approaches, Tools, and Outcomes

The main goal for treating pediatric obesity is the regulation of normal body weight, with consideration for growth and development [31]. Effective behavior change in children involves three primary components: (1) behavior therapy to foster healthier behavior change, (2) modification of diet, and (3) modification of physical activity habits. Tools for behavior change in children, just as in adults, often include reinforcement, stimulus control, behavioral contracting, self-monitoring, meal planning, modification of physical activity, problem solving, and social support. Intensive behavioral treatment programs generally yield weight losses of 6 to 10 kg during the initial weight loss induction phase that is completed in about 6 months [31]. Research studies have found that treatment spanning 1 year or more generally results in greater weight loss.

The Internet has also been utilized for the purpose of weight loss and maintenance in adolescents and children. Two studies related to pediatric obesity have been reported. A study reported by Baranowski et al. [32] tested the efficacy of an 8-week Internet-based intervention, for overweight 8-year-old African-American girls. The study did not yield significant weight changes in comparison to a control group. The second study, the Health Information Program for Teens (HIPTeens) project, is the only study that has reported the use of an Internet-based approach for weight *loss* in children or adolescents. The parents of these children were also overweight and were also targets of the Internet-based treatment. This study [33] yielded body fat loss for the adolescent girls and greater weight loss for their parents, providing further support for Internet-based interventions for weight loss. For more information on these approaches, see Williamson et al. [34].

4.2.   Reinforcement, Adherence, and Behavior Change

Frequent or daily reinforcement is necessary to foster motivation and adherence. This reinforcement most commonly comes from parents. From a behavioral viewpoint, positive reinforcement for healthy behavior is necessary to establish sustained behavior change. Over time, parents are likely to revert to punishment to influence children's behavior, which promotes negative parent–child interactions. Adherence to recommendations such as self-monitoring of diet and physical activity habits is extremely difficult for both the child and parent, and these records are frequently inaccurate. Therefore, the child and parent should work with the therapist to establish small attainable goals. They should establish clearly specified guidelines for treatment (called behavioral contracts) and, upon successful attainment of the goals, rewards should be provided. Children and adolescents can learn to monitor eating and exercise, but parents must assist by reminding and reinforcing completion of self-monitoring. Parents are also trained to use behavioral contracting, which generally includes some type of reinforcement contingency for successful attainment of the goal (e.g., child receives a music compact disc for meeting a weekly physical activity goal).

4.3.   Social Support and Parent Training

Parent involvement in treatment is recommended [22] to promote the enhancement of social support, which can be accomplished by inviting parents to treatment sessions. In these sessions, parents learn to be supportive of the child's progress (and reinforce healthy behavior change) and to avoid actions that sabotage progress. One reason for the significant impact of parental involvement on weight change is control over the home environment, including types and amounts of foods available, food preparation methods, and physical activity opportunities. Another reason for parental involvement and social support is to foster the morale and encourage the child in the behavior change process.

Research has provided support for not only parental involvement, but for specific types of parent training related to healthy eating and exercise. These findings support the inclusion of parents in childhood obesity treatment, even if the child is relatively unengaged in treatment.

4.4.   Problem-solving

In therapy sessions, parents and children are trained in problem-solving techniques to aid in identifying and solving potential situations that threaten success, particularly adherence in behavioral weight loss treatment. They learn to use these skills to promote adherence and to remove obstacles for successful weight management.

4.5.   Meal Planning

Several different dietary approaches have been reviewed with children including individualized dietary interventions, the diabetic exchange program, the "traffic-light" diet, and the protein-sparing modified fast (PSMF). Meal planning for children and adolescents relies on moderate calorie restriction (800 to 1000 kcal per day). More restrictive diets produce more weight loss in the short term. However, they produce long-term results similar to those of the less restrictive diets. It is important to note that the addition of nutrition education to the behavioral techniques of self-monitoring, behavioral contracting, positive reinforcement, and stimulus control procedures significantly improves reduction in percentage overweight, versus nutrition education alone [31].

4.6. Physical Activity

Exercise combined with dietary change improves childhood obesity greater than alteration of diet alone. Reduction of sedentary lifestyle behavior (versus programmed aerobic exercise), such as watching television, has been found to be a useful form of exercise prescription. When children are reinforced for less sedentary behavior they lose more weight and maintain better progress over time. However, it is important to note that reducing the duration of sedentary behavior may not necessarily promote children to allocate more time to physical activity.

Physical activity, combined with dietary changes, facilitates weight loss and long-term weight maintenance in children. Research on this topic has found that: (1) diet plus lifestyle groups maintained weight loss over time, whereas diet plus aerobic activity, diet plus callisthenic activity, and controls exhibited increases in weight over time, and (2) children reinforced for decreasing sedentary behavior and children reinforced for increasing physical activity showed comparable results in reduction of overweight. Thus, there may be a limit for the amount of physical activity that can be used to replace sedentary behavior.

4.7. Special Considerations

4.7.1. Health considerations. Once a child has been identified for weight control treatment, a medical evaluation is necessary to determine if a medical condition (e.g., hypothyroidism) is contributing to excess body weight or rapid weight gain. In addition, a child should receive medical clearance before increasing physical activity, a primary component of behavioral weight control interventions.

4.7.2. Cultural and family considerations. Special issues related to the treatment of pediatric weight problems include cultural factors, eating disorders, and motivation for lifestyle change. Ethnic and cultural factors should be considered when making recommendations. For example, dietary plans should take into consideration religious events or special dietary needs. Motivation for behavior change and adherence to recommendations are particularly problematic for children and adolescents, especially in an environment conducive to sedentary behavior and ingestion of large portions of energy-dense/high-calorie foods. In addition, motivation for lifestyle behavior change can be strongly impacted by culture. For example, some overweight African-American girls are relatively unconcerned about their weight status and may have fatalistic attitudes about the health risks associated with obesity.

The presence of child or parental psychopathology negatively affects weight loss and maintenance. Should psychopathology or family conflict be present, referrals for mental health treatment or family counseling to address these problems before initiating weight loss treatment may be appropriate. Finally, family support may not be universal and not all family members will support the behavioral changes necessary to promote weight loss for the child or adolescent who is the focus of therapy. For example, family members may offer poor food choices to the person in therapy, tease them, or reinforce their behavior with the provision of food.

4.7.3.   Eating disorders.   Another concern about dieting by children and adolescents is the development of eating disorder symptoms or the effect of dieting on the growth and development of children and adolescents. Research findings suggest that moderate calorie restriction might temporarily reduce growth rate, but there is no effect on long-term growth.

5.   CONCLUSIONS

In summary, research on weight control in children suggests that frequent or daily reinforcement facilitates behavior change and weight loss. In addition, weight loss is promoted by gradual or extended therapeutic contact. It is wise to present didactic information to the child at a pace that is flexible and promotes mastery of concepts. Providing children with perceived choices in therapy also promotes weight loss and longer therapy is generally associated with greater weight loss. Self-control training and cognitive therapy in the absence of parental support have not been found to promote long-term weight loss in children or adolescents. Therefore, the most effective treatment involves parents so that the child's environment is modified to promote healthy nutrition and physical activity, as well as the provision of adequate social support.

6.   SUMMARY

Behavioral weight control generally involves two phases: (1) weight loss induction and (2) weight maintenance. During the period of weight loss, energy intake via eating is reduced and energy expenditure resulting from physical activity is increased. During the period of weight maintenance, the person learns to match energy intake (eating habits) with energy expenditure (physical activity and exercise). The most effective behavioral weight loss programs have offered a combination of exercise, diet, and behavior modification. Specific treatment components can be used to enhance long-term successful weight management for adults and children. These components include, but are not limited to, (1) portion control and structured meal plans, (2) home-based and short-bout exercise prescriptions, (3) prolonged and regular therapeutic contact during weight loss induction, (4) utilization of social support throughout treatment, and (5) extended therapeutic contact or booster treatment to promote long-term weight maintenance. For long-term success, it is clear that the overweight person must sustain his or her efforts to change behavior patterns and prevent relapse by proactively modifying barriers to lifestyle behavior change. Further, behavioral weight management is most efficacious when the treatment plan is tailored to match an individual's cultural, social, and motivational circumstances.

REFERENCES

[1] Bray G, Bouchard C, James, P, eds. Handbook of Obesity. New York: Marcel Decker, 1999.
[2] U.S. Department of Health and Human Services. The Surgeon General's Call to Action to Prevent and Decrease Overweight and Obesity. Rockville, MD: U.S. Department of Health and Human Services, 2001.
[3] Flegal KM, Carroll MD, Ogden CL, Johnson CL. Prevalence and trends in obesity among US adults, 1999–2000. JAMA 2002;288:1723–1727.
[4] Ogden CL, Flegal KM, Carroll MD, Johnson CL. Prevalence and trends in overweight among children and adolescents, 1999–2000. JAMA 2002;288:1728–1732.
[5] Ogden CL, Fryar CD, Carroll MD, Flegal KM. Mean body weight, height, and body mass index, United States, 1960–2002. Advance data from vital and health statistics; no. 347. Hyattsville, MD: National Center for Health Statistics, 2004.
[6] Flegal KM, Carroll MD, Kuczmarski RJ, Johnson CL. Overweight and obesity in the United States: Prevalence and trends, 1960–1994. Int J Obes 1998;22:39–47.
[7] Flegal KM, Graubard BI, Williamson DF, Gail MH. Excess deaths associated with underweight, overweight, and obesity. JAMA 2005;293:1861–1874.
[8] Allison DB, Fontaine KR, Manson JE, Stevens J, VanItallie TB. Annual deaths attributable to obesity in the United States. JAMA 1999;282:1530–1538.
[9] Mokdad AH, Marks JS, Stroup DF, Geberding JL. Actual causes of death in the United States. JAMA 2000;291:1238–1245 [published correction appears in JAMA 2005; 293:298].
[10] Mark DH. Deaths attributable to obesity. JAMA 2005;293:1918–1919.
[11] Diabetes Prevention Program Research Group. Reduction in the incidence of type 2 diabetes with lifestyle intervention or metformin. N Engl J Med 2002;346:393–403.
[12] National Heart, Lung, and Blood Institute and the North American Association for the Study of Obesity. Practical Guide to the Identification, Evaluation, and Treatment of Overweight and Obesity in Adults, 1998.
[13] United States Department of Health and Human Services. Physical activity and health: A report of the Surgeon General, 1996.

[14] Wing RR. Behavioral weight control. In: Wadden T, Stunkard A, eds. Handbook of Obesity Treatment. New York: Guilford Press, 2002;301–316.

[15] Jeffrey RW, Drewnowski A, Epstein L, et al. Long-term maintenance of weight loss: Current status. Health Psychol 2000;19(1):5–16.

[16] Perri MG, Nezu AM, Viegener BJ, eds. Improving the Long-Term Management of Obesity: Theory, Research, and Clinical Guidelines. New York: John Wiley, 1992.

[17] Perri MG. The maintenance of treatment effects in the long-term management of obesity. Clin Psychol Sci Pract 1998;5:526–543.

[18] Ditschuneit HH, Fletchtner-Mors M, Johnson TD, et al. Metabolic and weight loss effects of a long-term dietary intervention in obese patients. Am J Clin Nutr 1999;69:198–204.

[19] Heymsfield SB, van Mierlo CA, van der Knaap HC, Heo M, Frier HI. Weight management using a meal replacement strategy: Meta and pooling analysis from six studies. Int J Obes Relat Metab Disord 2003;27(5):537–549.

[20] Wing RR. Physical activity in the treatment of the adulthood overweight and obesity: Current evidence and research issues. Med Sci Sports Exerc 1999;31:S547–S552.

[21] Klem ML, Wing RR, McGuire MT, et al. A descriptive study of individuals successful at long-term maintenance of substantial weight loss. Am J Clin Nutr 1997;66:39–246.

[22] McLean N, Griffin S, Toney K, Hardeman W. Family involvement in weight control, weight maintenance, and weight-loss interventions: A systematic review of randomized trials. Int J Obes 2003;27:987–1005.

[23] Wadden TA, Womble LG, Sarwer DB, et al. Great expectations: "I'm losing 25% of my weight no matter what you say". J Clin Consult Psychol 2003;71(6):1084–1089.

[24] Perri MG, Corsica JA. Improving the maintenance of weight loss in behavioral treatment of obesity. In: Wadden T, Stunkard A, eds. Handbook of Obesity Treatment. New York: Guilford Press, 2002;357–394.

[25] Tate D, Wing RR, Winett R. Development and evaluation of an Internet behavior therapy program for weight loss. JAMA 2001;285:1172–1177.

[26] Tate DF, Wing RR, Winett RA. Using Internet technology to deliver a behavioral weight loss program. JAMA 2001;285:1172–1177.

[27] Tate DF, Jackvony EH, Wing RR. Effects of Internet behavioral counseling on weight loss in adults at risk for type 2 diabetes: A randomized trial. JAMA 2003;289:1833–1836.

[28] Harvey-Berino J, Pintauro S, Buzzell P, et al. Does using the Internet facilitate the maintenance of weight loss? Int J Obes Metab Dis 2002;26:1254–1260.

[29] Harvey-Berino J, Pintauro S, Buzzell P, Gold EC. Effect of Internet support on the long-term maintenance of weight loss. Obes Res 2004;12:320–329.

[30] Perri MG, Nezu AM, McKelvey WF, Shermer RL, Renjilian DA, Viegener BJ. Relapse prevention training and problem-solving therapy in the long-term management of obesity. J Consult Clin Psychol 2001;69(4):722–726.

[31] Goldfield GS, Raynor HA, Epstein LH. Treatment of pediatric obesity. In: Wadden T, Stunkard A, eds. Handbook of Obesity Treatment. New York: Guilford Press, 2002;532–555.

[32] Baronowski T, Baronowski JC, Cullen KW, et al. The Fun, Food, and Fitness Project (FFFP): The Baylor GEMS pilot study. Ethnicity Dis 2003;13:S30–S39.

[33] White MA, Davis Martin P, Newton RL, et al. Mediators of weight loss in a family-based intervention presented over the internet. Obes Res 2004;12:1–10.

[34] Williamson DA, Walden H, York-Crowe E, Stewart TM. Internet-based treatment for pediatric obesity. In: Handbook of Pediatric Obesity: Vol. 2, Clinical Management. New York: Marcel Dekker (in press).

Chapter 14

Obesity Prevention

Shiriki K. Kumanyika[a] and Stephen R. Daniels[b]

[a]*Department of Biostatistics and Epidemiology, Department of Pediatrics, and Graduate Program in Public Health Studies, University of Pennsylvania School of Medicine, Philadelphia, PA 19104, USA*
[b]*Departments of Pediatrics and Environmental Health, Cincinnati Children's Hospital Medical Center and the University of Cincinnati College of Medicine, Cincinnati, OH 45267, USA*

1. INTRODUCTION

As of 2002, 30% of U.S. adults were obese and 16% of children and adolescents were overweight or obese,[1] reflecting increases in recent decades, with no sign of a decrease [1]. Obesity prevalence is even higher within some ethnic minority populations [2, 3]. Socioeconomic inequalities in obesity vary by age, ethnicity, and gender [4–6] and are changing over time [7, 8]. In the Coronary Artery Risk Development in Young Adults (CARDIA) study, men and women who were ages 18 to 30 years when enrolled in 1985–1986 were 7 to 12 kg (15 to 26 lb) heavier 10 years later, with larger weight gains observed in the younger part of the age range and among those who were heavier at baseline [9]. Obesity prevalence percentages increased from 24 to 42 in white women, from 48 to 72 in black women, from 35 to 60 in white men, and from 32 to 66 in black men. These statistics make a compelling case for obesity treatment and prevention.

Obesity treatment is difficult, costly, and often successful only over the short term [3, 10]. Hence, high priority is placed on preventing the progression of overweight into the obese range. The challenge of obesity prevention should not be underestimated [11, 12]. In 1990, national goals to reduce obesity prevalence were set for the year 2000, but the virtual impossibility of meeting these goals was evident even before 1995 [13]. Midway to the *Healthy People 2010* goals the situation has worsened [14]. Current obesity levels are double the target of 15% for adults and more than three times the target of 5% for children.

In this chapter, we review the scope and nature of the task of obesity prevention as it relates to both adults and children in the U.S. population. We provide a conceptual overview and some examples for different levels or types of prevention approaches, with comments on clinical implications.

2. DEFINING THE TASK

2.1. Individual Level Perspective

There is ultimately only one mechanism for achieving obesity prevention—enabling individuals to maintain energy balance such that inappropriate weight gain does not occur or small gains are quickly compensated [15, 16]. The relevant modifiable influences are determinants of caloric intake (food and beverage intake), energy expenditure (physical activity at work, home, and leisure), and the relationship between these variables. In the current environment, a gradual escalation of weight toward the obese end of the continuum has become typical. The challenge is to achieve energy balance in a manner compatible with good overall mental and physical health and (in children) also with healthy growth and development. Metabolic rate—the other main component of energy balance—is not under personal control and is, therefore, not targeted directly in preventive efforts.

Although there is some physiological ability to regulate the balance between caloric intake and caloric expenditure, this regulation is apparently not effective in the majority of individuals. Other than calculating energy consumed and expended based on food and activity diaries, a process that is relatively imprecise, there is no way for a person to assess the results of efforts to maintain day-to-day energy balance until weight changes. Theoretically, an error of an excess 100 calories (a difference equivalent to eating an entire large cookie vs. only two-thirds of it) in estimating daily energy balance could lead to a 1-pound weight gain if extended over about a month or 10 pounds over a year. This small excess can occur as a result of changes in eating or physical activity, or with altered energy needs due to changes in body composition or developmental stage. This small excess in calories can also occur as a result of environmental changes—increases in the portion size and caloric content of regularly consumed packaged food or being assigned a parking space that requires a shorter walk to and from the office. The substantial decreases in calorie intake or increases in expenditure required for weight reduction are difficult to achieve but relatively easy to identify when made. By contrast, in weight gain prevention the needed changes or day-to-day corrections in eating and activity may be small and difficult to track.

The obesity epidemic is driven by environmental and behavioral variables that predispose to overeating and inactivity [15]. These variables are the presumed targets of preventive interventions. The rapid increase in obesity prevalence over time is one type of evidence that genetic mechanisms, which evolve very slowly, are not driving the trends. The increases in weight associated with modernization and migration also show the important role of the environment in determining the expression of an underlying predisposition to excess weight gain [2, 15, 17, 18].

The prevention of obesity in children presents some unique challenges. From the onset of fetal growth through late adolescence, children are growing in height. This means that there is a consistent increase in lean body mass. Simultaneous with changes in lean body mass, there are also normal changes in adiposity. Hence, in children and youth the goal is to maintain appropriate amounts of fat accumulation in relation to growth of bone and muscle mass [16]. In practice this is complex. As in adults, children's energy intake and expenditure are difficult to measure precisely on a day-to-day basis. On a longer term basis, lean and fat mass are difficult to measure in the clinical setting. Clinicians can follow height, weight, and body mass index (BMI) as a more general guide to excess weight gain.

2.2. Population Perspective

Figure 1 shows the multiple layers of interacting individual, societal, and environmental variables that influence eating and physical activity behaviors in populations, as described elsewhere in detail [19, 20]. These variables are now heavily skewed toward overconsumption and inactivity [12, 21]. Influences in the "psychobiologic core" are geared to avoiding hunger but underdeveloped with respect to setting limits at the upper end of caloric intake. Psychosocial, ethnocultural, and lifestyle variables are entrenched; inherently resistant to change; and also continually reinforced by local, national, and global societal level variables acting through behavioral settings related to lifestyles, media, and marketing practices [12, 22–24].

As indicated by the continuing upward trajectory of population weight levels not only in the United States but also in many other countries [15, 23], the pervasive, societal level obesity promoting forces are not self correcting. The economic and technological drivers and related social and cultural patterns are not necessarily responsive to health issues. A social transformation will be needed to reshape these influences in a direction more favorable to population weight control, akin to the social movements that have resulted in an altered landscape with respect to tobacco use and automotive safety [25, 26]. Long-term obesity prevention strategies are geared to fostering such social transformations.

2.3. Goals and Priorities

"Obesity prevention" includes several complementary goals: (1) to prevent "healthy" or "normal" weight adults and children from crossing the threshold to overweight or obese; (2) to prevent overweight adults and children from becoming obese; (3) to prevent obese children from becoming obese adults; and (4) to maintain a nonobese state in those who have been obese but have lost weight [15]. Hence, prevention approaches are needed in the population

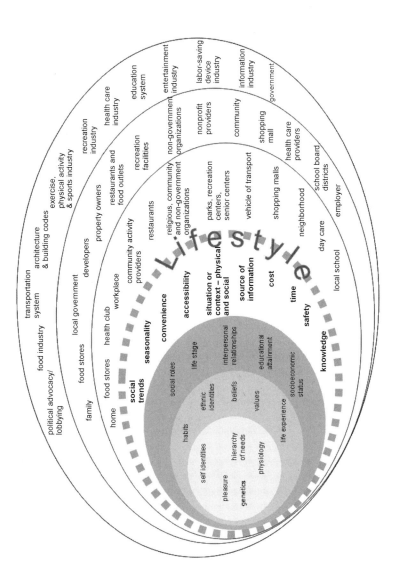

Figure 1. Framework for determinants of physical activity and eating behavior. Levels of influence, beginning with the innermost circle, are the Psychobiological Core, Cultural Influences, Social Influences, and Enablers of Choice, which together constitute "Lifestyle." Additional layers of influence are Behavioral Settings, Primary Leverage Points, and Secondary Leverage Points. See [19] and [20] for detailed explanations of these influences. (Reprinted with permission from [19]. Copyright, International Life Sciences Institute, 2001.)

at large, in groups or subpopulations at particularly high risk and in those with identified weight problems. Adapting terminology from the World Health Organization categorization of obesity prevention approaches [15], these approaches will be referred to, respectively, as "population-level" or "population wide," "selective," or "individually targeted."

Strong arguments can be made for giving priority to preventive interventions in both adults and children [26, 27]. Initiatives for children may be more socially or politically acceptable because, for children, it is clearer that society has a broad responsibility for health protection. However, the trajectory of weight gain during adulthood and the associated morbidity and mortality render prevention efforts directed to adults very cost effective [27]. In addition, these same adults may control the environments of children.

3.   POPULATION-WIDE APPROACHES

Population-level prevention attempts "to control the determinants of incidence, to lower the mean level of risk factors, to shift the whole distribution of exposure in a favorable direction" [28, p. 37]. These approaches are often termed "passive," i.e., they operate through systems or structures without requiring deliberate actions by individuals to have an effect. For obesity prevention, these approaches involve social marketing campaigns, policy development, and programmatic initiatives to change aspects of the social structure related to food access and physical activity options. Such approaches are most appropriate and most cost-effective where obesity prevalence is high [15]. They are cost-effective because they do not require time- and cost-intensive screening and counseling programs. The aim is to create trends in population behaviors that will ultimately decrease overeating and inactivity levels. Taken together these approaches can increase the motivation to bring eating and physical activity patterns in line with energy balance needs, make the targeted behaviors more normative, and make them easier to achieve. Population approaches, by definition, are impossible to link to benefit for any given individual [28]. Unfortunately, this makes them easy targets for opposition from those who argue that policy or environmental changes threaten personal freedoms.

Health care professionals may be skeptical about population-wide approaches, being more attuned to and skilled in individual level, interpersonal interventions than to social marketing and policy change approaches [29, 30] and equally unfamiliar with and unskilled in the sectors and disciplines that control many of the determinants of food intake and physical activity (see Figure 1). The political nature of taking on the powerful stakeholders who control these sectors may be another deterrent to the engagement of health professionals in this type of prevention.

The development of environmental and policy approaches to obesity prevention is an emerging field [31, 32]. Reviews of ongoing initiatives give a clear sense of the potential in this area, but few programs have been evaluated to date. Multiple, integrated changes are needed across multiple settings—some targeted to food and some to physical activity. However, when interventions are undertaken in entire communities it is difficult to match assessment of the impact of the changes to the specific population likely to have been affected by them. In the short term, success is measured by changes in the aspects of policy or resources that are directly targeted. Over the longer term, success is measured by downward shifts in the population BMI distribution [12].

3.1.   Initiatives Related to Food

Population-level strategies for improving access to healthful foods often focus on fruits and vegetables, for example, by establishing regular farmers' markets, subsidizing the provision of free fresh fruits and vegetables to school children, lowering the cost of fruits and vegetables while increasing the price of high-fat or high-sugar foods in school or worksite cafeterias, or changing marketing strategies in other ways that increase fruit and vegetable consumption [33–36]. Other initiatives seek to increase healthy food access by attracting supermarkets to areas in need, limiting low-nutrition foods in school vending machines or other food outlets, or taxing high-calorie, low-nutrition foods in the community at large [37]. There is concern that taxation approaches may selectively disadvantage low-income individuals who may depend on inexpensive sources of calories [38]. Incentives or regulation to reverse marketing practices such as "supersizing" food portions, targeting promotion of high-calorie, low nutrient density foods to children, or to require explicit labeling of the caloric content of packaged foods and restaurant or take-home meals are other potential strategies [26, 37].

3.2.   Initiatives Related to Physical Activity

Population-level approaches to improving options for physical activity include a range of strategies to reformulate and reengineer aspects of the "built environment" that predispose to sedentary behavior [19, 32]. The "built environment" refers to the way communities are designed, for example, types and configurations of housing, availability of sidewalks and bicycle paths, connectivity of streets and general pedestrian versus automobile friendliness, zoning regulations that determine the mix of residential and business uses in a given area, recreational facilities, transportation systems, and safety considerations. Built environment issues also apply to urban design and space use patterns that influence food access, but the term is used most often in relation to physical activity. The built environment refers also to physical layout and quality and quantity of facilities available at worksites or schools and policies governing access to these facilities. For example, at worksites, improving the attractiveness, safety, and accessibility of stairwells may be effective in increasing the use of stairs rather than elevators, particularly when accompanied by prompts (signs) encouraging stair use [39].

Approaches to improving the built environment for physical activity follow logically from the nature of the identified constraints, for example, instituting policies to limit or calm automobile traffic and build sidewalks and bicycle paths in order to favor walking or biking (termed "active transport") [40]. Efforts to increase the number of children who walk to school include programs such as "walking school buses" in which parents take turns walking groups of children to school, or "safe routes to school" which—as the name implies—focuses on addressing traffic and other issues to enable active transport of children to and from school on their own. Identifying or shaping the potential for some of these initiatives may be done synergistically, that is, related to public works projects undertaken for other reasons. Other interventions involve implementing policies that optimize aspects of new community development or construction projects from a physical activity perspective [32, 40].

3.3. Social Marketing

Social marketing is a key element of population level approaches because it increases the likelihood that structural changes will be acceptable to and taken advantage of by the general public. The National Cancer Institute's 5 A Day for Better Health program is a well recognized fruit and vegetable promotion, although its effectiveness in changing average fruit and vegetable intake has not been established [41]. VERB™—It's What you Do! is a CDC campaign designed to increase physical activity among ethnically diverse 9- to 13-year-olds (tweens) and, as a secondary audience, their parents [42]. Positive effects were seen relatively early in this campaign but final results of the evaluation have not yet been published. The "Healthier US" initiative http://www.healthierus.gov/ links a variety of federal government initiatives that promote healthier lifestyles directly to consumers as well as programs that support community level programming to promote healthful lifestyles. "America on the Move" (www.americanonthemove.org) is a social marketing initiative that encourages public–private partnerships to improve eating and activity patterns of the public.

4. PREVENTION TARGETED TO SELECTED POPULATION GROUPS

Candidates for selective prevention include (1) individuals who are overweight but not yet obese; (2) people at life stages associated with accelerated rates of weight gain, for example, young adults in general, women during pregnancy, the postpartum period, and the perimenopausal period; (3) ethnic and demographic groups with a higher than average obesity prevalence, such as several ethnic minority populations and some low-income populations; and (4) individuals at risk for accelerated weight gain for other reasons, for example, after smoking cessation [43] or during treatment with medications that are known to cause excess weight gain [44, 45]. Pregnancy and postpartum interventions can facilitate obesity prevention in children by encouraging more and longer breastfeeding [46]. Children of obese parents are also a high-risk group for obesity development and can potentially be identified through adult-oriented weight control programs. Selective approaches occur in settings that facilitate access to various audiences for obesity prevention activities and programs.

4.1.   Adults

The four studies in Table 1 are among the best available examples of obesity prevention addressing adults. Participants include nonobese young adults or young adults in general [47, 48] and women at risk of excess weight gain associated with reproductive stage [49–51]. The Pound of Prevention Study (see Table 1) [48, 52] is probably the largest and most general obesity prevention study reported to date. The design of this study reflects the principle that the public health impact of such programs will depend on reaching a relatively large number of people at relatively low cost. However, while this study demonstrated feasibility, some positive behavioral changes, and a lack of harm (i.e., there was no increase in unhealthful weight control practices), the interventions were not successful in preventing weight gain relative to the control condition. The finding that behavioral changes were in the expected direction suggests that this type of program might work, but perhaps at a higher intensity. Decreased fat intake and increased physical activity were the strongest predictors of weight maintenance [52]. The Leermakers et al. study [47] suggests the utility of well designed nutrition and physical activity behavior change programs for weight gain prevention, but it was not clear which of the effective interventions would be the least costly and potentially replicable for a larger audience. The short-term nature of this study is also a potential limitation in understanding its potential for obesity prevention, which is by nature a long-term prospect. A potentially effective approach to long-term weight gain prevention is illustrated in the 5-year results from the Healthy Women's Study [49, 50]. Behavioral counseling was effective at 6 months, preventing a net weight gain over the transition to menopause. The intervention program appears to have been well received, judging from retention rates, but it seems labor and cost-intensive to deliver.

Table 1. Examples of prevention studies in populations selected for high risk of obesity: adults

Reference	Study population	Study objective and design	Key results
Leermakers et al. [47]	Healthy men ($n = 67$); ethnicity 88% white; ages 25–40 years with a BMI of 22–30 kg/m² (mean ~ 26 kg/m²); recruited from a university setting; 75% had a graduate degree.	The study objective was to compare two 4-month treatments (clinic- or home-based version) to increase aerobic exercise and reduce fat intake with a delayed-treatment control group in a 4-month randomized trial. The clinic-based program was a group-based supervised diet and exercise program with eight week weekly and then four biweekly meetings. A similar home-based program involved one initial group meeting followed by mail and telephone contact. A fat intake of ~20% of kcal was targeted.	The treatment (both conditions) vs. control difference (−1.6 vs. +0.2 kg) was statistically significant for weight ($p < 0.01$) but not % body fat (assessed with BIA; $p = 0.12$). Results for the clinic- vs. home-based program were not significantly different for either variable.
Jeffery et al. [48]	Healthy adults ages 20 to 45 years ($n = 228$ men; 998 women); ethnicity 90% white; mean BMI 27 kg/m² (no BMI eligibility restriction); recruited from the general population, with special outreach to low socioeconomic status groups.	The Pound of Prevention Study objective was a randomized trial to test two low-cost, minimal contact educational interventions (education only or education plus incentives) to promote small dietary changes for weight gain prevention over a 3-year period, compared to a no-contact control condition. The primary intervention was a monthly mailed newsletter, with additional incentives and optional semi-annual low-cost activities.	Weight increased by 0.5–0.6 kg/year, with no significant differences between the three groups ($p = 0.75$ to 0.93 for years 1, 2, and 3).
Simkin-Silverman et al. [49], Kuller et al. [50]	Healthy premenopausal women ($n = 535$) ages 44–50 at enrollment; BMI 20–34 kg/m² (mean	The Women's Healthy Lifestyle Project was a randomized trial to test a behavioral, dietary, and physical activity program vs. an assessment-only	Weight change (kg) was −4.9 vs. −0.4 in intervention vs. control at 6 months and −0.1 vs. +2.4 at 54 months (both

Table 1. (Continued)

Reference	Study population	Study objective and design	Key results
	25 kg/m^2); 35% of women were postmenopausal by the end of the study).	control group to prevent peri-menopausal weight gain. The intervention targeted modest weight loss to prevent weight gain above baseline by the end of the study. Behavioral goals were calorie and fat reduction and increased physical activity. Initial contact was weekly for 15 weeks (group sessions), then less frequent, with refresher courses, mail and telephone contact for the duration of follow-up.	$p < 0.01$). A similar pattern was observed when results were stratified by normal weight, overweight, and obese status at baseline.
Olson et al. [51]	Rural, white population; Intervention cohort: healthy pregnant women ($n = 179$); 94% were ages 20–40 years; normal BMI or overweight; recruited from obstetrical clinics before the third trimester of pregnancy. Controls: similar women ($n = 381$) from an observational study conducted 3–5 years prior in the same health system.	Objective was to limit excess weight gain and decrease postpartum weight retention in the intervention cohort vs. the historical controls. The intervention consisted of clinical provider guidance and monitoring regarding weight gain supplemented by a mail-based educational component (tools for monitoring weight gain and diet and newsletters with return postcards that qualified the women for a prize drawing). Women were followed through 12 months postpartum.	No overall intervention vs. control difference in gestational weight gain was observed (14.1 vs. 14.8, respectively [$p = 0.09$]). However, among low-income women only (interaction $p = 0.02$, the percent with more than recommended weight gain was lower in intervention vs. control (33% vs. 52%, $p < 0.01$). For post partum weight retention, a significant benefit was observed in low-income overweight women and high-income, normal weight women (three-way interaction of BMI, income, and treatment group; $p = 0.008$).

BIA, bioelectrical impedance analysis; BMI, body mass index.

Mail-based or correspondence approaches similar to those used in the Pound of Prevention Study have been applied to obesity prevention in young women [53], including postpartum women [54], with some success. Olson [51] used such a correspondence approach in conjunction with clinic-based monitoring as a strategy to prevent excess pregnancy weight gain and postpartum weight retention (see Table 1). The program was effective in limiting pregnancy weight gain, but only in low-income women. For postpartum weight retention the effect was differential by initial weight status and income. Polley et al. [55] found an almost identical effect on prevention of excess weight gain in low-income women who were initially normal weight. This was in a different type of study population and with a more intensive intervention program and was accompanied by the potentially troubling suggestion of an opposite effect in the initially overweight women (i.e., more excess weight gain in those who received the intervention).

In spite of the lack of an evidence-base to clearly support guidelines as to how obesity prevention can be achieved in clinical settings, there appears to be support for the general concept of prevention and some straightforward minimum guidance that can be provided to adults. The National Heart, Lung and Blood Institute (NHLBI) Clinical Guidelines for the Identification, Evaluation and Treatment of Overweight and Obesity in Adults [3] recommend routine height and weight screening and BMI assessment. Adults with a BMI between 25 and 29.9 kg/m^2 who have one or no other cardiovascular risk factors should attempt to maintain their current weight rather than attempt weight loss. Regular moderate physical activity is identified as a critical component of a successful lifestyle to maintain weight after weight loss, which involves adjusting to lower energy needs than at the prior weight, along with consumption of a low-calorie/low-fat diet and frequent weight monitoring [56]. This is consistent with the recommendations for obesity prevention within the 2005 U.S. Dietary Guidelines [57]: (1) monitoring body fat, using BMI as a surrogate measure, (2) making small decreases in caloric intake to prevent gradual weight gain over time, and (3) obtaining 60 minutes of moderate-to-vigorous intensity physical activity per day. The basis for these guidelines is theoretical, i.e., these are simply more modest forms of the behaviors that have been proven to promote weight loss.

4.2. Children

Schools have been the primary venue for obesity prevention studies in children [58]. Children spend much time in school, learn about health behaviors, and engage in eating and physical activity behaviors in the school setting. School-based intervention studies have generally disappointing results, although more encouraging than in adults. While knowledge and behaviors have improved, weight status has often not been altered [59]. It is unclear after what duration a significant effect on body fat or body weight can occur. Some studies have had interventions as long as 3 years [60]. Community-based studies have also generally been ineffective in prevention of excess weight gain in children [23]. An issue with these studies is that it is hard to isolate the intervention and control groups. As with studies in adults, the control group may also improve knowledge and behaviors, reducing the treatment versus control group difference.

Four studies of prevention of obesity in children and youth in different settings are presented in Table 2 [61–64]. All of these studies found significant improvement in variables related to obesity or body composition and they represent the current best approaches with the strongest evidence base. On the other hand, none has been replicated and not all found consistent results across all subjects or consistent results regarding change in behaviors and measures of obesity.

Numerous organizations [16, 65] have recommended that primary care physicians follow BMI percentiles over time and implement both population based and individual-based strategies for obesity prevention. The population-based strategy is aimed at improving the diet and level of physical activity in all children, while the individual strategy identifies children at higher risk of obesity and implements a more aggressive intervention approach. BMI percentiles, available through the CDC, can also be used longitudinally to determine if a child is crossing percentiles to increasingly elevated levels [66].

There are benefits to primary care efforts for obesity prevention in childhood. First, the attention of the physician to the problem may be an important motivating factor for the patient or family. Second, the physician has longitudinal follow-up of patients and families. This places physicians in the optimum position for identifying those at higher risk for obesity development. Third, the pediatrician's office is a frequent venue for disease prevention such as immunizations, advice on safety, and so forth. Finally, pediatricians are an important source of information about diet and physical activity for children.

The optimum approach to prevention of childhood obesity in the primary care setting involves associated health professionals. There should be an overall emphasis on healthy diet, activity, growth, and development. This should include longitudinal monitoring of height, weight, and BMI. It should also include general counseling on diet starting with promotion of breast feeding, helping families make the transition to a healthy adult diet, and assisting adolescents in avoiding external pressures for less healthy eating. Primary care physicians should also provide counseling on developmentally appropriate physical activity and limits of sedentary time.

Primary care physicians can identify children at higher risk for obesity development, such as those with obese parents or siblings. Intervention for these

Table 2. Examples of prevention studies in populations selected for high-risk obesity: children

Reference	Study population	Study objective and design	Key results
Harvey-Berino et al. [61]	Native American mothers (St. Regis Mohawk Community) with BMI > 25 kg/m^2 and their toddlers ($n = 43$ dyads); mean age, mothers 26.5 years, toddlers 22 months; mean BMI in mothers 29.9; mean weight for height z score for toddlers 0.73.	The study objective was to determine whether maternal participation in an obesity prevention plus parenting support intervention would reduce the prevalence of obesity compared to a parenting support only intervention. Trained peer educators delivered the 16-week interventions one on one in the home. The obesity prevention intervention focused on improved parenting skills to facilitate children's development of appropriate eating and exercise behaviors.	Weight for height z scores decreased (-0.27 ± 1.1) in the combined intervention and increased (0.31 ± 1.1) in the parent support only group ($p = 0.06$). Children in the combined intervention had decreased energy intake (-316 ± 835 vs. 197 ± 608, $p < 0.05$).
Gortmaker et al. [62]	6th and 7th grade students ($n = 1295$), mean age 11.7 years, 48% female, 69% white, 11% African American, 11% Hispanic, 9% Asian Pacific, 2% American Indian; 5% other.	The objective of the study was to evaluate the impact of a school based health behavior intervention (Planet Health) on obesity. This was a randomized controlled field trial with five intervention and five control schools. The school based intervention occurred over 2 school years and included sessions on decreasing television viewing, high fat foods with increased fruit and vegetable intake and physical activity.	The prevalence of obesity decreased among girls in intervention schools compared to controls (odds ratio 0.47, 95% CI 0.24–0.93). There was also greater remission of obesity among intervention compared to control girls (odds ratio 2.16, 95% CI 1.07–4.35). The intervention resulted in reduced hours of television viewing in boys and girls and increased fruit and vegetable consumption in girls.

Table 2. (Continued)

Reference	Study population	Study objective and design	Key results
Robinson et al. [63]	3rd and 4th grade students ($n = 192$), mean age 8.9 years; parent ethnicity ~75% white.	The objective of the study was to assess the effects of reducing television, videotape and video game usage on changes in adiposity, physical activity and diet. This was a randomized controlled school based trial in two sociodemographically and scholastically matched schools. The intervention was an 18-lesson, 6-month classroom curriculum. Each intervention household received an electronic television time manager to aid with budgeting TV time.	Children in the intervention group had a statistically significant relative decrease in BMI compared to controls ($p = 0.002$). They also had significant improvement of triceps skin fold thickness, waist circumference and waist hip ratio and reductions in time viewing television and meals eaten in front of the television.
Fitzgibbon [64]	Children participating in Head Start ($n = 409$), mean age 48.6 months (intervention) and 50.8 months control; 99% of those in the intervention group were African American while 80.7% in the control group were African American, 12.7% Latino, 6.6% other.	The objective was to evaluate the effect of a culturally appropriate intervention (Hip-Hop to Health junior) on diet and physical activity and changes in BMI, with six Head Start Centers randomly assigned to the weight control intervention or a general health intervention. The 14-week intervention included a nutrition and physical activity curriculum and teacher-led aerobic exercise offered 3 times per week; parents received newsletters and information linked to the children's curriculum.	Children in the intervention group had a significantly smaller increase in BMI compared to control children at 1 year follow-up ($p = 0.01$) and at 2-year follow-up ($p = 0.02$). At year 1 follow-up there was a significant difference in percent of calories from fat (intervention 11.6% vs. control 12.8%, $p = 0.02$).

higher risk children should be more aggressive and may include involvement of dietitians, exercise specialists, social workers, and psychologists or behavioral therapists. The important role of the primary care physician is underscored by the medical complications of obesity that are now being seen in children and adolescents with obesity (e.g., type 2 diabetes mellitus, obstructive sleep apnea, and hypertension). Without an aggressive approach to prevention in high-risk children and adolescents, the primary care physician will have an increasing number of patients with chronic and sometimes debilitating problems.

Pediatricians and other primary care physicians are also important community advocates. This means that their opinions are respected and they are in a position to advocate for and support community and school-based efforts to improve diet and physical activity in children.

5.   INDIVIDUALLY TARGETED APPROACHES

Those appropriate for individually targeted prevention efforts include obese children, to prevent them from becoming obese adults, and adults who are already obese, to prevent their obesity from being more severe. Targeted prevention relies on the general screening and treatment strategies that apply to obese children [67] and adults [3, 10]. Targeted prevention for those with moderate obesity emphasizes behavioral strategies rather than invasive approaches such as drugs or surgery. Preventing weight regain in people who have lost weight can be included in this category. However, currently available guidelines for obesity treatment are uninformative with respect to long-term approaches to weight maintenance after weight loss [10]. Data from the National Weight Control Registry, although based on a very self-selected population, appear to be useful in this respect [56].

6.   MULTILEVEL APPROACHES

Combining interventions across two or three levels can be effective in a given community, although no definitive evidence of this has been reported to date. Some well designed and rigorously conducted multilevel interventions have been undertaken. However, these interventions have apparently not included the right mix or dose of a sufficient number of obesity determinants to be effective. For example, community-wide programs to prevent cardiovascular disease (CVD) conducted in the Minnesota, northern California, and Rhode Island areas constituted a first generation of sustained multilevel risk reduction approaches with a potential to impact on body weight. Two programs reported significantly less weight gain in the intervention versus control communities [68, 69] but a pooled analysis across all three programs concluded that there was essentially no intervention versus control difference in body weight trends, which increased at all sites [70].

Multilevel interventions have also been attempted in children. The Pathways study, conducted in 41 schools in 7 American Indian communities over a 3-year period, attempted to reduce percent body fat of 3rd, 4th, and 5th graders [60]. The intervention included a culturally adapted classroom based curriculum, changes to the school food service, physical education classes and increased physical activity in the classroom and at recess, and information and activities for the children's families. Some favorable knowledge and behavior changes were observed but neither percent body fat nor physical activity levels differed in intervention versus control schools.

7.   METHODOLOGICAL CONSIDERATIONS

There has been a recent upsurge in funding for research on obesity prevention [31, 32, 71]; also see http://www.obesityresearch.nih.gov. To date, only a handful of studies are available, and even fewer qualify for systematic reviews [23, 58, 71–73]. The slim evidence base led the U.S. Preventive Services Task Force to conclude that there is insufficient evidence for or against routine screening of children and adolescents for overweight in a primary care setting [67]. We could identify no controlled trials of obesity prevention research in a primary care setting in either adults or children. However, successful interventions on diet (e.g., to decrease fat intake or increase fruit and vegetable or fiber intake) or physical activity (to increase physical activity or decrease inactivity), undertaken to reduce or manage risk associated with cardiovascular diseases, diabetes, and cancer [39, 74–78] may also be relevant, although it is perhaps easier to alter dietary quality or physical activity than to align the two to achieve energy balance.

The difficulty of obesity prevention may be more with the nature of the task than with the quality of the available studies [71]. Periodic health-related advice to make and maintain small changes in eating and physical activity may be ineffective against a continuous stream of aggressive and sophisticated marketing of high-calorie food and sedentary entertainment products and lifestyles. Preventive interventions may be less intensive than in weight loss programs because the changes needed are smaller and also because the benefit to risk ratio of exhorting individuals to make major changes in eating and physical activity patterns is less clear than when obesity is already present. Concerns about inadvertently contributing to inappropriate dieting in a normal weight population may limit the specificity of advice about caloric restriction, particularly in programs for children and adolescents.

From a research perspective, several factors potentially bias obesity prevention studies toward findings of no effect. The changes desired are small—no weight gain versus the weight gain associated with gradual secular or aging-related trends—leading to a requirement for large sample sizes for statistical significance. Intervention and control group differences may be diminished by behavioral changes among control participants, either spontaneously (associated with the strong motivation that caused them to enroll in the study), because control groups receive advice and counseling offered to meet an ethical standard of care, or because they obtain advice through other means. For example, 23% of control group women who provided follow-up data in a study to reduce postpartum weight retention had enrolled in other formal weight loss programs during the study period [54]. Given the multiple determinants of eating and physical activity throughout the day, the effects of interventions that reach populations in only one setting (e.g., at school, work, or home) may be negated by compensatory changes in other settings or at other times.

8.   CONCLUSION

On the surface, weight maintenance may seem easier than weight loss because of the lower demand in terms of the number of calories to be reduced in the diet or added in energy expenditure through physical activity. However, the literature to date suggests that this reasoning may be deceptive. The prevention of obesity in childhood is particularly complex. Ultimately, to be successful, it will probably require broad efforts by families, schools, communities, and primary care physicians in concert with allied health professionals.

At present we lack definitive evidence to support specific approaches to obesity prevention. This means that a vigorous and ongoing research effort is needed to provide evidence which will drive the prevention strategies of the future. Clinicians will continue to play a pivotal role in all types of preventive strategies, either through direct intervention or as advocates for environmental and policy changes.

NOTE

1. Using definitions of body mass index (BMI) ≥ 30 kg/m^2 for adults and age–sex specific BMI above the 95th percentile of the Centers for Disease Control and Prevention (CDC) reference for children and adolescents. CDC uses the term "overweight" rather than obesity to describe children and adolescents in this weight category.

REFERENCES

[1] Hedley AA, Ogden CL, Johnson CL, Carroll MD, Curtin LR, Flegal KM. Prevalence of overweight and obesity among US children, adolescents, and adults, 1999–2002. JAMA 2004;291:2847–2850.

[2] Kumanyika S. Obesity in minority populations: An epidemiologic assessment. Obes Res 1994;2:166–182.

[3] Expert Panel on the Identification, Evaluation, and Treatment of Overweight and Obesity in Adults. Clinical Guidelines on the Identification, Evaluation, and Treatment of Obesity in Adults. The Evidence Report. National Institutes of Health, National Heart, Lung, and Blood Institute, 1998. Available at: http://www.nhlbi.nih.gov/guidelines/obesity/ob_home.htm

[4] Troiano RP, Flegal KM. Overweight children and adolescents: Description, epidemiology, and demographics. Pediatrics 1998;101(3 Pt 2):497–504.

[5] Gordon-Larsen P, Adair LS, Popkin BM. The relationship of ethnicity, socioeconomic factors, and overweight in US adolescents. Obes Res 2003;1:121–129. Erratum in: Obes Res 2003;11:597.

[6] Zhang Q, Wang Y. Socioeconomic inequality of obesity in the United States: Do gender, age, and ethnicity matter? Soc Sci Med 2004;58:1171–1180.

[7] Strauss RS, Pollack HA. Epidemic increase in childhood overweight, 1986–1998. JAMA 2001;12(286):2845–2848.

[8] Zhang Q, Wang Y. Trends in the association between obesity and socioeconomic status in U.S adults: 1971 to 2000. Obes Res 2004;12:1622–1632.

[9] Lewis CE, Jacobs DR Jr, McCreath H, et al. Weight gain continues in the 1990s: 10-year trends in weight and overweight from the CARDIA study. Coronary Artery Risk Development in Young Adults. Am J Epidemiol 2000;15(151):1172–1181.

[10] U.S. Preventive Services Task Force. Screening for obesity in adults. Recommendation and rationale. Ann Intern Med 2003;139:930–932.

[11] U.S. Department of Health and Human Services. The Surgeon General's Call to Action to Prevent and Decrease Overweight and Obesity. Rockville, MD: U.S. Department of Health and Human Services, Public Health Service, Office of the Surgeon General, 2001. Available from the U.S. Government Printing Office, Washington, DC.

[12] Kumanyika S, Jeffery RW, Morabia A, Ritenbaugh C, Antipatis VJ; Public Health Approaches to the Prevention of Obesity (PHAPO) Working Group of the International Obesity Task Force (IOTF). Obesity prevention: The case for action. Int J Obes Relat Metab Disord 2002;26:425–436. No abstract available.

[13] Russell CM, Williamson DF, Byers T. Can the year 2000 objective for reducing overweight in the United States be reached? A simulation study of the required changes in body weight. Int J Obes Relat Metab Disord 1995;19:149–153.

[14] U.S. Department of Health and Human Services. Healthy People 2010. Leading Health Indicators. Overweight and Obesity. Available at: http://www.healthypeople.gov/Document/html/uih/uih_4.htm#overandobese

[15] World Health Organization. Obesity: Preventing and managing the global epidemic. Report of a WHO consultation. World Health Organ Tech Rep Ser 2000;894:i–xii, 1–253.

[16] Daniels SR, Arnett DK, Eckel RH, et al. Overweight in children and adolescents: Pathophysiology, consequences, prevention, and treatment. Circulation 2005;111:1999–2012.

[17] Himmelgreen DA, Perez-Escamilla R, Martinez D, et al. The longer you stay, the bigger you get: Length of time and language use in the U.S. are associated with obesity in Puerto Rican women. Am J Phys Anthropol 2004;125:90–96.

[18] Kaplan MS, Huguet N, Newsom JT, McFarland BH. The association between length of residence and obesity among Hispanic immigrants. Am J Prev Med 2004;27:323–326.

[19] Booth SL, Sallis JF, Ritenbaugh C, et al. Environmental and societal factors affect food choice and physical activity rationale, influences, and leverage points. Nutr Rev 2001;59 (3 Pt 2):S21–S39.

[20] Wetter AC, Goldberg JP, King AC, et al. How and why do individuals make food and physical activity choices? Nutr Rev 2001;59(3 Pt 2):S11–S20.

[21] French SA, Story M, Jeffery RW. Environmental influences on eating and physical activity. Annu Rev Public Health 2001;22:309–335.

[22] Wadden TA, Brownell KD, Foster GD. Obesity: Responding to the global epidemic. J Consult Clin Psychol 2002;70:510–525.

[23] Lobstein T, Baur L, Uauy R. Obesity in children and young people: A crisis in public health. Obes Rev 2004;5(Suppl 1):4–104.

[24] Swinburn BA, Caterson I, Seidell JC, James WP. Diet, nutrition and the prevention of excess weight gain and obesity. Public Health Nutr 2004;7(1A):123–146.

[25] Economos CD, Brownson RC, DeAngelis MA, et al. What lessons have been learned from other attempts to guide social change? Nutr Rev 2001;59(3, Pt II);S40–S56.

[26] Koplan JP, Liverman CT, Kraak VI, eds.; Committee on Prevention of Obesity in Children in Youth. Food and Nutrition Board and Board of Health Promotion and Disease Prevention. Institute of Medicine. Preventing Childhood Obesity. Health in the Balance. Washington, DC: National Academy Press, 2005.

[27] Seidell JC, Nooyens AJ, Visscher TL. Cost-effective measures to prevent obesity: Epidemiological basis and appropriate target groups. Proc Nutr Soc 2005;64:1–5.

[28] Rose G. Sick individuals and sick populations. Int J Epidemiol 1985;14:32–38.

[29] Antipatis VJ, Kumanyika S, Jeffery RW, Morabia A, Ritenbaugh C. Confidence of health professionals in public health approaches to obesity prevention. Int J Obes Relat Metab Disord 1999;23:1004–1006.

[30] Kumanyika SK. Minisymposium on obesity. Overview and some strategic considerations. Annu Rev Public Health 2001;22:293–308.

[31] Kuczmarski R. Summary Report of July 2004 Workshop on Site Specific Approaches to Prevention or Management of Childhood Obesity. National Institute of Diabetes and Digestive and Kidney Diseases. National Institutes of Health. Available at: http://www.obesityresearch.nih.gov/news/meetings.htm

[32] League CA, Dearry A. Summary Report of May 2004 Workshop on Obesity and the Built Environment. Improving Public Health through Community Design. National Institute of Environmental Health Sciences. National Institutes of Health. Available at: www.niehs.nih.gov/drcpt/beoconf

[33] Buzby JC, Guthrie JF, Kantor LS. Evaluation of the USDA Fruit and Vegetable Pilot Program: Report to Congress. U.S. Department of Agriculture, Economic Research Service. E-FAN-03-006, May 2003. www.ers.usda.gov/publications/efan03006

[34] Glanz K, Hoelscher D. Increasing fruit and vegetable intake by changing environments, policy and pricing: Restaurant-based research, strategies, and recommendations. Prev Med 2004;39(Suppl 2):S88–S93.

[35] Glanz K, Yaroch AL. Strategies for increasing fruit and vegetable intake in grocery stores and communities: Policy, pricing, and environmental change. Prev Med 2004;39 (Suppl 2):S75–S80.

[36] French SA, Wechsler H. School-based research and initiatives: Fruit and vegetable environment, policy and pricing workshop. Prev Med 2004;39(Suppl 2):S101–S107.

[37] Nestle M, Jacobson MF. Halting the obesity epidemic: A public health policy approach. Public Health Rep 2000;115:12–24.

[38] Drewnowski A, Darmon N. The economics of obesity: Dietary energy density and energy cost. Am J Clin Nutr 2005;82(Suppl 1):265S–273S.

[39] Kahn EB, Ramsey LT, Brownson RC, et al. The effectiveness of interventions to increase physical activity. A systematic review. Am J Prev Med 2002;22(Suppl 4):73–107.

[40] Sallis JF, Moudon AV, Linton LS, Powell KE, eds. Active Living Research. Am J Prev Med 2005;28(Suppl 2), entire issue.

[41] Stables GJ, Subar AF, Patterson BH, et al. Changes in vegetable and fruit consumption and awareness among US adults: Results of the 1991 and 1997 5 A Day for Better Health Program surveys. J Am Diet Assoc 2002;102:809–817.

[42] Wong F, Huhman M, Heitzler C, et al. VERB—a social marketing campaign to increase physical activity among youth. Prev Chronic Dis 2004;1:A10. Epub 2004 Jun 15.

[43] Copeland AL, Martin PD, Geiselman PJ, Rash CJ, Kendzor DE. Smoking cessation for weight-concerned women: Group vs. individually tailored, dietary, and weight-control follow-up sessions. Addict Behav 2005; May 27 [Epub ahead of print].

[44] Littrell KH, Hilligoss NM, Kirshner CD, Petty RG, Johnson CG. The effects of an educational intervention on antipsychotic-induced weight gain. J Nurs Scholar 2003;35:237–241.

[45] Menza M, Vreeland B, Minsky S, Gara M, Radler DR, Sakowitz M. Managing atypical antipsychotic-associated weight gain: 12-month data on a multimodal weight control program. J Clin Psychiatry 2004;65:471–477.

[46] Arenz S, Ruckerl R, Koletzko B, von Kries R. Breast-feeding and childhood obesity—a systematic review. Int J Obes Relat Metab Disord 2004;28:1247–1256.

[47] Leermarkers EA, Jakicic JM, Viteri J, Wing RR. Clinic-based vs. home-based interventions for preventing weight gain in men. Obes Res 1998;6:346–352.

[48] Jeffery RW, French SA. Preventing weight gain in adults: The pound of prevention study. Am J Public Health 1999;89:747–751.

[49] Simkin-Silverman LR, Wing RR, Boraz MA, Kuller LH. Lifestyle intervention can prevent weight gain during menopause: Results from a 5-year randomized clinical trial. Ann Behav Med 2003;26:212–220.

[50] Kuller LH, Simkin-Silverman LR, Wing RR, Meilahn EN, Ives DG. Women's Healthy Lifestyle Project: A randomized clinical trial: Results at 54 months. Circulation 2001; 103:32–37.

[51] Olson CM, Strawderman MS, Reed RG. Efficacy of an intervention to prevent excessive gestational weight gain. Am J Obstet Gynecol 2004;191:530–536.

[52] Sherwood NE, Jeffery RW, French SA, Hannan PJ, Murray DM. Predictors of weight gain in the Pound of Prevention study. Int J Obes Relat Metab Disord 2000;24:395–403.

[53] Klem ML, Viteri JE, Wing RR. Primary prevention of weight gain for women aged 25–34: The acceptability of treatment formats. Int J Obes Relat Metab Disord 2000;24:219–225.

[54] Leermakers EA, Anglin K, Wing RR. Reducing postpartum weight retention through a correspondence intervention. Int J Obes Relat Metab Disord 1998;22:1103–1109.

[55] Polley BA, Wing RR, Sims CJ. Randomized controlled trial to prevent excessive weight gain in pregnant women. Int J Obes Relat Metab Disord 2002;26:1494–1502.

[56] Wing RR, Phelan S. Long-term weight loss maintenance. Am J Clin Nutr 2005;82 (Suppl 1):222S–225S.

[57] U.S. Department of Health and Human Services. U.S. Department of Agriculture Dietary Guidelines for Americans. HHS Publication number: HHS-ODPHP-2005-01-DGA-A. USDA Publication number: Home and Garden Bulletin No 232. Available at: http://www.healthiersus.gov/dietaryguidelines

[58] Summerbell C, Waters E, Edmunds L, Kelly S, Brown T, Campbell K. Interventions for preventing obesity in children. Cochrane Database Syst Rev 2005;20:CD001871.

[59] Luepker RV, Perry CL, McKinlay SM, et al.; The Child and Adolescent Trial for Cardiovascular Health. CATCH collaborative group. Outcomes of a field trial to improve children's dietary patterns and physical activity. JAMA 1996;275:768–776.

[60] Caballero B, Clay T, Davis SM, et al. Pathways: A school-based, randomized controlled trial for the prevention of obesity in American Indian schoolchildren. Am J Clin Nutr 2003;78:1030–1038.

[61] Harvey-Berino J, Rourke J. Obesity prevention in preschool Native-American children: A pilot study using home visiting. Obes Res 2003;11:606–611.

[62] Gortmaker SL, Peterson K, Wiecha J, et al. Reducing obesity via a school-based interdisciplinary intervention among youth: Planet health. Arch Pediatr Adolesc Med 1999; 153:409–418.

[63] Robinson TN. Reducing children's television viewing to prevent obesity: A randomized controlled trial. JAMA 1999;282:1561–1567.

[64] Fitzgibbon ML, Stolley MR, Schiffer L, Van Horn L, KauferChristoffel K, Dyer A. Two-year follow-up results for Hip-Hop to Health Jr.: A randomized controlled trial for overweight prevention in preschool minority children. J Pediatr 2005;146:618–625.

[65] Krebs NF, Jacobson MS. Prevention of pediatric overweight and obesity. Pediatrics 2003;112:424–430.

[66] Ogden CL, Flegal KM, Carroll MD, Johnson CL. Prevalence and trends in overweight among US children and adolescents, 1999–2000. JAMA 2002;288:1728–1732.

[67] Whitlock EP, Williams SB, Gold R, Smith PR, Shipman SA. Screening and interventions for childhood overweight: A summary of evidence for the US Preventive Services Task Force. Pediatrics 2005;116:e125–e144.

[68] Carleton RA, Lasater TM, Assaf AR, Feldman HA, McKinlay S. The Pawtucket Heart Health Program: Community changes in cardiovascular risk factors and projected disease risk. Am J Public Health 1995;85:777–785.

[69] Taylor CB, Fortmann SP, Flora J, et al. Effect of long-term community health education on body mass index. The Stanford Five-City Project. Am J Epidemiol 1991;134:235–249.

[70] Winkleby MA, Feldman HA, Murray DM. Joint analysis of three U.S. community intervention trials for reduction of cardiovascular disease risk. J Clin Epidemiol 1997;50:645–658.

[71] Kumanyika SK, Obarzanek E. Pathways to obesity prevention: Report of a National Institutes of Health workshop. Obes Res 2003;11:1263–1274.

[72] Glenny AM, O'Meara S, Melville A, Sheldon TA, Wilson C. The treatment and prevention of obesity: A systematic review of the literature. Int J Obes Relat Metab Disord 1997; 21:715–737.

[73] Hardeman W, Griffin S, Johnston M, Kinmonth AL, Wareham NJ. Interventions to prevent weight gain: A systematic review of psychological models and behaviour change methods. Int J Obes Relat Metab Disord 2000;24:131–143.

[74] Ammerman AS, Lindquist CH, Lohr KN, Hersey J. The efficacy of behavioral interventions to modify dietary fat and fruit and vegetable intake: A review of the evidence. Prev Med 2002;35:25–41.

[75] Eden KB, Orleans CT, Mulrow CD, Pender NJ, Teutsch SM. Does counseling by clinicians improve physical activity? A summary of the evidence for the U.S. Preventive Services Task Force. Ann Intern Med 2002;137:208–215.

[76] Pignone MP, Ammerman A, Fernandez L, et al. Counseling to promote a healthy diet in adults: A summary of the evidence for the U.S. Preventive Services Task Force. Am J Prev Med 2003;24:75–92.

[77] Pate RR, Trost SG, Mullis R, Sallis JF, Wechsler H, Brown DR. Community interventions to promote proper nutrition and physical activity among youth. Prev Med 2000;31(part 2 of 2):S138–S149.

[78] Sallis JF, Patrick K, Frank E, Pratt M, Wechsler H, Galuska DA. Interventions in health care settings to promote healthful eating and physical activity in children and adolescents. Prev Med 2000;31(part 2 of 2):S112–S120.

Chapter 15

Orlistat and Sibutramine in the Management of Obesity

Holly Wyatt

University of Colorado at Denver and Health Sciences Center, Denver, CO 80262, USA

1.   INTRODUCTION

More than one third of the adult population in the United States is obese (defined as a body mass index [BMI] $\geq$ 30 kg/m^2) and as a result of their excess body fat are at an increased risk of developing many associated chronic conditions such as cancer, cardiovascular disease, and type 2 diabetes as well as a reduced quality of life and early mortality [1, 2]. Small amounts of sustained weight loss can improve these serious health risks [1, 3]. Although lifestyle treatments directed at improving diet and physical activity are considered first-line treatment, many if not most obese patients do not sustain significant weight loss with lifestyle changes alone [3–9]. Based on the clinical guidelines for obesity management published by the National Institutes of Health (NIH), weight loss medications should be considered by health care providers as an evidence-based next step to be incorporated with the lifestyle interventions in appropriate patients [1]. The goal of adding weight loss medication to lifestyle changes is to improve the number of patients who can achieve and sustain a significant weight reduction and thus prevent or reduce obesity-associated morbidity and mortality by improving cardiovascular and metabolic risk factors in these patients.

2.   WHO IS APPROPRIATE? CRITERIA FOR USE OF WEIGHT LOSS MEDICATIONS

The NIH clinical guidelines advocate weight loss medications be prescribed for patients with BMIs $\geq$ 30 kg/m^2 or with BMIs $\geq$ 27 kg/m^2 if a comorbidity is present [1]. Comorbidities for the medication guideline include type 2 diabetes, hypertension, heart disease, sleep apnea, and dyslipidemia. These BMI cutoffs for prescribing medications are not arbitrary. They are based on large amounts of epidemiological data that illustrate a positive curvilinear relationship between increasing health risks such as the development of type 2 diabetes

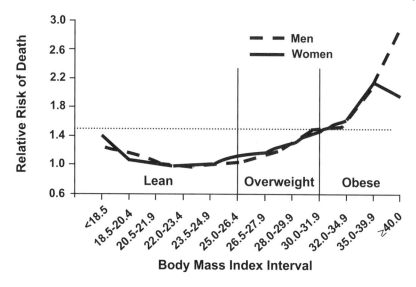

Figure 1. Relationship between BMI and cardiovascular disease mortality. Mortality risk begins to increase at a BMI of 25 kg/m^2 and continues to increase as BMI increases. The slope of the line is steeper as higher BMIs and represents a curvilinear relationship. The horizontal dotted line represents the relative risk of mortality at a BMI of 30 kg/m^2 and theoretically represents the point where the risk of obesity exceeds the risk of weight loss medications. (Data from Calle [10].)

and increasing BMI in the general population [10–12]. Figure 1 illustrates this relationship between BMI and cardiovascular mortality. The same basic relationship is seen for many if not most of the comorbidities associated with excess body fat. The guidelines chose a BMI of ≥ 30 kg/m^2 as the BMI cut point for medications because BMIs of this magnitude are associated with a general level of health risk that outweighs or exceeds the general medical risk of using medications for weight loss. It is felt, based on this relationship, that lower BMIs do not represent a sufficient health risk to merit the use of medications. In addition, it is generally believed that successful weight reduction starting from a BMI ≥ 30 kg/m^2 will produce a benefit that is worth the risk of the medication. The benefits of losing weight from a lower BMI are not considered to be worth the risk because the curvilinear relationship between BMI and health risk flattens or becomes less steep at lower BMIs (see Figure 1). For example, even though the data are cross-sectional, it is assumed that a greater health benefit would be obtained by reducing someone from a BMI of 30 kg/m^2 to a BMI of 27 kg/m^2 than from a BMI of 25 to 22 kg/m^2.

Individuals with obesity-related comorbidities are at even more risk from their excess weight and could potentially receive a greater benefit from weight reduction; therefore the NIH has lowered the guidelines to a BMI ≥ 27 kg/m^2 for the potential use of a weight loss medication in this higher risk population

[1]. In addition to the BMI criteria described in the preceding text, patients should have been unsuccessful at losing weight with diet and activity alone or have not sustained previous weight loss attempts to be appropriate for weight loss medications [1]. The continual assessment of efficacy and safety of weight loss medications is necessary once prescribed.

3. WHY DO HEALTH CARE PROVIDERS CHOOSE NOT TO USE WEIGHT LOSS MEDICATIONS?

Using these NIH evidenced-based criteria for potential candidates for drug treatment, more than 60 to 100 million adults may be eligible to receive drug therapy [2, 13]. Why is it then that weight loss medications are not widely used by the medical community? There are many reasons why physicians are reluctant and skeptical about using weight loss medications in their obese patients. Weight loss medications in general have a past history of poor outcomes and "unintended consequences" [14–18]. Past use of the amphetamine-derived addictive stimulant medications and the unexpected heart valve side effects of the "phen-fen" period have not helped to create confidence for use of weight loss medications. In addition only recently has obesity been recognized as a "legitimate" metabolic disease with both a physiologic and genetic basis [19–22]. In the past obesity was thought of as a social condition or character flaw stemming from a person's lack of will power or laziness, not a justifiable disease process deserving of true medical attention much less a medication. In addition, our previous lack of understanding of the chronic medical course of obesity and the benefit of modest weight loss led to unrealistic expectations for weight loss drugs [23] both from physicians and patients and created the general concept that they were not effective. More recently, the cost of these medications and lack of insurance coverage may also be major causes for the low levels for prescriptions written compared to the number of appropriate patients that could potentially benefit from a weight loss medications.

Fortunately, many of these misconceptions and prescribing barriers of the past are slowly changing as our knowledge about obesity and weight loss medications continues to grow and advance. Weight management and medications are becoming an important part of medical education and general office practice [24]. Physicians today know weight loss medications need to be prescribed long term to be effective and modest amounts of weight loss can produce a significant health benefit [1, 3]. There is a significant physiologic or biology component to obesity, and just like any other medical disease process, medications can be part of an effective treatment plan [25, 26]. Weight loss medications are now available that are as safe for long-term use and have no abuse potential [18]. There is still need to increase health care coverage for weight loss medications, but reimbursement for obesity treatment in general is increasing [27].

4.   WHAT WEIGHT LOSS DRUGS ARE AVAILABLE?

Only two prescription drugs are available for long-term use in treating obesity—sibutramine and orlistat. Short-term weight loss as well as long-term weight loss maintenance and safety have been demonstrated for both drugs in multiple randomized control trials [13, 18, 28–30]. These represent the two most-studied weight loss drugs in the literature to date [30]. Several other drugs are currently approved by the FDA for the indication of weight loss, but because they were approved before we understood the chronic nature of weight management and the necessity for long-term treatment protocols these drugs were studied only short term (see Table 1). Therefore these drugs have not undergone the rigorous evaluation in large, long-term studies to prove their efficacy and safety that the FDA now requires for long-term approval. Thus these drugs are approved only for short-term use (usually thought of as 3 months). This chapter focuses on the role of orlistat and sibutramine in the long-term management of obesity.

Table 1. Medications currently approved by the FDA for the treatment of obesity

Generic name	Trade name	DEA schedule	Mechanism	Approved use	Recommended dosage range
Benzphetamine	Didrex	III	NE release	Short term	25 mg to 50 mg/d
Phendimetrazine	Prelu-2 Bontril Plegine	III	NE release	Short term	35 mg TID or 105 mg SR/d
Mazindol	Maxanor Sanorex	IV	Blocks NE reuptake	Short term	1 mg TID
Phentermine	Adipex-P Fastin Ionamin Ionamin SR	IV	NE release	Short term	15–37.5 mg/d
Diethylpropion	Tenuate Tepanil Tenuate Dospan	IV	NE release	Short term	25 mg TID 25–75 SR mg/d
Sibutramine	Meridia Reductil	IV	Blocks serotinin and NE reuptake	Long term	5–15 mg/d
Orlistat	Xenical	Not scheduled	Lipase inhibitor	Long term	120 mg TID right before or with meals

NE, norepinepherine; TID, three times a day.

5. HOW SHOULD WEIGHT LOSS IN MEDICATION CLINICAL TRIALS BE EVALUATED?

Average weight loss is the most common outcome used to evaluate the efficacy of medication compared to placebo. It is important to understand its strengths and limitations when examining clinical trials. Average weight loss in obesity medication trials is significantly influenced by a variety of factors such as the dose of medication prescribed, the target patient population recruited (female vs. male, diabetics vs. nondiabetics, young vs. old) and the degree or intensity of the behavioral component. For example, with minimal behavioral intervention the weight loss in a study by Wadden and colleagues was about 5 kg for the medication group [31]. When group counseling was added to the medication, the weight loss increased to 10 kg and when a structured meal plan was added using meal replacements the weight loss increased to 15 kg. This illustrates that the absolute amount of weight loss that is reported (5 kg vs. 15 kg) is due in part to the intensity or "dose" of the behavioral prescription of the intervention. Figure 2 illustrates this concept. For this reason, average weight loss in one trial will differ from the next with the same medication.

Average weight loss data will inform the clinician about the difference in weight loss between the medication and placebo under the specific circumstances and patient population used in that specific trial. In addition, certain behavioral interventions may accentuate differences between placebo and medication arms while other behavioral protocols may minimize differences. Therefore different trials will report disparity in terms of the absolute or average amount of weight loss that the medication can achieve above placebo.

With this concept in mind, the efficacy of weight loss medications may not necessarily be best evaluated by measuring the production of a certain amount of weight loss above placebo given that the strength or "dose" of the placebo behavioral intervention can have a tremendous effect on outcomes. It also illustrates why different medications in different clinical trial protocols cannot be appropriately compared to each other in terms of average weight loss. Head-to-head comparison of weight loss medications can be made only within the same randomized protocol.

A different way to evaluate the efficacy of weight loss medications is to evaluate the proportion of subjects achieving different amount of weight loss in drug vs placebo (e.g., the percentage of subjects achieving a > 5% weight loss, or a > 10% weight loss). Weight loss medications may be particularly effective in helping more patients be successful at achieving a medical significant weight loss over time. This evaluation may be more informative to the general practitioner. Categorical analysis tells the provider how many of their patients he or she can expect to achieve a certain degree of weight loss with and without the medication in the same behavioral setting and population. Another

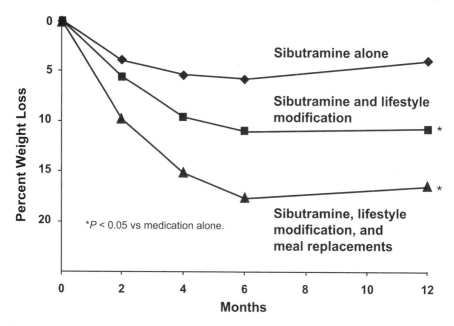

Figure 2. Percentage of weight changes for patients receiving sibutramine, sibutramine with lifestyle modification, and sibutramine with lifestyle modification and meal replacements. The figure represents the effect of the degree of intensity of behavioral treatment on mean weight loss data. (From Wadden et al. [31].)

point to consider is that it is also possible that some individuals will "respond" to a medication and others will "not respond" so that the average weight loss data may not accurately reflect the potential weight loss efficacy for a specific subgroup of patients. For these reasons it may be clinically meaningful to look at the weight loss medication data in terms of categorical weight loss both in the weight loss and weight maintenance phases in addition to the more traditional average weight reduction of medication compared to placebo. Both average weight loss data and categorical data are discussed in this chapter.

6. SIBUTRAMINE

Sibutramine (sold as Meridia in the United States and Reductil in Europe) was approved by the Federal Drug Administration (FDA) and available for use in the United States in 1997. It has undergone extensive testing in short- and long-term randomized clinical trials. It was first evaluated in clinical trials as an antidepressant with disappointing results. However, weight loss was an unexpected side effect in these clinical trials and the drug was subsequently evaluated and developed for its weight management potential [32].

Sibutramine is a selective reuptake inhibitor of norepinephrine, serotonin, and to a very small degree dopamine [28]. It has two active metabolites and a half-life of 14 to 16 hours which allows for once a day oral dosing [28, 33]. It currently is used at a dose of 10 to 15 mg/day and is available in 5-, 10-, and 15-mg pills. The currently recommended starting dose is 10 mg and doses greater than 15 mg are not recommended by the FDA. Similar to other medications used to treat chronic disorders, the disorder, in this case excess body weight, reoccurs when the medication is stopped.

6.1. Mechanism of Action

The principal mechanism of action for sibutramine is increasing feelings of satiation (the level of fullness during a meal) which results in a reduction in food intake for a meal and over time weight loss [34, 35]. Sibutramine mediates satiety by inhibiting the reuptake of the combination of serotonin and norepinephrine within the central nervous system [36]. Some studies have also demonstrated a mild increase in energy expenditure (thermogenesis) that may also contribute to its weight loss effects [37–39]. However, not all studies have confirmed this thermogenic finding in humans and its contribution to its mechanism of action if present is relatively small [40].

6.2. Therapeutic Potential for Obesity

Sibutramine has been evaluated extensively in multiple clinical trials lasting 8 weeks to 24 months in healthy obese adults and overweight and obese adults with a cardiovascular risk factor (hypertension, type 2 diabetes, or dyslipidemia [41–56]). Sibutramine causes a dose-dependent loss in body weight when given in doses ranging from 1 to 30 mg/day [41]. In a 6-month dosing ranging study of more than 1000 patients there is a very clear dose–response relationship, and regain of weight occurred as expected when the medication was stopped. Mean weight loss ranged from –1.2% for placebo to –7.4% loss from baseline for the 15-mg dose at 24 weeks [41]. The typical starting dose of sibutramine, 10 mg, produced a –6.1% weight loss. One can tell from the small amount of mean weight loss in the placebo arm (–1.2%) that the behavioral intervention or "dose" was weak in this study. Therefore total weight loss would be expected to be less in this study compared to other studies with a more intensive behavioral intervention.

Weight losses in the range of 5% to 10% from baseline are associated with meaningful health benefits and should be thought of as the current standard for medical care [1, 3]. In general, average weight loss in most sibutramine studies greater than 24 weeks in duration ranges from –3.1% to –10.4% in the sibutramine arms to –0.9% to –4.2% in the placebo arms [13]. Differences in weight loss between trials can be attributed to different doses of sibutramine, differences in the patient populations studied, and the "dose" of the behavioral intervention prescribed as described earlier. Table 2 summarizes several of the published longer-term randomized placebo-controlled studies (> 44 weeks) evaluating weight loss efficacy for sibutramine and illustrates the wide range of mean weight loss from trial to trial. Follow-up rates on most published trials ranged anywhere from 45% to 100% and make data difficult to interpret in some studies. In all the trials listed in Table 2 average weight loss was significantly greater ($p < 0.01$) in the sibutramine arms compared to placebo.

A meta-analysis of clinical trials published in 2004 by Arterburn and colleagues reported a mean difference in weight loss for sibutramine of –4.45 kg (95% CI, –3.62 to –5.29 kg) relative to placebo at 12 months [13]. It is important to understand that 4.45 kg represents the weight loss above placebo and not total average weight reduction achieved with sibutramine when combined with lifestyle or behavioral interventions. The authors of this meta-analysis and other systematic reviews have all concluded that sibutramine is effective in promoting weight loss [13, 30, 57, 58].

Table 2 also illustrates the categorical weight loss date for several long-term sibutramine studies. In general, three to four times as many subjects randomized to sibutramine therapy lost ≥ 5% of their initial body weight compared to those randomized to placebo. A meta-analysis of published studies concluded that adults taking sibutramine for 1 year are 19% to 34% more likely to achieve a 5% weight loss and 12% to 31% more likely to achieve 10% weight loss than those taking placebo [13]. What this means to a practicing physician is that while not everyone will achieve a significant weight loss, far more patients will be successful using sibutramine and a significant subgroup of almost 20% will be successful at achieving ≥ 10% weight reduction.

6.3.   Efficacy in Weight Loss Maintenance

Showing long-term maintenance of a weight loss may be more important than demonstrating weight loss itself. After all, many people succeed at losing weight with many different strategies but far fewer succeed at keeping it off long-term. Successful strategies to prevent weight regain are fewer in number than weight loss strategies. Several trials using sibutramine have addressed the specific issue of weight loss maintenance [48, 52, 53]. One of these studies the Multicenter European Sibutramine Trial of Obesity Reduction and Maintenance Trial (known as the STORM Trial) illustrates that sibutramine is effective in maintaining a weight loss for up to 2 years and represents the longest published use of sibutramine [53]. In this study obese subjects who lost ≥ 5% of their body weight after 6 months of sibutramine therapy were randomized to either sibutramine or placebo for the next 18 months. Ninety-four percent of the patients who completed the first 6 months of the study lost ≥ 5%

Table 2. Long-term (≥ 44 wks) randomized placebo controlled studies evaluating the mean and categorical weight loss and weight maintenance efficacy for sibutramine

Authors	Population	Dose (mg)	Cointervention or run-in	Duration	Percentage completing	Sibutramine- mwc	Placebo- mwc	Sibutramine cwl5	Placebo cwl5
Weight loss									
McNulty et al. [47]	Type 2 DM BMI > 27	15 20	Diet advice by dietitian	52 wks	74	−5.5 kg −8.0 kg	−0.2 kg	46% 65%	0%
Smith et al. [67]	Healthy BMI 27–40	10 15	Low-calorie diet	52 wks	53	−5.0% −7.3%	−1.8%	39% 52%	20%
McMahon et al. [46]	Hypertension BMI 27–40 36% African Americans	20	Minimal behavioral intervention	52 wks	54	−4.7% (−4.4 kg)	−0.7% (−0.5 kg)	40.1%	8.7%
Weight loss maintenance									
Apfelbaum et al. [48]	Healthy BMI >30	10	≥ 6 kg wt loss with 4 wks VLCD br	52 wks	68	−5.4% (−5.2 kg) from end of VLCD	+1% (+0.5 kg) from end of VLCD	86% fse	55% fse
James et al. [53]	Healthy BMI 30–45	10–20	≥ 5% wt loss with 6 months of sibutramine br	18 months	56	−8.9 kg fse	−4.9 kg fse	69% fse	42% fse
Wirth et al. [52]	Healthy BMI 30–40	15	≥ 2% or > 2 kg weight loss after 4 wks of sibutramine br	44 wks	79	−8.2% (−7.9 kg) fse	−3.9% (−3.8 kg) fse	65% fse	35% fse

BMI, body mass index in kg/m^2; wks, weeks; mwc, mean wt change; cwl5, categorical wt loss (>5%); fse, from study entry; br, before randomization.

and 18% withdrew from the study before 6 months so 467 patients or 77% (467/605) were randomized for weight loss maintenance. Placebo-treated subjects regained weight, maintaining only 20% of their 6-month weight loss at 24 months. Sibutramine-treated subjects maintained 80% of their initial weight loss. The completers in the sibutramine group averaged 10.2 kg weight loss at 2 years compared to a 4.7-kg loss for the placebo group. Fifty eight percent of the sibutramine group and 50% of the placebo group completed the 2-year study. This study proved sibutramine to be effective in both producing and maintaining weight loss for up to 2 years.

Another study by Apfelbaum and colleagues induced weight loss with a very low calorie diet (VLCD) for 4 weeks and then randomized those achieving a 6-kg or greater weight loss to placebo or sibutramine for 12 months [48]. On average the VLCD produced a 7.2% weight loss prior to randomization. One year later, 75% of patients in the sibutramine group maintained 100% of the weight lost achieved in the 4-week VLCD compared to 42% in the placebo arm. Mean weight changes for the sibutramine arm after initial weight loss was an additional –5.4% compared to +1% in the placebo group.

6.4.   Efficacy in Managing Obesity-related Risk Factors

The goal with weight reduction is to prevent or treat the comorbidities associated with excess body fat. Weight reduction in the range of 5% to 10% in general is associated with improvements in cholesterol, blood pressure, and glucose control. It is possible, however, that a medication that produces weight loss might alter physiology in such a way where the expected reductions or improvements in these health parameters would not be found. Therefore weight loss medication, in addition to proving weight loss efficacy, must also show data that risk factors improve with the weight reduction.

Sibutramine has been associated with small improvements in high-density lipoprotein (HDL), triglyceride levels, uric acid, waist circumference, and quality of life and among diabetic patients improvements in glycemic control [13, 28, 41, 59]. These improvements are all related to weight loss and improvements are proportional to the amount of weight loss. Sibutramine does not have an independent effect on any of the comorbidities. In a study with more than 300 men and women with high triglyceride levels (≥ 250 mg/dL) and low HDL levels, patients taking sibutramine who lost > 5% weight had a mean reduction in triglycerides of 33.4 mg/dL and increase in HDL of 4.9 mg/dL [43].

There are four large clinical trials that document sibutramine use in patients with diabetes and improvements in measures of glucose control [45, 54–56]. In general, it is important to remember that weight loss in patients with diabetes is not as great as the studies of nondiabetic individuals with any method of weight reduction including sibutramine. Mean weight loss in these studies was in the range of 2.4 to 9.6 kg. In all the studies the percentage of diabetic patients who achieve weight loss of at least 5% or greater is significantly greater than with placebo. Weight reduction corresponds to the degree of improvement in glycemic control and ranges from a reduction of 0.3% to 2.73% depending on level of baseline hemoglobin A1C and weight loss achieved. A meta-analysis by Vettor and colleagues confirmed a substantial effect of sibutramine on weight loss and glycemic control [58].

6.5. Tolerability and Safety

The most common adverse effects associated with the use of sibutramine are dry mouth, anorexia, constipation, and insomnia [28, 42]. There has been no evidence of any abuse potential or heart valve dysfunction [60–62]. The principal concerns with sibutramine safety involve potential increase in blood pressure and heart rate. Sibutramine can increase blood pressure and blood pressure response to sibutramine at an individual level varies [41, 42, 63]. The meta-analysis discussed earlier by Arterburn and colleagues reported that the effects of sibutramine on blood pressure in high-quality studies was highly varied and ranged from net reductions to net increases (–1.6 to 5.6 mm Hg) [13]. Blood pressure response does not appear to be augmented in mildly hypertensive patients [64]. Effects on heart rate, however, in the Arterburn meta-analysis were less variable and illustrated a mean difference in heart rate of +3.76 beats/min (95% CI, 2.70–4.82 beats/minute) for sibutramine treatment relative to placebo [13].

In clinical studies withdrawals for clinically significant blood pressure increases was low and in the range of 1% to 5% [53]. A recent meta-analysis found 1.1% of the sibutramine and 0.6% of placebo-treated patients withdrew because of hypertension [65]. In general, a small average increase in blood pressure in the range of 2 to 4 mm Hg in systolic and diastolic pressure occurs in sibutramine-treated patients versus controls [63, 66]. However, greater increases have been reported in a small number of individuals (> 2%) and therefore blood pressure and heart rate should be evaluated before starting sibutramine and 2–4 weeks after sibutramine is prescribed.

Because of the potential for increase in blood pressure and heart rate, sibutramine should not be used in patients with a history of coronary artery disease, congestive heart failure, uncontrolled or untreated hypertension, cardiac arrhythmias, or stroke [28]. Patients with treated and well controlled hypertension may be started on sibutramine and monitored. Patients on other selective serotonin reuptake inhibitors (SSRIs) may also be started on sibutramine. Initially concomitant use of another SSRI was an absolute contraindication owing to the theoretical possibility of serotoninergic syndrome; however, this potential complication has not been reported and SSRIs are now not viewed as an absolute contraindication. Caution and monitoring, however, are advised if the patient is taking another serotonergic agent or a drug that inhibits cytochrome P450(3a4), such as erythromycin. Sibutramine should not be used within 2 weeks of taking monoamine oxidase inhibitors (MAOIs).

6.6.   Special Considerations when Prescribing Sibutramine

The chance of achieving a meaningful weight loss with sibutramine can be determined by the response to treatment in the first 4 weeks of medication intervention. In a study by Bray and colleagues 60% of patients who lost 2 kg (about 4 lbs) in the first 4 weeks went on to lose more then 5% of starting body weight [42]. These data could be used to suggest that if a patient has not lost at least 4 pounds in about 4 weeks the chances of a meaningful weight loss are low and therefore the medication should be stopped to minimize risk.

Evaluation of blood pressure 2 to 4 weeks after starting sibutramine is recommended and important. Because about 1% to 5% of patients who take sibutramine may have an unacceptable increase in blood pressure and the medication will need to be stopped. For this reason, it is important to monitor blood pressure on all patients who are stared on this drug. In general, most experts feel if the blood pressure is less then 135/80 and there is less than a 10 mm Hg systolic and 5 mm Hg diastolic rise from baseline continued use of the medication is acceptable [28]. For patients who go on to have significant weight loss in the first month or longer the increase in blood pressure must be weighed against the amount of weight reduction and improvements in other risk factors when deciding if the medication should be continued long term.

7.   ORLISTAT

Orlistat (sold as Xenical in the United States and in Europe) was approved by the FDA in 1999 and has undergone extensive testing in short- and long-term randomized clinical trials [67–79]. Orlistat is a derivative of lipstatin and is a selective inhibitor of gastric and pancreatic lipase [80, 81]. It impairs the intestinal digestion and systemic absorption of dietary fat and vitamin esters. Orlistat is provided in 120-mg capsules and is administered orally with a 120-mg dosage at each meal three times a day. Systemic absorption is very low (< 3%) and elimination half life through feces is 1 to 2 hours [82]. Small amounts of metabolites of orlistat have been found in plasma and are eliminated through the urine [82].

7.1. Mechanism of Action

The principal mechanism of action for orlistat is decreasing absorption of dietary fat in the gut through its interaction with gastric and pancreatic lipases. Orlistat decreases the hydrolysis of triglycerides by binding to the lipases and thus limits the production of absorbable free fatty acids and monoglycerol. It can block the absorption of about 30% of the fat consumed in a meal that contains approximately 30% fat. It is presumed that by blocking 30% of the fat from being absorbed, total caloric intake will be reduced and weight loss will result over a longer period of time. Orlistat at a dose of 120 mg three times a day with meals will block absorption of one third of ingested fat [83]. Higher doses of orlistat will not increase the fat malabsorption.

A different potential mechanism of action may center on how taking this drug may affect subsequent eating behavior. Because 30% of fat is not absorbed while taking orlistat the effects of the fat that has not been absorbed involve gastrointestinal (GI) side effects such as loose stools and fecal urgency. The more fat in the diet, the more likely patients will experience unpleasant GI effects. Some patients may decrease the amount of fat they consume to prevent these GI side effects. In this sense the drug may also decrease the amount of fat consumed prior to absorption and make patients aware of what they are eating and what foods are high in fat. In addition to blocking absorption of the fat consumed, orlistat may function as a behavioral tool for self-monitoring of intake and for reducing the consumption of high-fat foods.

7.2. Therapeutic Potential for Obesity

Orlistat has been evaluated extensively in multiple randomized trials in the United States and Europe lasting 6 months to 4 years [67–79]. Drent and colleagues evaluated the efficacy of various doses of orlistat in combination with a low-fat diet in 188 patients [69]. Patients were randomly assigned to receive 10-, 60-, or 120-mg doses of orlistat three times a day for 12 weeks. Average weight loss in the placebo group was 2.98 kg and ranged between 3.61 kg and 4.74 kg in the orlistat arms for doses of orlistat of 30 mg, 180 mg, and 360 mg [69].

Table 3 summarizes results of several long-term randomized placebo-controlled studies that have evaluated orlistat for weight loss. In general, average weight loss in these studies range from –5 to –10% in the orlistat arms to –2 to –6% in the placebo arms [66]. Differences in weight loss can be attributed to different doses of orlistat, differences in patient populations studied and the "dose" of the behavioral intervention prescribed. Weight regain was significantly less for those patients who remained on drug versus those who were rerandomized to placebo in the second year of trials [68, 72]. Almost 35% to 70% of orlistat treated subjects lost ≥ 5% of their body weight compared to

Table 3. Long-term (≥ 44 weeks) randomized placebo-controlled studies evaluating the mean and categorical weight loss and weight maintenance efficacy for orlistat

Authors	Population	Dose (mg TID)	Cointervention or run-in	Duration	Percentage completing	Orlistat-mwc	Placebo-mwc	Orlistat cwl5	Placebo cwl5
Weight loss									
Kelley et al. [78]	Type 2 DM BMI 28–40 HbA1c 7.5–12%	120	Reduced calorie diet	52 wks	49	−3.9% (−3.9 kg)	−1.3% (−1.3 kg)	32.7%	13.0%
Davidson et al. [68]	US women only, BMI 30–43	120	Reduced calorie diet 1st yr, wt maintenance diet 2nd yr	2 yrs	66 (1 yr) 45 (2 yrs)	−8.8% (−8.8 kg) at 1 yr −7.6% at 2 yrs	−5.8% (−5.8 kg) at 1 yr −4.5% at 2 yrs	65.7% at 1 yr	43.6% at 1 yr
Hollander et al. [76]	Type 2 DM BMI 28–40 HbA1c 6.5–10%	120	Reduced calorie diet	52 wks	79	−6.2% (6.2 kg)	−4.3% (4.3 kg)	49%	23%
Miles et al. [77]	Type 2 DM BMI 28–43 HbA1c 7.5–12%	120	Reduced calorie diet	1 yr	60.2	−4.6% (−4.7 kg)	−1.7% (−1.8 kg)	39%	15.7%

Table 3. (Continued)

Authors	Population	Dose (mg TID)	Cointervention or run-in	Duration	Percentage completing	Orlistat-mwc	Placebo-mwc	Orlistat cwl5	Placebo cwl5
Rossner et al. [71]	European BMI 28–43	60 120	Reduced calorie diet 1st yr, wt maintenance diet 2nd yr	2 yrs	71.5 (1 yr) 59.7 (2 yrs)	−9.4 kg (9.7%) at 1 yr −7.4 kg (7.6%) at 2 yrs (120 mg group)	−6.4 kg (6.6%) at 1 yr −4.3 kg (4.5%) at 2 yrs	∼63% at 1 yr (120 mg group)	∼43% at 1 yr
Togerson et al. [75]	Swedish BMI > 30 21% IGT	120	Lifestyle intervention	4 yrs	43	−5.8 kg at 4 yrs (ITT)	−3.0 kg at 4 yrs (ITT)	52.8% at 4 yrs (compl)	37.3% at 4yrs (compl)
Weight loss maintenance									
Hill et al. [84]	BMI 28–43	30 60 120	≥ 8% wt loss with low-calorie diet at 6 months before randomization	1 yr	74% from randomization	−8.2% (−7.2 kg) fse (120-mg group)	−6.4% (−5.9 kg) fse	61.8% fse (120-mg group)	49.8% fse

BMI, body mass index in kg/m^2; IGT, impaired glucose tolerance; ITT, intent to treat; wks, weeks; yrs, years; mwc, mean wt change; cwl5, categorical wt loss (<5%); fse, from study entry; compl, completers.

20% to 50% of the placebo group. Data from Torgerson and colleagues in a 4-year trial in more than 3000 subjects demonstrated orlistat therapy and lifestyle intervention resulted in weight loss of 11% and 7% at 1 and 4 years compared to 6% and 4% in the placebo and lifestyle group [75]. A meta-analysis of weight loss medications by Li and colleagues reported a mean weight loss difference of 2.89 kg (CI, 2.27 to 3.51 kg) at 12 months in orlistat groups relative to placebo [30]. The 2.89 kg represents the amount of weight loss greater than placebo, not the total amount of weight loss achieved with the drug.

7.3.   Efficacy in Weight Loss Maintenance

Weight loss maintenance with orlistat was evaluated in a 1-year study published by Hill and colleagues [84]. More than 700 subjects who lost more than 8% of their body weight over a 6-month period eating a calorie-reduced diet were randomized to receive either placebo or 30-, 60-, or 120-mg of orlistat three times a day for an additional 12 months [84]. At the end of the 12-month maintenance phase the placebo group had regained 58.7% of their body weight compared with 32.8% regain of body weight in the group treated with 120 mg of orlistat three times a day. Almost half (47.5%) of the 120-mg Orlistat group regained < 25% of their initial weight loss compared to 30% of the placebo group. Improvements in cardiovascular risk factors were also noted. This study illustrated that partial inhibition of dietary fat absorption enhanced long-term weight maintenance following a significant weight loss.

7.4.   Efficacy in Managing Obesity-related Risk Factors

The role of orlistat in the prevention of type 2 diabetes was studied in a large prospective multicenter randomized double-blinded placebo-controlled 4-year study in Sweden called the Xenical Diabetes Outcome Study (Xendos) [75]. This study is the longest trial to date with weight loss medications. Approximately 3200 obese subjects were enrolled in a lifestyle plus placebo or orlistat treatment protocol. Twenty-one percent of participants had impaired glucose tolerance (IGT). At year 4 the placebo group had maintained a loss of 4.1 kg and the orlistat group had maintained a loss of 6.9 kg. The incidence of diabetes was 6.2% in the orlistat-treated group and 9.0% in the patient treated with placebo. Therapy with orlistat in this trial resulted in a 37% reduction in the incidence of new onset type 2 diabetes. The difference in the rate was seen because of a decrease in conversion of the IGT group to type 2 diabetes.

Several studies have evaluated the effect of orlistat on glycemic control in patients with type 2 diabetes [76–78]. In all these studies, the average weight loss was greater and HbA1c decreased more in the orlistat groups compared to placebo. In general two to three times more diabetic patients in these trials achieved a 5% or 10% decrease in body weight. A meta-analysis of seven randomized control trials of orlistat in overweight and obese patients with type 2 diabetes found 23% of orlistat patients achieved a weight reduction $\geq$ 5% [79]. These patients showed a mean decrease in HbA1c of 1.16%, a weight reduction of 8.6 kg, a reduction in total cholesterol of 5.3%, and a reduction in systolic blood pressure of 5.2 mm Hg [79].

Heymsfield and colleagues analyzed all the orlistat trials that lasted longer than 1 year and found that conversion of normal glucose tolerance to diabetes occurred in 6.6% of orlistat patients and 11% of placebo-treated patients. Conversion of IGT to diabetes was also less frequent in the orlistat group then placebo (3.0% and 7.5%) [85]. These data show that modest weight reduction with orlistat may lead to an important risk reduction for the development of type 2 diabetes.

One unique feature of orlistat is its beneficial effect on serum cholesterol concentration that is independent of weight loss alone [68, 72, 86]. The decrease in low-density lipoprotein (LDL) cholesterol concentrations after weight reduction with orlistat therapy is greater than after placebo therapy even when statistically adjusted for differences in the amount of weight reduction [68, 72]. The mechanism responsible for this lipid-lowering effect may be related to the ability of orlistat to block dietary cholesterol and triglyceride absorption [86]. Patients treated with orlistat had almost twice as much reduction in LDL cholesterol as the placebo-treated groups for the same amount of weight reduction at the end of 12 months.

7.5.   Tolerability and Safety

Orlistat has not been associated with a serious event profile. The drug is very safe and little if any monitoring requirements are necessary from a safety standpoint. It is not absorbed to any significant degree. The tolerability of orlistat, however, is not as good as its safety profile. About 75% of subjects treated with orlistat experience one or more gastrointestinal (GI) side effects [66]. This is not surprising because the mechanism of action of orlistat involves the malabsorption of fat. These GI adverse effects are manageable if patients control the amount of fat in their diet. The more dietary fat orlistat-treated patients eat, the more likely they are to have GI side effects. For this reason, patients must be informed of how to decrease the amount of fat in their diet.

The most common GI adverse events associated with the use of orlistat include abdominal pain, liquid stool, nausea, vomiting, and flatulence [81]. These adverse effects usually occurred early in treatment (first 4 weeks of therapy) and were mild or moderate in intensity and resolved spontaneously without intervention. However, 20% to 40% of patients will have at least one major GI event. Approximately 4% of subjects treated with orlistat withdrew from treatment compared to 1% in the placebo group [66]. Because of the mechanism of action, small decreases in fat-soluble vitamin concentrations are possible but usually remain in the normal range without vitamin supplementation. Orlistat has also been shown to block beta-carotene absorption by one third [87].

7.6. Special Considerations when Prescribing Orlistat

About 5% of patients taking orlistat may experience larger decreases in vitamin levels than the general population. Because those patients cannot be predicted and vitamin levels can be difficult to measure routinely, all patients are recommended to take a daily multivitamin supplement at a time when orlistat is not being consumed. Orlistat can also impair the absorption of lipophilic medications. Therefore absorption of drugs such as cyclosporine can be impaired and levels of cyclosporine have dropped in obese patients that began orlistat after organ transplantation [88, 89]. Nonlipophilic drugs (antihypertensives, warfarin, digoxin, phenytoin, oral contraceptives) are not blocked from absorption and dosages do not need to be adjusted [90–96]. Patients on blood thinners such as warfarin, however, who are keeping their INRs in a narrow therapeutic window, usually for important health reasons should have their INRs followed carefully when starting orlistat. This is not because orlistat blocks absorption of the medication but because changes in vitamin K level could in theory affect the dose of the medication needed to keep the INR in the therapeutic window.

8.   THE FUTURE OF WEIGHT LOSS MEDICATIONS

8.1. Sibutramine and Orlistat Usage in Adolescents

The increasing prevalence of obesity among children and adolescents is of great concern. The use of weight loss medications for obesity in the adolescent population is largely investigational. However, a few studies have been published that evaluated the efficacy and safety in this population [97–99]. Godoy-Matos and colleagues evaluated the efficacy and safety of sibutramine versus placebo in 60 adolescents (14 to 17 years) for 6 months [97]. Patients in the sibutramine group lost an average 10.3 kg and patients in the placebo group lost on average 2.4 kg at 6 months ($p < 0.001$) [97]. Berkowitz and colleagues randomized 82 adolescents aged 13 to 17 years with a BMI of 32 to 44 to behavioral therapy plus placebo or sibutramine 15 mg for 6 months followed by an open label sibutramine only period of 6 months [98]. Adolescents in the sibutramine arm lost 7.8 kg and had a 8.5% reduction in BMI compared to the placebo group that lost 3.2 kg and reduced BMI by 4% at the end of 6 months. Ten adolescents in the study had sustained marked increases in blood pressure

($\geq$ 10 mm Hg) that required discontinuation of the medication and 23 required a reduction in dosage.

A large study by Chanoine and colleagues evaluated the use of orlistat in 539 obese adolescents in a randomized multicenter 54-week double-blinded study evaluating the use of orlistat [99]. They found a decrease in BMI in both treatment groups up to 12 weeks, thereafter stabilizing with orlistat but increasing above baseline with placebo [99]. Twenty-six percent of the orlistat group had 5% or higher decrease in BMI compared with 15.7% of the placebo group. No major safety concerns were noted in this study; however, gastrointestinal adverse events were more common in the orlistat group.

8.2. Combination Therapy

Because sibutramine and orlistat work to reduce weight be completely different mechanisms combining them might produce synergy in terms of weight reduction. Wadden and colleges evaluated this possibility and randomly assigned patients to orlistat or placebo following a year of treatment with sibutramine [100]. Unfortunately, over the next 4 months of treatment no additional weight loss was seen with the addition of orlistat when compared to placebo.

8.3. Continuous vs. Episodic Medication Usage

Although experts agree that weight loss medications should be considered as long-term interventions similar to hypertension or diabetes medications, obesity medications may turn out to be slightly different in how they can be prescribed. Unlike elevated blood pressure and blood sugar, total weight regain does not occur in a few days or even weeks after stopping medications. It is possible that weight loss medications may need to be chronic but not necessarily constant to be effective long-term. Sibutramine (15 mg) given continuously for one year has been compared with placebo and sibutramine (15 mg) given intermittently [52]. In this study responders (patients losing an initial 2% of body weight or 2 kg) after 4 weeks of treatment with sibutramine 15 mg were randomized to continuous sibutramine, placebo, or intermittent sibutramine (dosed for 11 weeks, then discontinued for 7 weeks). There was small regain in weight during periods when the drug was not given followed by weight loss when the drug was resumed. Overall intermittent sibutramine therapy and continuous sibutramine therapy produced similar weight loss results and were both significantly better than placebo (see Figure 3). In clinical practice, it is sometimes difficult to obtain long-term compliance with medications. This study supports a novel concept that intermittent use may be an effective option and may once again change how we view and prescribe medication therapy in the future.

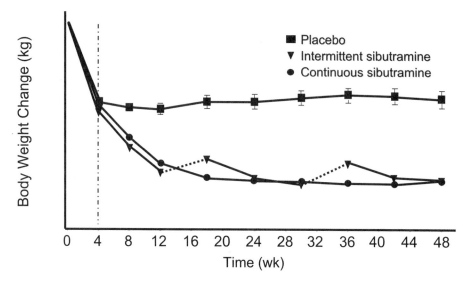

Figure 3. Weight loss results for intermittent sibutramine therapy and continuous sibutramine therapy. (From Wirth and Krause [52].)

9.   SUMMARY

Obesity is a chronic medical disease that is not going away any time soon. Physicians need all the education, tools, and resources possible to successfully help the overweight and obese patients in their practices. Weight loss medications alone are clearly not the answer. They represent, however, one evidence-based tool physicians can use in combination with lifestyle changes to increase long-term weight loss success in appropriate patients. Multiple studies have shown more patients can achieve a significant weight loss when they combine lifestyle and weight loss medications than either alone. Both sibutramine and orlistat have demonstrated effectiveness for obesity treatment and represent evidence-based tools physicians should consider using in appropriate patients. In the future, using combinations of weight loss medications along with new drugs in development may yield additional safe and long-term treatments to treat this serious metabolic disease.

REFERENCES

[1] National Institutes of Health: Clinical guidelines on the identification, evaluation, and treatment of overweight and obesity in adults—the Evidence Report. Obes Res 1998;6(Suppl 2):51S–210S.

[2] Flegal KM, Carroll MD, Ogden CL, Johnson CL. Prevalence and trends in obesity among US adults, 1999–2000. JAMA 2002;288:1723–1727.

[3] Diabetes Prevention Program Research Group. Reduction in the incidence of type 2 diabetes with lifestyle intervention or metformin. N Engl J Med 2002;346:393–403.

[4] Wadden TA, Sternberg JA, Letizia KA, Stunkard AJ, Foster GD. Treatment of obesity by very low calorie diet, behavior therapy, and their combination: A five-year perspective. Int J Obes 1989;13(Suppl 2):39–46.

[5] Wadden TA. Treatment of obesity by moderate and severe caloric restriction in weight loss and control: Results of clinical research trials. Ann Intern Med 1993;119:688–693.

[6] Kramer FM, Jeffery RW, Forster JL, Snell MK. Long-term follow-up of behavioral treatment for obesity: Patterns of weight regain among men and women. Int J Obes 1989; 13:123–136.

[7] Skunkard AJ, McLaren-Hume M. The results of treatment for obesity. Arch Int Med 1959; 103:79–85.

[8] Pavlou KN, Krey S, Steffee WP. Exercise as an adjunct to weight loss and maintenance in moderately obese subjects. Am J Clin Nutr 1989;49:1115–1123.

[9] Perri MG, McAllister DA, Gange JJ, Jordan RC, McAdoo WG, Nezu AM. Effects of four maintenance programs on the long-term management of obesity. J Consult Clin Psychol 1988;56(4):529–534.

[10] Calle EE, Thum MJ, Petrelli JM, et al. Body mass index and mortality in a prospective cohort of US adults. N Engl J Med 1999;341:1097–1105.

[11] Colditz GA, Willett WC, Stampfer MJ, et al. Weight as a risk factor for clinical diabetes in women. Am J Epidemiol 1990;132:501.

[12] Manson JE, Willet WC, Stampfer MJ, et al. Body weight and mortality among women. N Eng J Med 1995;333:677–685.

[13] Arterburn DE, Crane PK, Veenstra DL. The efficacy and safety of sibutramine for weight loss: A systematic review. Arch Intern Med 2004;164(9):994–1003.

[14] Bray GA. Uses and misuses of the new pharmacotherapy of obesity [editorial]. Ann Med 1999;31:1–3.

[15] Connolly HM, Crary J, McGoon MD, et al. Valvular heart disease associated with fenfluramine-phentermine. N Engl J Med 1997;337:581–588.

[16] Yanovski SZ, Yankovski JA. Obesity. N Engl J Med 2002;346:591–602.

[17] Bray GA, Greenway FL. Current and potential drugs for the treatment of obesity. Endocrinol Rev 1999;20:805–875.

[18] Bray GA. Drug treatment of obesity. Psychiatr Clin N Am 2005;28:193–217.

[19] World Health Organization. Obesity: Preventing and managing the global epidemic. WHO Technical Report Series 894. Albany, NY: World Health Organization, 2000.

[20] Peters JC, Wyatt HR, Donahoo WT, Hill JO. From instinct to intellect: The challenge of maintaining healthy weight in the modern world. Obes Rev 2002;3:69–74.

[21] Comuzzie AG, Allison DB. The search for human obesity genes. Science 1998;280: 1374–1377.

[22] Levine JA, Eberhardt NL, Jensen MD. Role of nonexercise activity thermogenesis in resistance to fat gain in humans. Science 1999;283:212–214.

[23] Foster GD, Wadden TA, Vogt RA. What is a reasonable weight loss? Patients' expectations and evaluations of obesity treatment outcomes. J Consult Clin Psychol 1997;65:79–85.

[24] Kushner RF. Roadmaps for Clinical Practice: Case Studies in Disease Prevention and Health Promotion—Assessment and Management of Adult Obesity: A Primer for Physicians. Chicago: American Medical Association, 2003.

[25] Bray GA. Barriers to the treatment of obesity. Ann Intern Med 1991;115:152–153.

[26] Wyatt HR, Hill JO. What role for weight-loss medication? Weighing the pros and cons for obese patients. Postgrad Med 2004;115(1):38–40, 43–35, 58.

[27] Downey M. Insurance coverage for obesity treatments. In: Bessesen DH, Kushner R, eds. Evaluation and Management of Obesity. Philadelphia, PA: Hanley & Belfus, 2002.

[28] Ryan DH. Use of sibutramine to treat obesity. Prim Care Clin Office Pract 2003;30:405–426.

[29] Hollander P. Orlistat in the treatment of obesity. Prim Care Clin Office Pract 2003;30: 427–440.

[30] Li Z, Maglione M, Tu W, et al. Meta-analysis: Pharmacologic treatment of obesity. Anna Intern Med 2005;142(7):532–546.

[31] Wadden TA, Berkowitz RI, Sarwer DB, et al. Benefits of lifestyle modification in the pharmacologic treatment of obesity: A randomized trial. Arch Intern Med 2001;161(2): 218–227.

[32] Kelly F, Jones SP, Lee IK. Sibutramine; weight loss in depressed patients [abstract]. Int J Obes Related Metab Dis 1995;19(Suppl 2):145.

[33] Luque CA, Rey JA. Sibutramine: A serotonin–norepinephrine reuptake-inhibitor for the treatment of obesity. Ann Pharmacother 1999;33:968–978.

[34] Chapelot D, Marmonier C, Thomas F, et al. Modalities of the food intake-reducing effect of sibutramine in humans. Physiol Behav 2000;68(3):299–308.

[35] Rolls BJ, Shide DJ, Thorwart ML, et al. Sibutramine reduces food intake in non-dieting women with obesity. Obes Res 1998;6(1):1–11.

[36] Heal DJ, Aspley S, Prow MR, et al. Sibutramine: A novel anti-obesity drug. A review of the pharmacological evidence to differentiate it from d-amphetamine and d-fenfluramine. Int J Obes Relat Metab Disord 1998;22(Suppl 1):S18–S28; discussion S29.

[37] Connoley IP, Liu YL, Frost I, et al. Thermogenic effects of sibutramine and its metabolites. Br J Pharmacol 1999;126(6):1487–1495.

[38] Walsh KM, Leen E, Lean ME. The effect of sibutramine on resting energy expenditure and adrenaline-induced thermogenesis in obese females. Int J Obes Relat Metab Disord 1999;23(10):1009–1015.

[39] Hansen DL, Toubro S, Stock MJ, et al. Thermogenic effects of sibutramine in humans. Am J Clin Nutr 1998;68(6):1180–1186.

[40] Seagle HM, Bessesen DH, Hill JO. Effects of sibutramine on resting metabolic rate and weight loss in overweight women. Obes Res 1998;6:115–121.

[41] Bray GA, Blackburn GL, Ferguson JM, et al. Sibutramine produces dose-related weight loss. Obes Res 1999;7(2)189–198.

[42] Bray GA, Ryan DH, Gordon D, et al. A double-blind randomized placebo-controlled trial of sibutramine. Obes Res 1996;4(3):263–270.

[43] Dujovne CA, Zavoral JH, Rowe E, et al. Effects of sibutramine on body weight and serum lipids: A double-blind, randomized, placebo-controlled study in 322 overweight and obese patients with dyslipidemia. Am Heart J 2001;142(3):489–497.

[44] Fanghanel G, Cortinas L, Sanchez-Reyes L, et al. A clinical trial of the use of sibutramine for the treatment of patients suffering essential obesity. Int J Obes Relat Metab Disord 2000;24(2):144–150.

[45] Finer N, Bloom SR, Frost GS, et al. Sibutramine is effective for weight loss and diabetic control in obesity with type 2 diabetes: A randomised, double-blind, placebo-controlled study. Diabetes Obes Metab 2000;2(2):105–112.

[46] McMahon FG, Fujioka K, Singh BN, et al. Efficacy and safety of sibutramine in obese white and African American patients with hypertension: A 1-year, double-blind, placebo-controlled, multicenter trial. Arch Intern Med 2000;160(14):2185–2191.

[47] McNulty SJ, Ur E, Williams G. A randomized trial of sibutramine in the management of obese type 2 diabetic patients treated with metformin. Diabetes Care 2003;26(1):125–131.

[48] Apfelbaum M, Vague P, Ziegler O, et al. Long-term maintenance of weight loss after a very-low-calorie diet: A randomized blinded trial of the efficacy and tolerability of sibutramine. Am J Med 1999;106(2):179–184.

[49] Cuellar GE, Ruiz AM, Monsalve MC, et al. Six-month treatment of obesity with sibutramine 15 mg; a double-blind, placebo-controlled monocenter clinical trial in a hispanic population. Obes Res 2000;8(1):71–82.

[50] Philip W, James T, Astrup A, et al. Effect of sibutramine on weight maintenance after weight loss: A randomized trial. Lancet 2000;356(9248):2119–2125.

[51] Vettor R, Serra R, Fabris R, et al. Effect of sibutramine on weight management and metabolic control in type 2 diabetes: A meta-analysis of clinical studies. Diabetes Care 2005;28(4):942–949.

[52] Wirth A, Krause J. Long-term weight loss with sibutramine: A randomized controlled trial. JAMA 2001;286(11):1331–1339.

[53] James WP, Astrup A, Finer N, et al. Effect of sibutramine on weight maintenance after weight loss: A randomised trial. Storm study group. Sibutramine trial of obesity reduction and maintenance. Lancet 2000;356(9248):2119–2125.

[54] Fujioka K, Seaton TB, Rowe E, et al. Weight loss with sibutramine improves glycaemic control and other metabolic parameters in obese patients with type 2 diabetes mellitus. Diabetes Obes Metab 2000;2(3):175–187.

[55] Gokcel A, Karakose H, Ertorer EM, et al. Effects of sibutramine in obese female subjects with type 2 diabetes and poor blood glucose control. Diabetes Care 2001;24(11):1957–1960.

[56] Serrano-Rios M, Melchionda N, Morenao-Carretero E. Spanish investigators. Role of sibutramine in the treatment of obese type 2 diabetic patients receiving sulfonylurea therapy. Diabet Med 2002;19:119–124.

[57] O'Meara S, Riemsma R, Shirran L, et al. The clinical effectiveness and cost effectiveness of sibutramine in the management of obesity. Health Technol Assess 2002;6:1–97.

[58] Vettor R, Serra R, Fabris R, Pagano C, Federspil G. Effect of sibutramine on weight management and metabolic control in type 2 diabetes: A metaanalysis of clinical studies. Diabetes Care 2005;28:942–949.

[59] Samsa GP, Kolotkin RL, Williams GR, et al. Effect of moderate weight loss on health-related quality of life: An analysis of combined data from 4 randomized trials of sibutramine vs placebo. Am J Manag Care 2001;7(9):875–883.

[60] Bach DS, Rissanen AM, Mendel CM, et al. Absence of cardiac valve dysfunction in obese patients treated with sibutramine. Obes Res 1999;7(4):363–369.

[61] Zannad F, Gille B, Grentzinger A, et al. Effects of sibutramine on ventricular dimensions and heart valves in obese patients during weight reduction. Am Heart J 2002;144(3):508–515.

[62] Cole JO, Levin A, Beake B, et al. Sibutramine: A new weight loss agent without evidence of the abuse potential associated with amphetamines. J Clin Psychopharmacol 1998; 18(3):231–236.

[63] Lean ME. Sibutramine—a review of clinical efficacy. Int J Obes Relat Metab Disord 1997; 21(Suppl 1):S30–S36; discussion 37–39.

[64] Jordan J, Scholze J, Matiba B, Wirth A, Hauner H, Sharma AM. Influence of sibutramine on blood pressure: Evidence from placebo-controlled trials. Int J Obes 2005;29:509–516.

[65] Narkiewicz K. Sibutramine and its cardiovascular profile. Int J Obes Relat Metab Disord 2002;26(Suppl 4):S38–S41.

[66] Klein S. Long-term pharmacotherapy for obesity. Obes Res 2004;12(Suppl):163S–166S.

[67] Smith IG, Goulder MA. Randomized placebo-controlled trial of long-term treatment with sibutramine in mild to moderate obesity. J Fam Pract 2001;50(6):505–512.

[68] Davidson MH, Hauptman J, DiGirolamo M, et al. Weight control and risk factor reduction in obese subjects treated for 2 years with orlistat: A randomized controlled trial. JAMA 1999;281(3):235–242.

[69] Drent ML, Larsson I, William-Olsson T, et al. Orlistat (Ro 18-0647), a lipase inhibitor, in the treatment of human obesity: Multiple dose study. Int J Obes Relat Metab Disord 1995;19:221–226.

[70] Van Gaal LF, Broom JI, Enzi G, et al. Efficacy and tolerability of orlistat in the treatment of obesity: A 6-month dose-ranging study. Orlistat dose-ranging study group. Eur J Clin Pharmacol 1998;54(2):125–132.

[71] Rossner S, Sjostrom L, Noack R, et al. Weight loss, weight maintenance, and improved cardiovascular risk factors after 2 years treatment with orlistat for obesity. European orlistat obesity study group. Obes Res 2000;8(1):49–61.

[72] Sjostrom L, Rissanen A, Andersen T, et al. Randomised placebo-controlled trial of orlistat for weight loss and prevention of weight regain in obese patients. European multicentre orlistat study group. Lancet 1998;352(9123):167–172.

[73] Finer N, James WP, Kopelman PG, Lean ME, Williams G. One-year treatment of obesity: A randomized, double blinded placebo-controlled, multicenter study of orlistat, a gastrointestinal lipase inhibitor. Int J Obes Metab Disord 2000;24:306–313.

[74] Hauptman J, Lucas C, Boldrin MN, Collins HG, Seagal KR. Orlistat in the long-term treatment of obesity in primary care settings. Arch Fam Med 2000;9:160–167.

[75] Torgerson JS, Hauptman J, Boldrin MN, Sjostrom L. XENical in the prevention of diabetes in obese subjects (XEN-DOS) study: A randomized study of orlistat as an adjunct to lifestyle changes for the prevention of type 2 diabetes in obese patients. Diabetes Care 2004;27:155–161.

[76] Hollander PA, Elbein SC, Hirsch IB, et al. Role of orlistat in the treatment of obese patients with type 2 diabetes. A 1-year randomized double-blind study. Diabetes Care 1998; 21(8):1288–1294.

[77] Miles JM, Leiter L, Hollander P, et al. Effect of orlistat in overweight and obese patients with type 2 diabetes treated with metformin. Diabetes Care 2002;25(7):1123–1128.

[78] Kelley DE, Bray GA, Pi-Sunyer FX, et al. Clinical efficacy of orlistat therapy in overweight and obese patients with insulin-treated type 2 diabetes: A 1-year randomized controlled trial. Diabetes Care 2002;25(6):1033–1041.

[79] Ruof J, Golay A, Berne C, et al. Orlistat in responding obese type 2 diabetic patients: Meta-analysis findings and cost-effectiveness as rationales for reimbursement in Sweden and Switzerland. Int J Obes Relat Metab Disord 2005;29(5):517–523.

[80] Guerciolini R. Mode of action of orlistat. Int J Obes Relat Metab Disord 1997;21 (Suppl 3):S12–S23.

[81] Drent ML, van der Veen EA. Lipase inhibition; a novel concept in the treatment of obesity. Int J Obes 1993;17:241–244.

[82] Zhi J, Melia AT, Funk C, et al. Metabolic profiles of minimally absorbed orlistat in obese/overweight volunteers. J Clin Pharmacol 1996;36(11):1006–1011.

[83] Zhi J, Melia AT, Guerciolini R, et al. Retrospective population-based analysis of the dose-response (fecal fat excretion) relationship of orlistat in normal and obese volunteers. Clin Pharmacol Ther 1994;56(1):82–85.

[84] Hill JO, Hauptmann J, Andersen JW, et al. Orlistat, a lipase inhibitor, for weight maintenance after conventional dieting: A 1 year study. Am J Clin Nutr 1999;69:1108–1116.

[85] Heymsfield S, Segal K, Hauptman J, et al. Effects of weight loss with orlistat on glucose tolerance and progression of type 2 diabetes in obese adults. Arch Intern Med 2000; 160:1321–1326.

[86] Mittendorfer B, Ostlund RE Jr, Patterson BW, et al. Orlistat inhibits dietary cholesterol absorption. Obes Res 2001;9(10):599–604.

[87] Zhi J, Melia AT, Koss-Twardy SG, et al. The effect of orlistat, an inhibitor of dietary fat absorption, on the pharmacokinetics of beta-carotene in healthy volunteers. J Clin Pharmacol 1996;36(2):152–159.

[88] Coleman E, Fossler M. Reduction in blood cyclosporine concentrations by orlistat. N Engl J Med 2000;342:1141–1142.

[89] LeBeller C, Bezie Y, Chabatte C, Guillemain R, Amrein C, Billaud EM. Co-administration of orlistat and cyclosporin in heart transplant recipient. Transplantation. 2000; 70:1541–1542.

[90] Schnetzler B, Kondo-Oe Weber C, et al. Effect of the lipase inhibitor orlistat on the pharmacokinetics of four different antihypertensive agents in healthy volunteers. Eur J Clin Parmacol 1996;51:87–90.

[91] Melia AT, Mulligan TE, Zhi J. Lack of effect of orlistat on the bioavailability of a single-dose of nifedipine extended-release tablets (Procardia XL) in healthy volunteers. J Clin Pharmacol 1996;36:352–355.

[92] Zhi J, Melia AT, Guerciolini R, et al. The effect of orlistat on the pharmacokinetics and pharmacodynamics of warfarin in healthy volunteers. J Clin Parmacol 1996;36:659–666.

[93] Melia AT, Zhi J, Koss-Twardy SG, et al. The influence of reduced dietary fat absorption induced by orlistat on the pharmacokinetics of digoxin in healthy volunteers. J Clin Pharmacol 1995;35:840–843.

[94] Melia AT, Mulligan TE, Zhi J. The effect of orlistat on the pharmacokinetics of phenytoin in healthy volunteers. J Clin Pharmacol 1996;36:654–658.

[95] Zhi J, Melia AT, Koss-Twardy SG, et al. The influence of orlistat on the pharmacokinetics and pharmacodynamics of glyburide in healthy volunteers. J. Clin Pharmacol 1995;35:521–525.

[96] Hartman D, Guzelhan C, Zuiderwijk PMB, Odink J. Lack of interaction between orlistat and oral contraceptives. Eur J Clin Pharmacol 1996;50:421–424.

[97] Godoy-Matos A, Carraro L, Vieira A, et al. Treatment of obese adolescents with sibutramine: A randomized, double-blind, controlled study. J Clin Endocrinol Metab 2005; 90(3):1460–1465.

[98] Berkowitz RI, Wadden TA, Tershakovec AM, et al. Behavior therapy and sibutramine for the treatment of adolescent obesity: A randomized controlled trial. JAMA 2003;289 (14):1805–1812.

[99] Chanoine JP, Hamptl S, Jensen C, Boldrin M, Hauptman J. Effect of orlistat on weight and body composition in obese adolescents: A randomized controlled trial. JAMA 2005; 293(23):2873–2883.

[100] Wadden TA, Berkowitz RI, Womble LG, et al. Effects of sibutramine plus orlistat in obese women following 1 year of treatment by sibutramine alone: A placebo controlled trail. Obes Res 2000;8(6):431–437.

Chapter 16

A Status of Drugs on the Horizon for Obesity and the Metabolic Syndrome— a Comprehensive Review 2005

Frank Greenway and George Bray

Pennington Biomedical Research Center, Louisiana State University System, Baton Rouge, LA 70808, USA

1. INTRODUCTION

Although the drug treatment of obesity has a long history, progress was given an impetus by the discovery of leptin. This particular peptide demonstrated that obesity can be caused by a hormone deficiency and be reversed by replacement of that hormone [1, 2]. In fact, at the NIH conference of 1985, obesity was declared to be a chronic disease, not a consequence of bad habits as it was formerly considered [3]. Because bad habits can be extinguished over a 12-week period, obesity medications approved before 1985 were approved for periods up to 12 weeks as an adjunct to a lifestyle change program. The stigma associated with obesity and the public's equating it with bad habits slowed the chronic use of obesity medications as is done with other chronic diseases [4]. Therefore, although thyroid hormone was used in the treatment of obesity from the late 19th century, there have been medications approved for the chronic treatment of obesity only since 1995 [5, 6].

Although only two medications have been approved for the long-term treatment of obesity—sibutramine and orlistat—there is a great deal of activity in the pharmaceutical industry to develop new drugs or discover old ones to treat this disease. The prevalence of obesity continues to grow and new obesity drugs are clearly needed.

The public health significance of treating obesity cannot be understated. In susceptible individuals obesity will lead to the development of traditional and nontraditional cardiovascular risk factors and to the development of a condition referred to as the "metabolic syndrome." The "metabolic syndrome" describes coexisting traditional risk factors for cardiovascular disease (CVD) such as hypertension, dyslipidemia, glucose intolerance, obesity, and insulin resistance, in addition to nontraditional CVD risk factors such as inflammatory processes and abnormalities of the blood coagulation system [7–13]. Although the etiology of the metabolic syndrome is not specifically known, it is well established that central obesity and insulin resistance are generally present. The components of the metabolic syndrome contribute greatly to increased morbidity and mortality in humans on several levels. First, metabolic syndrome can be considered to be a "prediabetic" condition. A second reason why obesity and metabolic syndrome contribute to increased morbidity and mortality is the association with CVD. Coexisting CVD risk factors such as dyslipidemia, hypertension, inflammatory markers and coagulopathy are highly associated with the "pre-diabetic" state as defined by central obesity and insulin resistance [11, 14–16]. Each risk factor, when considered alone, increases CVD risk, but in combination they provide a "synergistic" or "additive" effect [16]. The presence of the "metabolic syndrome" may increase the relative risk of CVD by 3- to 4-fold, and the increase in relative risk for CVD precedes the diagnosis of diabetes by as much as 15 years [17, 18].

Approximately 7% to 8% of the United States population have adult-onset diabetes, and approximately 40% are obese and 25% have the metabolic syndrome [19–21]. Minority ethnic groups are at even greater risk. Although lifestyle interventions consisting of weight loss and exercise will greatly improve insulin sensitivity and can delay the progression to type 2 diabetes [22], maintenance of lifestyle changes in humans over a long-term period is poor, and pharmacologic approaches for treatment of obesity hold greater promise for success.

We review the information about presently available drugs for other purposes that produce weight loss, discuss the drugs in late development with an emphasis on rimonabant which seems likely to be approved, and then cover in less depth the drugs in earlier stages of development.

2. DRUGS APPROVED FOR INDICATIONS OTHER THAN OBESITY AND THAT CAUSE WEIGHT LOSS

2.1. Bupropion

Bupropion is a norepinephrine and dopamine reuptake inhibitor that is approved for the treatment of depression and for smoking cessation. Gadde et al. reported a clinical trial in which 50 obese subjects were randomized to bupropion or placebo for 8 weeks with a blinded extension for responders to 24 weeks. The dose of bupropion was increased to a maximum of 200 mg twice daily in conjunction with a calorie-restricted diet. At 8 weeks, 18 subjects in the bupropion group lost $6.2 \pm 3.1\%$ of body weight compared to $1.6 \pm 2.9\%$ for the 13 subjects in the placebo group ($p < 0.0001$). After 24 weeks, the 14 responders to bupropion lost $12.9 \pm 5.6\%$ of initial body weight, of which 75% was fat, as determined by dual-energy X-ray absorptiometry (DEXA) [23].

Two multicenter clinical trials, one in obese subjects with depressive symptoms and one in uncomplicated obesity, followed this study. The study in obese patients with depressive symptom ratings of 10 to 30 on a Beck Depression Inventory [24] randomized 213 subjects to 400 mg of bupropion per day and 209 subjects to placebo for 24 weeks. The 121 subjects in the bupropion group that completed the trial lost $6.0 \pm 0.5\%$ of initial body weight compared to $2.8 \pm 0.5\%$ in the 108 subjects in the placebo group ($p < 0.0001$) [25]. The study in uncomplicated obese subjects randomized 327 subjects to bupropion 300 mg/day, bupropion 400 mg/day or placebo in equal proportions. At 24 weeks, 69% of those randomized remained in the study and the percent losses of initial body weight were $5 \pm 1\%$, $7.2 \pm 1\%$, and $10.1 \pm 1\%$ for the placebo, bupropion 300 mg, and bupropion 400 mg groups, respectively ($p < 0.0001$). At 24 weeks the placebo group was randomized to receive either 300 mg or 400 mg and the trial was extended to week 48. By the end of the trial the dropout rate was 41%, and the weight losses in the bupropion 300 mg and bupropion 400 mg groups were $6.2 \pm 1.25\%$ and $7.2 \pm 1.5\%$ of initial body weight, respectively [26].

2.2. Fluoxetine/Sertraline

Fluoxetine and sertraline are both selective serotonin reuptake inhibitors (SSRI) approved for the treatment of depression. Sertraline produced an average weight loss of 0.45 to 0.91 kg in 8- to 16-week clinical trials for depression. Fluoxetine at a dose of 60 mg per day was evaluated by the Lilly Company in clinical trials for the treatment of obesity. Goldstein et al. reviewed these trials, which included one 36-week trial in type 2 diabetic subjects, a 52-week trial in subjects with uncomplicated obesity, and two 60-week trials in subjects with dyslipidemia, diabetes, or both [27]. A total of 1441 subjects were randomized to fluoxetine (719) or placebo (722). Five hundred and twenty-two subjects on fluoxetine and 504 subjects on placebo completed 6 months of treatment. Weight loss in the placebo and fluoxetine groups at 6 months and 1 year were 2.2, 4.8, and 1.8, 2.4 kg, respectively. The regain of 50% of the lost weight during the second 6 months of treatment on fluoxetine made it inappropriate for the treatment on obesity that requires chronic treatment. Fluoxetine and sertraline, although not good obesity drugs, may be preferred in obese individuals over some of the tricyclic antidepressants that are associated with significant weight gain.

2.3.   Zonisamide

Zonisamide is an antiepileptic drug that has serotonergic and dopaminergic activity in addition to inhibiting sodium and calcium channels. Weight loss was noted in the trials for the treatment of epilepsy. Zonisamide has been studied in one 16-week randomized control trial in 60 obese subjects. Subjects were placed on a calorie-restricted diet and randomized to zonisamide or placebo. The zonisamide was started at 100 mg/day and increased to 400 mg/day. At 12 weeks, those subjects who had not lost 5% of initial body weight were increased to 600 mg/day. The zonisamide group lost 6.6% of initial body weight at 16 weeks compared to 1% in the placebo group. Thirty-seven subjects completing the 16-week trial elected to continue to week 32–20 in the zonisamide group and 17 in the placebo group. At the end of 32 weeks, the 19 subjects in the zonisamide group lost 9.6% of their initial body weight compared to 1.6% for the 17 subjects in the placebo group [28].

2.4.   Topiramate

Topiramate is an antiepileptic drug that was observed to give weight loss in the clinical trials for epilepsy. Weight losses of 3.9% of initial weight were seen at 3 months and losses of 7.3% of initial weight were seen at 1 year [29]. Bray et al. reported a 6-month, placebo-controlled, dose-ranging study. Three hundred and eighty-five obese subjects were randomized to placebo or topiramate at 64 mg/day, 96 mg/day, 192 mg/day, or 384 mg/day. These doses were gradually reached by a tapering increase and were reduced in a similar manner at the end of the trial. Weight loss from baseline to 24 weeks was 2.6%, 5%, 4.8% 6.3%, and 6.3% in the placebo, 64-mg, 96-mg, 192-mg, and 384-mg groups, respectively. The most frequent adverse events were paresthesia; somnolence; and difficulty with concentration, memory, and attention [30]. This trial was followed by two multicenter trials. The first trial randomized 1289 obese subjects to topiramate 89 mg/day, 192 mg/day, or 256 mg/day. This trial was terminated early because of the sponsor's decision to pursue a time-release form of the drug. The 854 subjects who completed 1 year of the trial before it was terminated by the sponsor lost 1.7%, 7%, 9.1%, and 9.7% of their initial body weight in the placebo, 89-mg, 192-mg, and 256-mg groups, respectively. Subjects in the topirmate groups had significant improvement in blood pressure and glucose tolerance [31]. The second trial enrolled 701 subjects who were treated with a very low calorie diet to induce an 8% loss of initial body weight. The 560 subjects who achieved an 8% weight loss were randomized to topiramate 96 mg/day, 192 mg/day, or placebo. The sponsor terminated the study early to pursue a time-released formulation of the drug. At the time of early termination, 293 subjects completed 44 weeks. The topiramate 96-mg and 192-mg groups lost 15.4% and 16.5%, respectively, of their baseline weight while the placebo group lost 8.9% [32]. Although topiramate is still available as an antiepileptic drug, the development program to pursue an indication for obesity was terminated by the sponsor in December 2004 because of the associated adverse events.

Topiramate has also been evaluated in the treatment of binge-eating disorder. Thirteen women with binge-eating disorder were treated with a mean dose of 492 mg/day of topiramate. The binge-eating disorder symptoms improved and a weight loss was observed [33]. This open-label study was followed by a randomized controlled trial of 14 weeks in subjects with binge-eating disorder. Sixty-one subjects were randomized to 25–600 mg/day of topiramate or placebo in a 1:1 ratio. The topiramate group had improvement in binge eating symptoms and lost 5.9 kg at an average topiramate dose of 212 mg/day [34]. The 35 completers of this trial were given the opportunity to participate in an open-label extension. The topiramate treated subjects continued to maintain improvement in binge-eating symptoms and weight [35].

Topiramate has also been used to treat patients with the Prader–Willi syndrome. Three subjects with Prader–Willi syndrome were treated with topiramate and had a reduction in the self-injurious behavior that is associated with this uncommon genetic disease [36]. A second study in seven additional subjects confirmed these findings [37]. A third study evaluated appetite, food intake and weight in patients with Prader–Willi syndrome. Although the self-injurious behavior improved, there was no effect on these other parameters [38]. Topiramate was also used to treat two subjects with nocturnal eating syndrome and two subjects with sleep-related eating disorder. There was an improvement in all four subjects and there was an 11-kg mean weight loss over 8.5 months with an average topiramate dose of 218 mg/day [39].

2.5. Metformin

Metformin is a biguanide that is approved for the treatment of diabetes mellitus, a disease that is exacerbated by obesity and weight gain. This drug reduces hepatic glucose production, decreases intestinal absorption from the gastrointestinal tract and enhances insulin sensitivity. In clinical trials where metformin was compared with sulfonylureas, it produced weight loss [40]. In BIGPRO, a 1-year French multicenter study, metformin was compared to placebo in 324 middle-aged subjects with upper body obesity. The subjects on metformin lost significantly more weight (1 to 2 kg) than the placebo group, and the study concluded that metformin may have a role in the primary prevention of type 2 diabetes [41].

The best trial of metformin in terms of evaluating weight loss effects is the Diabetes Prevention Program study of individuals with impaired glucose tolerance. This study included three treatment arms to which participants were randomly assigned, if they were older than 25 years of age, had a body mass index (BMI) above 24 kg/m^2 (except Asian Americans, who needed only a BMI $\geq$ 22 kg/m^2) and had impaired glucose tolerance. The three primary arms included lifestyle ($N = 1079$ participants), metformin ($N = 1073$) and placebo ($N = 1082$). At the end of 2.8 years on average, the Data Safety Monitoring Board terminated the trial because the advantages of lifestyle and metformin were clearly superior to placebo. During this time the metformin-treated group lost 2.5% of their body weight ($p < 0.001$ compared to placebo), and the conversion from impaired glucose tolerance to diabetes was reduced by 31% compared to placebo. In the DPP trial, metformin was more effective in reducing the development of diabetes in the subgroup who were most overweight, and in the younger members of the cohort [22]. Although metformin does not produce enough weight loss (5%) to qualify as a "weight-loss drug" using the FDA criteria, it would appear to be a very useful choice for overweight individuals newly diagnosed with diabetes. Another area where metformin has found use is in treating women with the polycystic ovary syndrome where the modest weight loss may contribute the increased fertility and reduced insulin resistance [42].

2.6.   Somatostatin

Hypothalamic obesity has been associated with insulin hypersecretion [43]. Lustig treated eight children with obesity due to hypothalamic damage with octreotide injections to decrease insulin hypersecretion. These children gained 6 kg in the 6 months prior to octreotide treatment and lost 4.8 kg in the 6 months on octreotide, an analog of somatostatin. The weight loss was correlated with the reduction of insulin secretion on a glucose tolerance test [44]. This open-label trial was followed by a randomized controlled trial of octreotide treatment in children with hypothalamic obesity. The subjects received octreotide 5 to 15 mcg/kg per day or placebo for 6 months. The children on octreotide gained 1.6 kg compared to 9.1 kg for those in the placebo group [45]. This same group of investigators postulated that there might be a subset of obese subjects who were insulin hypersecretors and that these subjects would respond with weight loss to treatment with octreotide. Following an oral glucose tolerance test in which glucose and insulin were measured, 44 subjects were treated with octreotide-LAR 40 mg/month for 6 months. These subjects lost weight, reduced food intake and a reduced carbohydrate intake. Weight loss was greatest in those with insulin hypersecretion and the amount of weight loss was correlated with the reduction in insulin hypersecretion [46]. A controlled trial of octreotide LAR randomized 172 obese subject screened for insulin hypersecretion to doses of 20 mg/mo, 40 mg/month, 60 mg/month or placebo for 6 months. The greatest weight loss was 3.8% of initial body weight in the high-dose group, an amount that does not meet the criteria for approval by the FDA [47].

Octreotide has been shown to decrease gastric emptying [48]. Octreotide treatment of patients with the Prader–Willi syndrome who have elevated ghrelin levels does not cause weight loss but ghrelin levels are normalized. The reason for the lack of weight loss has been postulated to be the reduction of PYY, a satiating gastrointestinal hormone that also decreased [49].

2.7. Pramlintide

Amylin is secreted from β-cells along with insulin, and amylin is deficient in type 1 diabetes where β-cells are immunologically destroyed. Pramlintide, a synthetic amylin analog, was recently approved by the FDA for the treatment of diabetes. Unlike insulin and many other diabetes medications, pramlintide is associated with weight loss. In a study in which 651 subjects with type 1 diabetes were randomized to placebo or subcutaneous pramlintide 60 mcg three or four times a day along with an insulin injection, the hemoglobin A1c decreased 0.29% to 0.34% and weight decreased 1.2 kg relative to placebo [50]. Maggs et al. analyzed the data from two 1-year studies in insulin-treated type 2 diabetic subjects randomized to pramlintide 120 mcg twice a day or 150 mcg three times a day [51]. Weight decreased by 2.6 kg and hemoglobin A1c decreased 0.5%. When weight loss was then analyzed by ethnic group, African Americans lost 4 kg, Caucasians lost 2.4 kg, and Hispanics lost 2.3 kg and the improvement in diabetes correlated with the weight loss, suggesting that pramlintide is effective in ethnic groups with the greatest obesity burden. The most common adverse event was nausea, which was usually mild and confined to the first 4 weeks of therapy.

2.8. Exenatide

Glucagon-like peptide-1 (GLP-1) or enteroglucagon is a protein derived from proglucagon and secreted by L-cells in the terminal ileum in response to a meal. GLP-1 decreases food intake and has been postulated to be responsible for the superior weight loss and superior improvement in diabetes seen with obesity bypass surgery [52, 53]. Increased GLP-1 inhibits glucagon secretion, stimulates insulin secretion, stimulates glycogenesis, and delays gastric emptying [54]. GLP-1 is rapidly degraded by dipeptidyl peptidase-4 (DPP-4), an enzyme that is elevated in the obese. Obesity bypass operations increase GLP-1, but do not change the levels of DPP-4 [55].

Exendin-4 is a 39-amino-acid peptide that is produced in the salivary gland of the Gila monster lizard. It has 53% homology with GLP-1, and has a much longer half-life. Exendin-4 decreases food intake and body weight gain in Zucker rats while lowering HgbA1c [56]. Exendin-4 increases β-cell mass to a greater extent than would be expected for the degree of insulin resistance [57]. Exendin-4 induces satiety and weight loss in Zucker rats with peripheral administration and crosses the blood–brain barrier to act in the central nervous system (CNS) [58, 59]. In humans, exendin-4 reduces fasting and postprandial glucose levels, slows gastric emptying, and decreases food intake by 19% [60]. The side effects of exendin-4 in humans are headache, nausea, and vomiting, which are lessened by gradual dose escalation [61]. Exendin-4 at 10 mcg subcutaneously per day or a placebo was given to 377 type 2 diabetic subjects for 30 weeks who were failing maximal sulfonylurea therapy. The HgbA1c fell 0.74% more than placebo, fasting glucose decreased, and there was a progressive weight loss of 1.6 kg [62]. Thus, exendin-4 shows promise of being an effective treatment for diabetes with a favorable weight loss profile.

3.   DRUGS IN PHASE III CLINICAL TRIALS WITH NO APPROVAL

3.1.   Rimonabant

The endocannabinoid system appears to be a good target for obesity treatment. There are two known cannabinoid receptors, CB-1 (470 amino acids in length) and CB-2 (360 amino acids in length). CB-1 receptors are distributed through the brain in the areas related to feeding, on fat cells, in the GI tract and on immune cells. Marijuana and tetrahydrocannabinol, which stimulate the CB-1 receptor, increase high fat and high sweet food intake, and fasting increases the levels of endocannabinoids. The rewarding properties of cannabinoid agonists are mediated through the mesolimbic dopaminergic system. Rimonabant is a specific antagonist of the CB-1 receptor, and inhibits sweet food intake in marmosets as well as high fat food intake in rats but not in rats fed standard chow. In addition to being specific in inhibiting highly palatable food intake, pair feeding experiments in diet-induced obese rats show that the rimonabant-treated animals lost 21% of their body weight compared to 14% in the pair-fed controls. This suggests, at least in rodents, that rimonabant increases energy expenditure in addition to reducing food intake. CB-1 knockout mice are lean and resistant to diet-induced obesity. CB-1 receptors are upregulated on adipocytes in diet-induced obese mice, and rimonabant increases adiponectin, a fat cell hormone associated with insulin sensitivity [63]. Thus, rimonabant holds promise for potential efficacy not just in weight loss, but also in the lipotoxicity-mediated comorbidities associated with obesity.

The results of four phase III trials of rimonabant for the treatment of obesity have been announced. These reports are posted on the Sanofi Internet Web site, and only one exists in the form of a peer-reviewed publication at the time of this writing [64, 65]. The first trial to be published was the RIO-Europe trial in which 1507 obese subjects were randomized in a 1:2:2 ratio to receive placebo, 5 mg rimonabant, or 20 mg rimonabant once daily for 1 year. Weight loss was 3.5% in the placebo group and 8.5% in the 20 mg rimonabant group. The 20 mg rimonabant group lost 8 cm from the waist, triglycerides decreased 10%, and high-density lipoprotein (HDL) cholesterol rose 28% compared to loss of 4 cm, a rise of 7%, and a rise 16%, respectively, in the placebo group. The prevalence of metabolic syndrome decreased by 34% in the placebo group compared to a 65% decrease in the 20 mg rimonabant group. There was no increase in depression or anxiety as measured by the Hospital Anxiety Depression scale, and there was no increase in pulse or blood pressure, in contrast to sibutramine. The most common side effects were nausea, dizziness, arthralgia, and diarrhea. Forty percent of the study dropped out by 1 year and 14.5% dropped in the high-dose group for an adverse event.

3.2.   Axokine

Axokine is an analog of ciliary neurotrophic factor that, like leptin, acts through the STAT signaling pathway in the brain [66]. Axokine has been tested in two phase II studies, one in obesity and one in diabetes, in addition to one phase III study in obesity. The first multicenter 12-week phase II study randomized 170 obese subjects with a BMI between 35 and 50 kg/m^2. The optimal dose was 1 mcg/kg, and this group lost 4.6 kg compared to a weight gain of 0.6 kg in the placebo group [67]. The second 12-week phase II study randomized 107 overweight and obese type 2 diabetic subjects with a BMI between 35 and 50 kg/m^2 [68]. Subjects treated with the 1.0 mcg/kg dose of axokine lost 3.2 kg compared to 1.2 kg in the placebo group ($p < 0.01$).

The 1-year phase III trial with a 1-year open label extension randomized 501 subjects to placebo and 1467 subjects to axokine at a dose of 1 mcg/kg per day [68]. Subjects had a BMI between 30 and 55 kg/m^2, if their obesity was uncomplicated, or between 27 and 55 kg/m^2, if their obesity was complicated by hypertension or dyslipidemia. At the end of 1 year, the axokine group lost 3.6 kg compared to 2.0 kg in the placebo group ($p < 0.001$), a difference that does not meet the FDA efficacy criteria for approval. The most common adverse events were mild and included injection site reactions, nausea, and cough. The most concerning finding, however, was that two thirds of people receiving axokine developed antibodies after 3 months that limited weight loss, and there was no way to prospectively predict those who would develop the antibodies. Development of axokine has been terminated.

3.3.   Leptin

The lack of leptin, a hormone derived from the fat cell, causes massive obesity in animals and humans. Its replacement reverses the obesity associated with the deficiency state. The discovery of leptin generated hope that leptin would be an effective treatment for obesity. Leptin at subcutaneous doses of 0, 0.01 mg/kg, 0.05 mg/kg, 0.1 mg/kg, and 0.3 mg/kg daily were tested in lean [54] and obese [73] humans of both sexes. Lean subjects were treated for 4 weeks and lost 0.4–1.9 kg. Obese subjects were treated for 24 weeks and a dose–response relationship for weight loss was seen with the 0.3 mg/kg group losing 7.1 kg [69]. Pegylated leptin allows for weekly, rather than daily, injections. Although pegylated leptin at 20 and 60 mg/week in obese subjects over 8 to 12 weeks did not give any weight loss above placebo, pegylated leptin at 80 mg weekly combined with a very low calorie diet for 46 days gave 2.8 kg more weight loss in 12 subjects randomized to leptin compared to the 10 randomized to placebo ($p < 0.03$) [70].

4.   DRUGS IN THE EARLY PHASES OF DEVELOPMENT

4.1.   Growth Hormone Fragment

AOD9604 is a modified fragment of the amino acids in growth hormone from 177 to 191, and is orally active. This growth hormone fragment is said to bind to the fat cell stimulating lipolysis and inhibiting reesterification without stimulating growth. A 12-week multicenter trial randomized 300 obese subjects to one of 5 daily doses (1, 5, 10, 20, and 30 mg) of AOD9604 or placebo. The 1-mg dose was the most effective for weight loss. Subjects on the 1-mg dose lost 2.6 kg compared to 0.8 kg in the placebo group and the rate of weight loss was constant throughout the trial [71]. Phase III trials are being planned.

4.2.   Cholecystokinin

Cholecystokinin decreases food intake by causing subjects to stop eating sooner [72]. Although the relationship between cholecystokinin and satiety has been known for many years, development as a weight loss agent has been slow due to concerns regarding pancreatitis. Because the human pancreas has no cholecystokinin-A receptors, an orally active compound that is a selective agonist of the cholecystokinin-A receptor is being evaluated in clinical trials, but no reports of those trials have yet appeared.

4.3.   PYY 3-36

PYY 3-36 is a hormone produced by the L-cells in the gastrointestinal tract and is secreted in proportion to the caloric content of a meal. PYY 3-36 levels are lower fasting and after a meal in the obese compared to lean subjects. Caloric intake at a lunch buffet was reduced by 30% in 12 obese subjects and by 29% in 12 lean subjects after 2 h of PYY 3-36 infused intravenously [73]. Thrice daily nasal administration over 6 days was well tolerated and reduced caloric intake by about 30% while producing 0.6-kg weight loss [74].

4.4. Oleoylestrone

Oleoylestrone is a weakly estrogenic compound that is produced in fat cells, carried in the blood on HDL particles, and feeds back to the CNS to reduce food intake while maintaining energy expenditure. Oleolyestrone is orally active and has been used to treat one morbidly obese male without an accompanying weight loss program. Oleoylestrone was given in doses of 150 to 300 micromoles/day in 10 consecutive 10-day courses of treatment separated by at least 2 months. Weight dropped 38.5 kg and BMI dropped from 51.9 to 40.5 kg/m^2 over 27 months, and weight was still declining at the time of the report [75]. Oleoylestrone was well tolerated and there were no estrogenic side effects observed. Phase I trials are presently in progress.

4.5. Serotonin 2C Receptor Agonist

Mice lacking the 5-hydroxytryptamine-2c (5HT-2c) receptor have increased food intake, because they take longer to be satiated. These mice also are resistant to fenfluramine, a serotonin agonist that causes weight loss. A human mutation of the 5HT-2c receptor has been identified that is associated with early-onset human obesity [76, 77]. Arena Pharmaceuticals recently announced the results of a 4-week obesity trial of its 5HT-2c agonist compound APD356. Three hundred and fifty-two obese subjects were randomized to placebo, 1 mg, 5 mg, and 15 mg of APD356. The high-dose group lost 1.32 kg and the placebo group lost 0.32 kg ($p < 0.0002$), and the drug was well-tolerated. Longer studies are being planned [78].

4.6. Neuropeptide Y Receptor Antagonists

Neuropeptide Y (NPY) is a widely distributed neuropeptide that has six receptors, Y-1 through Y-6. NPY stimulates food intake, inhibits energy expenditure, and increases body weight by activating Y-1 and Y-5 receptors in the hypothalamus [79]. Levels of NPY in the hypothalamus are temporally related to food intake and are elevated with energy depletion. Surprisingly, NPY knockout mice have no phenotype. NPY-5 receptor antagonists fall into two categories—those that reduce food intake and those that do not, but of those that do seem to do so through a mechanism separate from Y-5. Thus, Y-5 receptor antagonists do not appear promising as antiobesity agents [80].

Y-1 receptor antagonists appear to have greater potential as antiobesity agents. A dihydropyridine neuropeptide Y-1 antagonist inhibited NPY-induced feeding in satiated rats [81]. Another Y-1 receptor antagonist, J-104870, suppressed food intake when given orally to Zucker rats [82]. A study measuring NPY in obese humans casts doubt on the importance of the NPY antagonists in the treatment of obesity in humans. Obese women had lower NPY levels than lean women and weight loss with a 400 kcal/day diet and adrenergic agonists (caffeine and ephedrine or caffeine, ephedrine and yohimbine) did not change NPY levels at rest or after exercise [83].

4.7.   Melanin Concentrating Hormone Receptor-1 Antagonist

Melanin concentrating hormone and alpha-melanocyte-stimulating hormone (α-MSH) have opposite effects on skin coloration in fish, and excess melanin concentrating hormone blocks the effects of α-MSH when both are injected into the cerebral ventricles of rats [84]. Melanin concentrating hormone has two receptors, MCH-1 and MCH-2. Mice without the MCH-1 receptor have increased activity, increased temperature, and increased sympathetic tone [85]. Overexpression of the MCH-1 receptor and chronic infusion of an MCH-1 agonist cause enhanced feeding, caloric efficiency, and weight gain while an MCH-1 antagonist reduces food intake and body weight gain without an effect on lean tissue [86]. MCH-1 antagonists reduce food intake by decreasing meal size, and also act as antidepressants and anxiolytics [87, 88]. An orally active MCH-1 receptor antagonist that has good plasma levels and CNS exposure induced weight loss in obese mice with chronic treatment [89]. A number of other MCH-1 antagonists reduce food intake and body weight in experimental animals [90]. No human studies have been reported.

4.8.   Pancreatic Lipase Inhibitor

Although orlistat, a lipase inhibitor, is already approved for the treatment of obesity, ATL-962, another gastrointestinal lipase inhibitor is also in development. A 5-day trial of ATL-962 in 90 normal volunteers was conducted on an inpatient unit. There was a three–sevenfold increase in fecal fat that was dose dependent, but only 11% of subjects had more than one oily stool. It was suggested that this lipase inhibitor may have fewer gastrointestinal adverse events than orlistat [91].

4.9.   Glucagon-like Peptide-1 Agonists and Dipeptidyl Peptidase-4 Inhibitors

Liraglutide is an analog of GLP-1 that stimulates the GLP-1 receptor and is more resistant to degradation than GLP-1. When given to rats by subcutaneous injection, liraglutide caused a 10% lower body weight and a 19% increase in

β-cell mass by inhibiting apoptosis [92]. A 12-week study in 193 type 2 diabetic subjects gave a 0.75% reduction in HgbA1c, a decrease in fasting glucose and a 1.2-kg weight loss [93].

Another way to prolong the effect of GLP-1 is to inhibit the enzyme that breaks it down, DPP-4. One such inhibitor, LAF237, was tested in 107 type 2 diabetic subjects over 12 weeks with an extension to 1 year using daily oral doses of 50 mg. The HgbA1c dropped 0.7% compared to placebo, fasting glucose declined, but weight did not go down [94]. Thus, DPP-4 inhibitors may have usefulness in the treatment of diabetes and the metabolic syndrome, but their potential in the treatment of obesity has yet to be demonstrated.

5. DRUGS NO LONGER UNDER INVESTIGATION OR WITHDRAWN

5.1. β3-adrenergic Agonists

In the early 1980s the β3-adrenergic receptor was identified and shown, when stimulated, to increase lipolysis, fat oxidation, energy expenditure, and insulin action. Selective β-adrenergic agonists based on the rodent β3-adrenergic receptor were not selective in humans, and the human β3-adrenergic receptor was subsequently cloned and found to be only 60% homologous with rodents [95]. A β3-adrenergic agonist selective for the human β3 receptor, L-796568, increased lipolysis and energy expenditure when given as a single 1000-mg dose to obese men without significant stimulation of the β2-adrenergic receptor [96]. A 28-day study with the same compound at 375 mg/day versus a placebo in obese men gave no significant increase in energy expenditure, reduction in respiratory quotient, or changes in glucose tolerance. There was a significant reduction of triglycerides, however. This lack of a chronic effect was interpreted as either a lack of recruitment of β3-responsive tissues, a downregulation of β3 receptors or both [97]. Thus, despite encouraging results from rodent trials, human trials of selective β3 agonists have been disappointing.

5.2. Ephedra

Ephedrine combined with methylxanthines was used in the treatment of asthma for decades. A physician in Denmark noted weight loss in his patients taking this combination drug for asthma. The combination of caffeine 200 mg and ephedrine 20 mg given three times a day was subsequently approved as a prescription obesity medication in Denmark, where it enjoyed commercial success for more than a decade [98]. In 1994, legislation in the United States declared ephedra and caffeine to be foods, eligible to be sold as dietary herbal supplements. The use of this combination as an unregulated dietary supplement for the treatment of obesity was accompanied by reports of cardiovascular and neuropsychiatric adverse events, leading to the FDA declaring ephedra, the herbal form of ephedrine, as an adulterant [99]. Recently, courts in the United States have overturned the FDA decision to withdraw ephedra from the herbal market, at least in regard to ephedra doses of 10 mg or less, and the implications this legal decision may have on the availability of ephedra in the herbal dietary supplement market remains to be determined.

5.3.   Phenylpropanolamine

Short-term studies with phenylpropanolamine were reviewed in 1992, and weight loss was similar to the short-term weight loss seen with prescription obesity drugs [100]. The longest study of phenylpropanolamine lasted 20 weeks. There was a 5.1-kg weight loss in the drug group and 0.4-kg weight loss in the placebo group meeting the FDA criteria for a prescription weight loss drug of a greater than 5% weight loss compared to placebo [101]. Although phenylpropanolamine had a long history of safety in clinical trials dating to the 1930s, it was taken off the market because of an association with hemorrhagic stroke in women [102].

5.4.   Bromocriptine

Hibernating and migratory animals change their ability to store and burn fat based on circadian rhythms, and these circadian rhythms are controlled by prolactin secretion. It has been postulated that obese and diabetic individuals have abnormal circadian rhythms. These abnormal rhythms favor fat storage and insulin resistance. Rapid-release bromocriptine (Ergocet®), given at 8:00 am, has been postulated to reverse this abnormal circadian rhythm and effectively treat diabetes and obesity. An uncontrolled trial of quick-release bromocriptine given orally for 8 weeks significantly decreased 24-hour plasma glucose, free fatty acid, and triglyceride levels from baseline [103]. This was followed by a controlled trial in which 22 diabetic subjects were randomized to quick-release bromocriptine or placebo. The hemoglobin $A1_c$ fell from 8.7% to 8.1% in the bromocriptine group and rose from 8.5% to 9.1% in the placebo group, a statistically significant difference [104]. In an uncontrolled trial, 33 obese postmenopausal women reduced their body fat by 11.7%, measured via skinfold thickness over 6 weeks of treatment with quick-release bromocriptine [105]. This was followed by a controlled trial in which 17 obese subjects were randomized to rapid-release bromocriptine (1.6 to 2.4 mg/day) or a placebo for 18 weeks. The bromocriptine group lost significantly more weight (6.3 kg vs. 0.9 kg) and more fat as measured by skinfolds (5.4 kg vs. 1.5 kg) [106]. The company developing Ergocet® received an approvable determination by the

FDA for quick-release bromocriptine to treat diabetes, but were asked to do additional safety studies. These studies were never performed, and the obesity development program proceeded no further.

5.5. Ecopipam

Ecopipam is a dopamine 1 and 5 receptor antagonist that was originally studied for the treatment of cocaine addiction [107]. Ecopipam was in development as an obesity drug but its development was recently terminated [108].

6. NEW AREAS WHERE DRUGS ARE BEING DEVELOPED

6.1. Histamine-3 Receptor Antagonists

Histamine and its receptors can affect food intake. Among the antipsychotic drugs that produce weight gain, binding to the H-1 receptor is higher than with any other monoamine receptor and histamine reduces food intake by action on this receptor [109]. The search for drugs that can modulate food intake through the histamine system has focused on the histamine H3 receptor which is an autoreceptor, that is, activation of this receptor inhibits histamine release whereas blockade of the receptor increases histamine release. Both imidazole and non-imidazole antagonists of the H3 receptor have been published and shown to reduce food intake and body weight gain in experimental animals [77, 110].

6.2. Ghrelin Antagonist

The search for small orally absorbed peptides that could release growth hormone led to the identification in 1996 of the growth hormone secretogogue (GHS) receptor, and the isolation in 1998 of ghrelin, the natural ligand for this GHS receptor. Ghrelin stimulates food intake in human subjects. Moreover, clinical trials with the small GH-stimulating peptides produced weight gain in humans, suggesting that antagonists to this receptor might be useful in the treatment of obesity [111]. No clinical data are yet available.

6.3. 11β-hydroxysteroid Dehydrogenase Type I Inhibitor

Cortisol, the glucocorticoid secreted by the adrenal gland can be inactivated through conversion to cortisone in peripheral tissues. Cortisone can be reactivated by the enzyme 11β-hydroxysteroid dehydrogenase type 1. In mice, where this enzyme is overexpressed, there are increased amounts of fat in the abdomen, suggesting that modulation of this enzyme could be a target to selectively modulate visceral or central adiposity.

6.4.   Modulators of Energy Sensing in the Brain (Acetyl Co-A Carboxylase 2 Inhibitor; Fatty Acid Synthase; Carnitine Palmitoyltransferase-3)

Recent developments suggest that the ratio of AMP to ATP in selected regions of the brain may play a role in modulating food intake and energy balance. The discovery that blockade of the fatty acid synthase with cerulenin, a naturally occurring product, or a synthetic molecule (C-75) opened the door to these insights. Fatty acid synthesis and oxidation are coordinately regulated. Adenosine 5-monophosphate activated kinase (AMPK) phosphorylates acetyl-Co-A-carboxylase to inhibit the enzyme that converts acetyl-CoA to malonyl-CoA in the first step toward long-chain fatty acid synthesis. AMPK dephosphorylates malonyl Co-A decarboxylase, which activates this enzyme that lowers malonyl-CoA concentration. The net effect of these phosphorylations by AMPK is to convert substrate to oxidation rather than fatty acid synthesis. Cerulenin or C-75 blocks fatty acid synthase, which also blocks fat synthesis and activates fatty acid oxidation by activating carnitine palmitoyl Co-A transferase-I. Injection of these fatty acid synthase inhibitors into animals produces a reduction in food intake and weight loss, suggesting the potential for future clinical drugs.

6.5.   Adiponectin

Adiponectin, also called adipocyte complement-related protein, is produced exclusively in fat cells, and is their most abundant protein. It has a long half-life in the blood and is of interest because its production and secretion by the fat cell is decreased as the fat cell increases in size. Higher levels of adiponectin are associated with insulin sensitivity and lower levels of adiponectin, as seen in obesity, are associated with insulin resistance. In experimental studies, adiponectin has been shown to reduce food intake when administered into the brain. Although a large molecule, drugs that modulate its production, release, or action may be potential candidates for treating obesity.

6.6.   Melanocortin-4 Receptor (MC4R) Agonists

Of the potential targets for drugs to treat obesity, the biological data favoring this receptor are among the strongest. There are five melanocortin receptors that belong to the G-protein coupled 7-transmembrane family of receptors. The MC1 receptor is located primarily in skin and modulates pigmentation changes in response to α-MSH. The MC2 receptor is in the adrenal gland, where it responds to adrenocorticotropic hormone (ACTH) modulating steroid production. The MC3 and MC4 receptors are primarily in the brain, where they are both involved in energy homeostasis. The final receptor, MC5, is located in exocrine tissues. The MC4 receptors in the brain are located in sites that affect feeding. In the hypothalamus, leptin-responsive neurons modulate MC4 expression, modifying energy balance. The MC4 receptor responds to α-MSH with a decrease in food intake. When animals are genetically engineered to remove expression of MC4 receptors, they become massively obese. The effect of α-MSH on the MC4 receptor can be blocked by agouti-related peptide (AgRP). Mice that overexpress AgRP or its equivalent agouti peptide (Yellow Mice) are obese. Numerous genetic variants of the MC4 receptor have been identified in humans that are associated in variable degrees of overweight and taller stature.

These biological observations have led to the search for agonists and antagonists to this receptor. The first two, an agonist called Melanotan-II (MT-II) and an antagonist called SHU-9119, are modifications of the core sequence of α-MSH. They demonstrate the viability of this strategy, because MT-II reduces food intake and body weight, while SHU-9119 as well as AgRP block this effect. Both peptide and nonpeptide agonists for the MC4 receptor have been developed, but no reports have yet emerged of clinical studies [112].

7. NATURAL PRODUCTS (OVER-THE-COUNTER PREPARATIONS)

7.1. Chromium

Chromium is a trace mineral and a cofactor to insulin. It has been claimed that chromium can cause weight loss and fat loss while increasing lean body mass. A recent meta-analysis of 10 double-blind randomized controlled obesity trials showed a statistically significant weight loss of 1.1 to 1.2 kg over a 6- to 14-week treatment period. There were no adverse events, but the authors pointed out that this weight loss, although statistically significant, was not clinically significant [113].

7.2. *Garcinia cambogia*

Garcinia cambogia contains hydroxycitric acid, an inhibitor of citrate cleavage enzyme that inhibits fatty acid synthesis from carbohydrate. Hydroxycitrate was studied by Roche in the 1970s and was shown to reduce food intake and cause weight loss in rodents [114]. Although there have been reports of successful weight loss in humans with small studies, some of which were combined other herbs, the largest and best designed placebo-controlled study demonstrated no difference in weight loss compared to a placebo [113, 115]. Thus, there is no evidence for efficacy.

7.3.   Chitosan

Chitosan or acetylated chitin is a dietary fiber derived from crustaceans that
has been advocated as a weight loss agent. A recent systematic review of the
randomized clinical trials of chitosan concluded, based on 14 trials longer than
4 weeks involving 1071 subjects, that chitosan gives 1.7-kg weight loss that is
statistically significant [116]. This degree of weight loss falls far short of the
5 kg felt to be clinically significant, however.

7.4.   *Hoodia*

Hoodia gordonii is a cactus that grows in Africa. It has been eaten by bush-
men to decrease appetite and thirst on long treks across the desert. The active
ingredient is steroidal glycoside, called P57AS3 or just P57. P57 injected into
the third ventricle of animals increases the ATP content of hypothalamic tissue by 50% to 150% and decreases food intake by 40% to 60% over 24 hours
[117]. Phytopharm is developing P57 in partnership with Unilever. Information
on the Phytopharm Web site describes a double-blind 15-day trial in which 19
overweight males were randomized to P57 or placebo. Nine subjects in each
group completed that study. There was a statistically significant decrease in
calorie intake and body fat with good safety. Since *Hoodia* is a rare cactus in
the wild and cultivation is difficult, it is not clear what the dietary herbal supplements claiming to contain *Hoodia* actually contain or if they are effective
in causing weight loss.

7.5.   *Stevia*

Stevia rebaudiana is a South American plant that contains stevosides that act
as noncaloric sweeteners. In fact, *Stevia* has been used as a sweetener in Brazil
and Japan for more than 20 years. *Stevia* is sold as a dietary herbal supplement
and has been said to be useful in the treatment of obesity [118]. There are
three clinical trials testing *Stevia*. The first trial was a randomized multicenter,
placebo-controlled trial that enrolled 106 hypertensive subjects for 1 year of
treatment. Subjects took stevoside 250 mg three times a day or a placebo. By
3 months the systolic blood pressure dropped from 166 to 153 mm Hg and
the diastolic blood pressure fell from 105 to 90 mm Hg, and this statistically
significant reduction was maintained for the rest of the year-long trial [119].
The second trial enrolled 12 diabetic subjects in a crossover design. Glucose
and insulin were measured around a standard meal with 1 g of stevioside or
1 g of corn starch was given just prior to the meal. There was a statistically
significant 18% reduction in the glucose area under the curve and an increase in
insulin sensitivity [120]. The third trial randomized 174 hypertensive subjects
to stevioside 500 mg three times a day or placebo for 2 years. The systolic
blood pressure fell from 150 to 140 mm Hg and the diastolic pressure fell from

95 to 89 mm Hg by the end of the first week, and this statistically significant difference persisted for the rest of the 2-year study. The stevoside group was protected from left ventricular hypertrophy, and like in the other two trials, there were no adverse events or laboratory abnormalities [121]. There was no weight loss in this 2-year trial. Thus, stevia does not appear to produce weight loss, but may be useful in the treatment of the metabolic syndrome.

7.6. *Citrus aurantium*

Since the withdrawal of ephedra from the dietary herbal supplement market, manufacturers of dietary herbal supplements for weight loss have turned to *Citrus aurantium*, which contains phenylephrine. A recent systematic review found only one randomized, placebo-controlled trial involving 20 subjects treated with *Citrus aurantium* for 6 weeks. This trial demonstrated no statistically significant benefit for weight loss [122]. There have been reports of cardiovascular events associated with the use of *Citrus aurantium* including a prolonged QT interval with syncope and an acute myocardial infarction [123, 124]. Thus, there is no evidence for efficacy of *Citrus aurantium* in the treatment of obesity, but concern does exist regarding its safety.

8.   SUMMARY AND CONCLUSIONS

Obesity is increasing in prevalence and its medical liabilities are, in large measure, related to the metabolic syndrome, a syndrome of insulin resistance. The drugs available at present for the treatment of obesity and the metabolic syndrome are few in number and limited in efficacy. This chapter reviewed the drugs approved for other indications that cause weight loss, drugs in the late development process that have not been approved, drugs in earlier stages of drug development for which clinical information is limited, drugs that have been dropped from development, and new potential drug targets for which essentially no clinical data yet exist. We also reviewed the nonprescription products sold for the treatment of obesity and the metabolic syndrome. The development pipeline of drugs for the treatment of obesity and the metabolic syndrome is rich. Because drugs to treat obesity are being developed in an era characterized by more sophisticated drug development tools than existed when hypertension drugs were being developed, much faster progress in developing safe and effective drugs for obesity and the metabolic syndrome is anticipated. With safe and effective drugs available, we anticipate that the chronic treatment of obesity with weight loss medication will become as well accepted and prevalent as is the chronic drug treatment of hypertension and diabetes in the medical practice of today.

REFERENCES

[1] Maffei M, Fei H, Lee GH, et al. Increased expression in adipocytes of ob RNA in mice with lesions of the hypothalamus and with mutations at the db locus. Proc Natl Acad Sci USA 1995;92:6957–6960.

[2] Halaas JL, Gajiwala KS, Maffei M, et al. Weight-reducing effects of the plasma protein encoded by the obese gene. Science 1995;269:543–546.

[3] NIH Consensus Development Conference Statement. Health implications of obesity. Ann Intern Med 1985:1973–1977.

[4] Puhl RM, Brownell KD. Psychosocial origins of obesity stigma: Toward changing a powerful and pervasive bias. Obes Rev 2003;4:213–227.

[5] Putnam J. Cases of myxedema and acromegalia treated with benefit by sheep's thyroids: Recent observations respecting the pathology of the cachexias following disease of the thyroid; clinical relationships of Grave's disease and acromegalia. Am J Med Sci 1893;106:125–148.

[6] Anonymous. Dexfenfluramine for obesity. Med Lett Drugs Ther 1996;38:64–65.

[7] Liese AD, Mayer-Davis EJ, Haffner SM. Development of the multiple metabolic syndrome: An epidemiologic perspective. Epidemiol Rev 1998;20:157–172.

[8] DeFronzo RA. Insulin resistance, hyperinsulinemia, and coronary artery disease: A complex metabolic web. J Cardiovasc Pharmacol 1992;20(Suppl 11):S1–S16.

[9] Reaven GM. Banting lecture 1988. Role of insulin resistance in human disease. Diabetes 1988;37:1595–1607.

[10] Haffner SM. The insulin resistance syndrome revisited. Diabetes Care 1996;19:275–277.

[11] Isomaa B, Almgren P, Tuomi T, et al. Cardiovascular morbidity and mortality associated with the metabolic syndrome. Diabetes Care 2001;24:683–689.

[12] Devaraj S, Rosenson RS, Jialal I. Metabolic syndrome: An appraisal of the proinflammatory and procoagulant status. Endocrinol Metab Clin North Am 2004;33:431–453, table of contents.

[13] Caballero AE. Endothelial dysfunction, inflammation, and insulin resistance: A focus on subjects at risk for type 2 diabetes. Curr Diab Rep 2004;4:237–246.

[14] McLaughlin T, Allison G, Abbasi F, Lamendola C, Reaven G. Prevalence of insulin resistance and associated cardiovascular disease risk factors among normal weight, overweight, and obese individuals. Metabolism 2004;53:495–499.

[15] Shirai K. Obesity as the core of the metabolic syndrome and the management of coronary heart disease. Curr Med Res Opin 2004;20:295–304.

[16] Executive Summary of the Third Report of the National Cholesterol Education Program (NCEP) Expert Panel on Detection, Evaluation, and Treatment of High Blood Cholesterol in Adults (Adult Treatment Panel III). JAMA 2001;285:2486–2597.

[17] Lakka HM, Laaksonen DE, Lakka TA, et al. The metabolic syndrome and total and cardiovascular disease mortality in middle-aged men. JAMA 2002;288:2709–2716.

[18] Hu FB, Stampfer MJ, Haffner SM, Solomon CG, Willett WC, Manson JE. Elevated risk of cardiovascular disease prior to clinical diagnosis of type 2 diabetes. Diabetes Care 2002; 25:1129–1134.

[19] Diabetes prevalence among American Indians and Alaska Natives and the overall population—United States, 1994-02. Morb Mortal Wkly Rep Surveill Summ 2003; 52:702–704.

[20] Mokdad AH, Ford ES, Bowman BA, et al. Prevalence of obesity, diabetes, and obesity-related health risk factors, 2001. JAMA 2003;289:76–79.

[21] Ford ES, Giles WH, Dietz WH. Prevalence of the metabolic syndrome among US adults: Findings from the third National Health and Nutrition Examination Survey. JAMA 2002;287:356–359.

[22] Knowler WC, Barrett-Connor E, Fowler SE, et al. Reduction in the incidence of type 2 diabetes with lifestyle intervention or metformin. N Engl J Med 2002;346:393–403.

[23] Gadde KM, Parker CB, Maner LG, et al. Bupropion for weight loss: An investigation of efficacy and tolerability in overweight and obese women. Obes Res 2001;9:544–551.

[24] Beck A, Rial W, Rickels K. Short form of depression inventory: Cross-validation. Psychol Rep 1974;34:1184–1186.

[25] Jain AK, Kaplan RA, Gadde KM, et al. Bupropion SR vs. placebo for weight loss in obese patients with depressive symptoms. Obes Res 2002;10:1049–1056.

[26] Anderson JW, Greenway FL, Fujioka K, Gadde KM, McKenney J, O'Neil PM. Bupropion SR enhances weight loss: A 48-week double-blind, placebo-controlled trial. Obes Res 2002;10:633–641.

[27] Goldstein DJ, Rampey AH Jr, Roback PJ, et al. Efficacy and safety of long-term fluoxetine treatment of obesity—maximizing success. Obes Res 1995;3(Suppl 4):481S–490S.

[28] Gadde KM, Francisy DM, Wagner HR 2nd, Krishnan KR. Zonisamide for weight loss in obese adults: A randomized controlled trial. JAMA 2003;289:1820–1825.

[29] Ben-Menachem E, Axelsen M, Johanson EH, Stagge A, Smith U. Predictors of weight loss in adults with topiramate-treated epilepsy. Obes Res 2003;11:556–562.

[30] Bray GA, Hollander P, Klein S, et al. A 6-month randomized, placebo-controlled, dose-ranging trial of topiramate for weight loss in obesity. Obes Res 2003;11:722–733.

[31] Wilding J, Van Gaal L, Rissanen A, Vercruysse F, Fitchet M. A randomized double-blind placebo-controlled study of the long-term efficacy and safety of topiramate in the treatment of obese subjects. Int J Obes Relat Metab Disord 2004;28:1399–1410.

[32] Astrup A, Caterson I, Zelissen P, et al. Topiramate: Long-term maintenance of weight loss induced by a low-calorie diet in obese subjects. Obes Res 2004;12:1658–1669.

[33] Shapira NA, Goldsmith TD, McElroy SL. Treatment of binge-eating disorder with topiramate: A clinical case series. J Clin Psychiatry 2000;61:368–372.

[34] McElroy SL, Arnold LM, Shapira NA, et al. Topiramate in the treatment of binge eating disorder associated with obesity: A randomized, placebo-controlled trial. Am J Psychiatry 2003;160:255–261.

[35] McElroy SL, Shapira NA, Arnold LM, et al. Topiramate in the long-term treatment of binge-eating disorder associated with obesity. J Clin Psychiatry 2004;65:1463–1469.

[36] Shapira NA, Lessig MC, Murphy TK, Driscoll DJ, Goodman WK. Topiramate attenuates self-injurious behaviour in Prader–Willi syndrome. Int J Neuropsychopharmacol 2002;5:141–145.

[37] Smathers SA, Wilson JG, Nigro MA. Topiramate effectiveness in Prader–Willi syndrome. Pediatr Neurol 2003;28:130–133.

[38] Shapira NA, Lessig MC, Lewis MH, Goodman WK, Driscoll DJ. Effects of topiramate in adults with Prader–Willi syndrome. Am J Ment Retard 2004;109:301–309.

[39] Winkelman JW. Treatment of nocturnal eating syndrome and sleep-related eating disorder with topiramate. Sleep Med 2003;4:243–246.

[40] Bray GA, Greenway FL. Current and potential drugs for treatment of obesity. Endocr Rev 1999;20:805–875.

[41] Fontbonne A, Charles MA, Juhan-Vague I, et al. The effect of metformin on the metabolic abnormalities associated with upper-body fat distribution. BIGPRO Study Group. Diabetes Care 1996;19:920–926.

[42] Ortega-Gonzalez C, Luna S, Hernandez L, et al. Responses of serum androgen and insulin resistance to metformin and pioglitazone in obese, insulin-resistant women with polycystic ovary syndrome. J Clin Endocrinol Metab 2005;90:1360–1365.

[43] Bray GA, Gallagher TF Jr. Manifestations of hypothalamic obesity in man: A comprehensive investigation of eight patients and a review of the literature. Medicine (Baltimore) 1975;54:301–330.

[44] Lustig RH, Rose SR, Burghen GA, et al. Hypothalamic obesity caused by cranial insult in children: Altered glucose and insulin dynamics and reversal by a somatostatin agonist. J Pediatr 1999;135:162–168.

[45] Lustig RH, Hinds PS, Ringwald-Smith K, et al. Octreotide therapy of pediatric hypothalamic obesity: A double-blind, placebo-controlled trial. J Clin Endocrinol Metab 2003;88:2586–2592.

[46] Velasquez-Mieyer PA, Cowan PA, Arheart KL, et al. Suppression of insulin secretion is associated with weight loss and altered macronutrient intake and preference in a subset of obese adults. Int J Obes Relat Metab Disord 2003;27:219–226.

[47] Lustig R, Greenway F, Velasquez D, et al. Weight loss in obese adults with insulin hypersecretion treated with Sandostatin LAR Depot. Obes Res 2003;11(Suppl):A25.

[48] Foxx-Orenstein A, Camilleri M, Stephens D, Burton D. Effect of a somatostatin analogue on gastric motor and sensory functions in healthy humans. Gut 2003;52:1555–1561.

[49] Tan TM, Vanderpump M, Khoo B, Patterson M, Ghatei MA, Goldstone AP. Somatostatin infusion lowers plasma ghrelin without reducing appetite in adults with Prader–Willi syndrome. J Clin Endocrinol Metab 2004;89:4162–4165.

[50] Ratner RE, Dickey R, Fineman M, et al. Amylin replacement with pramlintide as an adjunct to insulin therapy improves long-term glycaemic and weight control in Type 1 diabetes mellitus: A 1-year, randomized controlled trial. Diabet Med 2004;21:1204–1212.

[51] Maggs D, Shen L, Strobel S, Brown D, Kolterman O, Weyer C. Effect of pramlintide on A1C and body weight in insulin-treated African Americans and Hispanics with type 2 diabetes: A pooled post hoc analysis. Metabolism 2003;52:1638–1642.

[52] Small CJ, Bloom SR. Gut hormones as peripheral anti obesity targets. Curr Drug Targets CNS Neurol Disord 2004;3:379–388.

[53] Greenway SE, Greenway FL, Klein S. Effects of obesity surgery on non-insulin-dependent diabetes mellitus. Arch Surg 2002;137:1109–1117.

[54] Patriti A, Facchiano E, Sanna A, Gulla N, Donini A. The enteroinsular axis and the recovery from type 2 diabetes after bariatric surgery. Obes Surg 2004;14:840–848.

[55] Lugari R, Dei Cas A, Ugolotti D, et al. Glucagon-like peptide 1 (GLP-1) secretion and plasma dipeptidyl peptidase IV (DPP-IV) activity in morbidly obese patients undergoing biliopancreatic diversion. Horm Metab Res 2004;36:111–115.

[56] Szayna M, Doyle ME, Betkey JA, et al. Exendin-4 decelerates food intake, weight gain, and fat deposition in Zucker rats. Endocrinology 2000;141:1936–1941.

[57] Gedulin BR, Nikoulina SE, Smith PA, et al. Exenatide (exendin-4) improves insulin sensitivity and beta-cell mass in insulin-resistant obese fa/fa Zucker rats independent of glycemia and body weight. Endocrinology 2005;146:2069–2076.

[58] Rodriquez de Fonseca F, Navarro M, Alvarez E, et al. Peripheral versus central effects of glucagon-like peptide-1 receptor agonists on satiety and body weight loss in Zucker obese rats. Metabolism 2000;49:709–717.

[59] Kastin AJ, Akerstrom V. Entry of exendin-4 into brain is rapid but may be limited at high doses. Int J Obes Relat Metab Disord 2003;27:313–318.

[60] Edwards CM, Stanley SA, Davis R, et al. Exendin-4 reduces fasting and postprandial glucose and decreases energy intake in healthy volunteers. Am J Physiol Endocrinol Metab 2001;281:E155–E161.

[61] Fineman MS, Shen LZ, Taylor K, Kim DD, Baron AD. Effectiveness of progressive dose-escalation of exenatide (exendin-4) in reducing dose-limiting side effects in subjects with type 2 diabetes. Diabetes Metab Res Rev 2004;20:411–417.

[62] Buse JB, Henry RR, Han J, Kim DD, Fineman MS, Baron AD. Effects of exenatide (exendin-4) on glycemic control over 30 weeks in sulfonylurea-treated patients with type 2 diabetes. Diabetes Care 2004;27:2628–2635.

[63] Bensaid M, Gary-Bobo M, Esclangon A, et al. The cannabinoid CB1 receptor antagonist SR141716 increases Acrp30 mRNA expression in adipose tissue of obese fa/fa rats and in cultured adipocyte cells. Mol Pharmacol 2003;63:908–914.

[64] Web site. http://en.sanofi-aventis.com/investors/p_investors.asp.

[65] Van Gaal LF, Rissanen AM, Scheen AJ, Ziegler O, Rossner S. Effects of the cannabinoid-1 receptor blocker rimonabant on weight reduction and cardiovascular risk factors in overweight patients: 1-year experience from the RIO-Europe study. Lancet 2005; 365:1389–1397.

[66] Anderson KD, Lambert PD, Corcoran TL, et al. Activation of the hypothalamic arcuate nucleus predicts the anorectic actions of ciliary neurotrophic factor and leptin in intact and gold thioglucose-lesioned mice. J Neuroendocrinol 2003;15:649–660.

[67] Ettinger MP, Littlejohn TW, Schwartz SL, et al. Recombinant variant of ciliary neurotrophic factor for weight loss in obese adults: A randomized, dose-ranging study. JAMA 2003;289:1826–1832.

[68] Web site. http://www.regeneron.com/.

[69] Heymsfield SB, Greenberg AS, Fujioka K, et al. Recombinant leptin for weight loss in obese and lean adults: A randomized, controlled, dose-escalation trial. JAMA 1999; 282:1568–1575.

[70] Hukshorn CJ, Westerterp-Plantenga MS, Saris WH. Pegylated human recombinant leptin (PEG-OB) causes additional weight loss in severely energy-restricted, overweight men. Am J Clin Nutr 2003;77:771–776.

[71] Website. http://www.metabolic.com.au/files/T5SH4035T6/ASX_%20AOD9604_result %20announcement.pdf.

[72] Pi-Sunyer X, Kissileff HR, Thornton J, Smith GP. C-terminal octapeptide of cholecystokinin decreases food intake in obese men. Physiol Behav 1982;29:627–630.

[73] Batterham RL, Cohen MA, Ellis SM, et al. Inhibition of food intake in obese subjects by peptide YY3-36. N Engl J Med 2003;349:941–948.

[74] Brandt GAS, Quay S. Intranasal peptide YY 3-36: Phase 1 dose ranging and dose sequencing studies. Obes Res 2004;12(Suppl):A28.

[75] Alemany M, Fernandez-Lopez JA, Petrobelli A, Granada M, Foz M, Remesar X. Weight loss in a patient with morbid obesity under treatment with oleoyl-estrone. Med Clin (Barc) 2003;121:496–499.

[76] Gibson WT, Ebersole BJ, Bhattacharyya S, et al. Mutational analysis of the serotonin receptor 5HT2c in severe early-onset human obesity. Can J Physiol Pharmacol 2004; 82:426–429.

[77] Nilsson BM. 5-hydroxytryptamine 2C (5-HT2C) receptor agonists as potential antiobesity agents. J Med Chem 2006;49:4023–4034.

[78] Web site. http://investor.arenapharm.com/phoenix.zhtml?c=121703&p=irolnewsArticle &ID=708471&highlight=.

[79] Parker E, Van Heek M, Stamford A. Neuropeptide Y receptors as targets for anti-obesity drug development: Perspective and current status. Eur J Pharmacol 2002;440:173–187.

[80] Levens NR, Della-Zuana O. Neuropeptide Y Y5 receptor antagonists as anti-obesity drugs. Curr Opin Investig Drugs 2003;4:1198–1204.

[81] Poindexter GS, Bruce MA, LeBoulluec KL, et al. Dihydropyridine neuropeptide Y Y(1) receptor antagonists. Bioorg Med Chem Lett 2002;12:379–382.

[82] Kanatani A, Hata M, Mashiko S, et al. A typical Y1 receptor regulates feeding behaviors: Effects of a potent and selective Y1 antagonist, J-115814. Mol Pharmacol 2001;59:501–505.

[83] Zahorska-Markiewicz B, Obuchowicz E, Waluga M, Tkacz E, Herman ZS. Neuropeptide Y in obese women during treatment with adrenergic modulation drugs. Med Sci Monit 2001;7:403–408.

[84] Ludwig DS, Mountjoy KG, Tatro JB, et al. Melanin-concentrating hormone: A functional melanocortin antagonist in the hypothalamus. Am J Physiol 1998;274:E627–E633.

[85] Astrand A, Bohlooly YM, Larsdotter S, et al. Mice lacking melanin-concentrating hormone receptor 1 demonstrate increased heart rate associated with altered autonomic activity. Am J Physiol Regul Integr Comp Physiol 2004;287:R749–R758.

[86] Shearman LP, Camacho RE, Sloan Stribling D, et al. Chronic MCH-1 receptor modulation alters appetite, body weight and adiposity in rats. Eur J Pharmacol 2003;475:37–47.

[87] Kowalski TJ, Farley C, Cohen-Williams ME, Varty G, Spar BD. Melanin-concentrating hormone-1 receptor antagonism decreases feeding by reducing meal size. Eur J Pharmacol 2004;497:41–47.

[88] Borowsky B, Durkin MM, Ogozalek K, et al. Antidepressant, anxiolytic and anorectic effects of a melanin-concentrating hormone-1 receptor antagonist. Nat Med 2002;8:825–830.

[89] Souers AJ, Gao J, Brune M, et al. Identification of 2-(4-benzyloxyphenyl)-N-[1-(2-pyrrolidin-1-yl-ethyl)-1H-indazol-6-yl]acetamide, an orally efficacious melanin-concentrating hormone receptor 1 antagonist for the treatment of obesity. J Med Chem 2005;48:1318–1321.

[90] Handlon A, Zhou H. Melanin-concentrating hormone-1 receptor antagonists. J Med Chem 2005 (in press).

[91] Dunk C, Enunwa M, De La Monte S, Palmer R. Increased fecal fat excretion in normal volunteers treated with lipase inhibitor ATL-962. Int J Obes Relat Metab Disord 2002;26(Suppl):S135.

[92] Bock T, Pakkenberg B, Buschard K. The endocrine pancreas in non-diabetic rats after short-term and long-term treatment with the long-acting GLP-1 derivative NN2211. Apmis 2003;111:1117–1124.

[93] Madsbad S, Schmitz O, Ranstam J, Jakobsen G, Matthews DR. Improved glycemic control with no weight increase in patients with type 2 diabetes after once-daily treatment with the long-acting glucagon-like peptide 1 analog liraglutide (NN2211): A 12-week, double-blind, randomized, controlled trial. Diabetes Care 2004;27:1335–1342.

[94] Ahren B, Gomis R, Standl E, Mills D, Schweizer A. Twelve- and 52-week efficacy of the dipeptidyl peptidase IV inhibitor LAF237 in metformin-treated patients with type 2 diabetes. Diabetes Care 2004;27:2874–2880.

[95] de Souza CJ, Burkey BF. Beta 3-adrenoceptor agonists as anti-diabetic and anti-obesity drugs in humans. Curr Pharm Des 2001;7:1433–1449.

[96] van Baak MA, Hul GB, Toubro S, et al. Acute effect of L-796568, a novel beta 3-adrenergic receptor agonist, on energy expenditure in obese men. Clin Pharmacol Ther 2002;71:272–279.

[97] Larsen TM, Toubro S, van Baak MA, et al. Effect of a 28-d treatment with L-796568, a novel beta(3)-adrenergic receptor agonist, on energy expenditure and body composition in obese men. Am J Clin Nutr 2002;76:780–788.

[98] Greenway FL. The safety and efficacy of pharmaceutical and herbal caffeine and ephedrine use as a weight loss agent. Obes Rev 2001;2:199–211.

[99] Shekelle PG, Hardy ML, Morton SC, et al. Efficacy and safety of ephedra and ephedrine for weight loss and athletic performance: A meta-analysis. JAMA 2003;289:1537–1545.

[100] Greenway FL. Clinical studies with phenylpropanolamine: A metaanalysis. Am J Clin Nutr 1992;55:203S–205S.

[101] Schteingart DE. Effectiveness of phenylpropanolamine in the management of moderate obesity. Int J Obes Relat Metab Disord 1992;16:487–493.

[102] Kernan WN, Viscoli CM, Brass LM, et al. Phenylpropanolamine and the risk of hemorrhagic stroke. N Engl J Med 2000;343:1826–1832.

[103] Kamath V, Jones CN, Yip JC, et al. Effects of a quick-release form of bromocriptine (Ergoset) on fasting and postprandial plasma glucose, insulin, lipid, and lipoprotein concentrations in obese nondiabetic hyperinsulinemic women. Diabetes Care 1997;20:1697–1701.

[104] Pijl H, Ohashi S, Matsuda M, et al. Bromocriptine: A novel approach to the treatment of type 2 diabetes. Diabetes Care 2000;23:1154–1161.

[105] Meier AH, Cincotta AH, Lovell WC. Timed bromocriptine administration reduces body fat stores in obese subjects and hyperglycemia in type II diabetics. Experientia 1992;48:248–253.

[106] Cincotta AH, Meier AH. Bromocriptine (Ergoset) reduces body weight and improves glucose tolerance in obese subjects. Diabetes Care 1996;19:667–670.

[107] Nann-Vernotica E, Donny EC, Bigelow GE, Walsh SL. Repeated administration of the D1/5 antagonist ecopipam fails to attenuate the subjective effects of cocaine. Psychopharmacology (Berl) 2001;155:338–347.

[108] Bays H, Dujovne C. Anti-obesity drug development. Expert Opin Investig Drugs 2002;11:1189–1204.

[109] Kroeze WK, Hufeisen SJ, Popadak BA, et al. H1-histamine receptor affinity predicts short-term weight gain for typical and atypical antipsychotic drugs. Neuropsychopharmacology 2003;28:519–526.

[110] Leurs R, Bakker RA, Timmerman H, de Esch IJ. The histamine H3 receptor: From gene cloning to H3 receptor drugs. Nat Rev Drug Discov 2005;4:107–120.

[111] Svensson J, Lonn L, Jansson JO, et al. Two-month treatment of obese subjects with the oral growth hormone (GH) secretagogue MK-677 increases GH secretion, fat-free mass, and energy expenditure. J Clin Endocrinol Metab 1998;83:362–369.

[112] Nargund RP, Strack AM, Fong TM. Melanocortin-4 receptor (MC4R) agonists for the treatment of obesity. J Med Chem 2006;49:4035–4043.

[113] Pittler MH, Ernst E. Dietary supplements for body-weight reduction: A systematic review. Am J Clin Nutr 2004;79:529–536.

[114] Sullivan C, Triscari J. Metabolic regulation as a control for lipid disorders. I. Influence of (–)-hydroxycitrate on experimentally induced obesity in the rodent. Am J Clin Nutr 1977;30:767–776.

[115] Heymsfield SB, Allison DB, Vasselli JR, Pietrobelli A, Greenfield D, Nunez C. Garcinia cambogia (hydroxycitric acid) as a potential antiobesity agent: A randomized controlled trial. JAMA 1998;280:1596–1600.

[116] Mhurchu CN, Dunshea-Mooij C, Bennett D, Rodgers A. Effect of chitosan on weight loss in overweight and obese individuals: A systematic review of randomized controlled trials. Obes Rev 2005;6:35–42.

[117] Web site. http://www.phytopharm.co.uk/press/P57%20Third%20Stage%20final.htm.

[118] Web site. http://www.primalnature.com/stevia.html.

[119] Chan P, Tomlinson B, Chen YJ, Liu JC, Hsieh MH, Cheng JT. A double-blind placebo-controlled study of the effectiveness and tolerability of oral stevioside in human hypertension. Br J Clin Pharmacol 2000;50:215–220.

[120] Gregersen S, Jeppesen PB, Holst JJ, Hermansen K. Antihyperglycemic effects of stevio-side in type 2 diabetic subjects. Metabolism 2004;53:73–76.

[121] Hsieh MH, Chan P, Sue YM, et al. Efficacy and tolerability of oral stevioside in patients with mild essential hypertension: A two-year, randomized, placebo-controlled study. Clin Ther 2003;25:2797–2808.

[122] Bent S, Padula A, Neuhaus J. Safety and efficacy of citrus aurantium for weight loss. Am J Cardiol 2004;94:1359–1361.

[123] Nasir JM, Durning SJ, Ferguson M, Barold HS, Haigney MC. Exercise-induced syn-cope associated with QT prolongation and ephedra-free xenadrine. Mayo Clin Proc 2004; 79:105962.

[124] Nykamp DL, Fackih MN, Compton AL. Possible association of acute lateral-wall my-ocardial infarction and bitter orange supplement. Ann Pharmacother 2004;38:812–816.

Chapter 17

Surgical Treatment of the Overweight Patient

George A. Bray

Pennington Biomedical Research Center, Baton Rouge, LA 70808, USA

1.   INTRODUCTION

Treatment of overweight patients with surgery is increasing at a rapid rate The Nationwide Inpatient Sample from 1998 to 2002 has provided one quantitative estimate of bariatric surgical procedures. Between 1998 and 2002 the number of operations increased from 13,365 to 72,177, a more than 5-fold increase. More than 80% of these were the so-called gastric bypass operation. Several other trends were also noted in this paper: An increase in women being operated on rising from 81 to 84%; a rise in the percent of privately insured patients increasing from 75 to 83%; and an increase in the number of older patients aged 50 to 64 being operated on rising from 15% to 24%. The length of hospitalization decreased from 4.5 to 3.3 days, and operative mortality ranged from 0.1 to 0.2%. Serious consideration of this growing form of treatment for overweight is thus important both for the patient and for the physicians and other health professionals who will take care of these patients.

Interest in bariatric surgery results from the positive results for weight loss and for maintaining weight loss. This has impacted health care for this group of people. On February 21, 2006, the Center for Medicare and Medicaid Services agreed to expand the coverage for bariatric surgery in the treatment of obesity. We can thus expect even more procedures to be done in the future (Figure 1). This chapter will cover the types of bariatric surgery available for overweight patients, the effectiveness of these operations and some of the problems associated with them. There are several sources of information that the reader can consult for additional details [1–6].

The operations used to treat obesity are generally referred to as "bariatric" procedures, a word derived from the Greek meaning "heavy". All of them involve some manipulation of the plumbing that we call the gastro-intestinal track. Figure 2 shows some of the operations that are or have been used to treat the overweight patient. They are grouped into those that are "restrictive" and those that have a component of malabsorption in them.

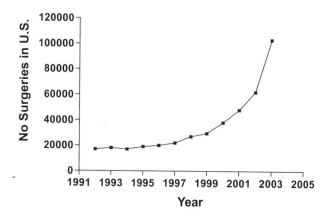

Figure 1. Growth in number of bariatric operations performed each year.

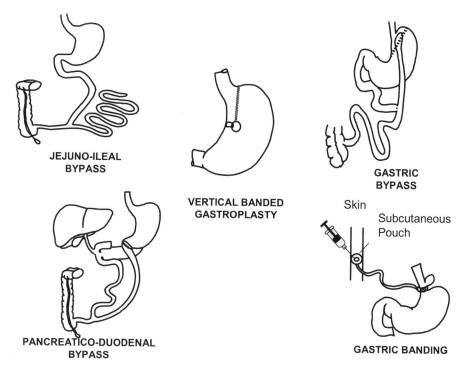

Figure 2. Illustrations of operative procedures. The jejuno-ileal by-pass operation on the upper left is no longer performed due to its complications. The pancreaticoduodenal procedure is technically difficult and is performed at a smaller number of centers. The lap-banding procedures, gastric bypass and vertically banded gastroplasty are the most widely performed operations.

2. SURGICAL APPROACHES TO OBESITY AND THEIR HISTORICAL CONTEXT

The earliest systematic use of surgery to treat obesity was published in 1963 by Payne et al. [7]. They separated the intestine at the mid-jejunum and connected the proximal end to the colon so that the contents of the upper GI track were emptied into the colon. Weight loss with this procedure was rapid and subjects returned to nearly normal weight. However, there were serious problems with diarrhea and loss of potassium and other minerals. Believing that their patients had been "cured" of their obesity, the operations were reversed. To their dismay, there was a rapid regain of the lost weight. The next approach was by the same group [8] who pioneered a less drastic rearrangement of the GI-track by coupling the jejunum to the distal segment of the ileum. These operations were very popular during the 1970's but fell into disuse as the number of complications continued to rise, and alternative gastric operations came into use.

Restrictive operations involving reducing the volume of the stomach with various stapling procedures, but leaving the flow of food from esophagus to duodenum appeared in 1979 [9] and 1980 [10]. They consisted of both transverse staple lines as well as vertical staple lines. One version that in effect prolonged the esophagus is a procedure called the vertical-banded gastroplasty [11].

An alternative restrictive procedure consists of placing a plastic band around the stomach and, in some of the systems providing a way to inflate it from a subcutaneous reservoir. The initial procedure was performed in 1976, but not published until 8 years later [12]. This procedure is now widely used in Europe and has been approved by the Food and Drug Administration in the United States.

Three procedures have been developed that involve combinations of gastric and intestinal operations. The first of these is the gastric bypass originally developed by Mason and Ito [13, 14]. In this procedure a small gastric pouch is anastamosed to the distal limb of the jejunum, while the proximal limb is attached to the side of this loop a short ways below the connection of the jejunum to the stomach. This is thus a restrictive and modest malabsorptive procedure. The next procedure is the biliopancreatic diversion which was developed by Scopinaro and consists of two long intestinal segments, one draining contents from the stomach and the other the duodenal juices. They are connected near the ileo-cecal valve thus reducing the length of intestine where food and intestinal juices are together and reducing absorption. The final procedure in this group is the distal gastric bypass where the jejunum replaces the duodenum in draining the lower stomach—the so-called biliopancreatic diversion with duodenal switch [15].

All of these operations can now be done by laparoscopy which has significantly reduced the operative morbidity and allowed more patients to have this procedures. Laparoscopic procedures were first undertaken by Fried and Peskova [16] and by Belachew et al. [17]. Gradually these techniques have spread and will probably dominate the surgical treatment of obesity, if they have not already done so.

3.   INDICATIONS AND CONTRAINDICATIONS

3.1.   Indications in Adults

Indications and contraindications for bariatric surgical procedures were outlined by a consensus conference at the National Institutes of Health (NIH) in 1991 and are summarized in Table 1 [18, 19]. Adult patients may be considered for these procedures if they have a BMI > 40 kg/m^2 or a BMI > 35 kg/m^2

Table 1. Indications and contraindications for bariatric surgery

Indications	Contraindications
1. BMI > 40 kg/m^2 or BMI 35–39.9 kg/m^2 and life-threatening cardiopulmonary disease, severe diabetes, or lifestyle impairment 2. Failure to achieve adequate weight loss with nonsurgical treatment	1. History of noncompliance with medical care 2. Certain psychiatric illnesses: personality disorder, uncontrolled depression, suicidal ideation, substance abuse 3. Unlikely to survive surgery

if they have serious co-morbidities such as sleep apnea, diabetes mellitus, or joint disease. For individuals less than 16 years of age, surgical and pediatric consultants should review each case separately [4], since operations that reduce caloric intake can slow weight gain when performed before an individual has achieved adult height. Similarly, bariatric surgery for individuals older than 65 years of age should also be considered on an individual basis, since the adaptation to the procedure may be more troublesome and difficult. Potential patients must have tried and failed non-surgical weight loss procedures. The patient and their significant others must understand the procedure and its complications. A recent paper suggests that for some patients with a BMI below 35 kg/m^2 may benefit from laparoscopic insertion of an adjustable gastric band [20].

3.2.   Contraindications for Adults

Patients with major depression or psychosis should be carefully reviewed before being accepted. Patients with binge-eating disorders, abuse of drugs or alcohol, severe cardiac disease, prohibitive anesthetic risks, severe coagulopathy, or inability to comply with nutritional requirements including life-long vitamin replacement should be reviewed very carefully by a team approach or declined. A large number of complications can occur in the post-operative period and it is thus desirable to have bariatric operations performed by a team with comprehensive surgical, medical and nutritional support. To provide guidance in how to do this, The American Society of Bariatric Surgeons (ASBS) has developed guidelines for establishing Centers of Excellence (COE) for bariatric clinics that are desirable to have in place [21]. In addition, a number of NIH-funded Surgical Centers have been established to advance the science and care of patients needing bariatric surgery.

3.3. Bariatric Surgery for the Pediatric Age Group

The rising prevalence of overweight among children and adolescents has seen an increased interest in bariatric surgery for this age group [4]. The principal concern in this age group is the potential for reducing linear growth if a patient is operated on before their adult height is reached. Criteria for adolescent patients are shown in Table 2. The largest study in adolescents contained

Table 2. Criteria for batriatric surgery in adolescents

Adolescents being considered for bariatric surgery should:

1. Have failed $\geq$ 6 months of organized attempts at weight management, as determined by their primary care provide
2. Have attained or nearly attained physiologic maturity
3. Be very severely overweight (BMI $\geq$ 40 kg/m^2) with serious obesity-related comorbidities or have a BMI of $\geq$ 50 with less severe comorbidities
4. Demonstrate commitment to comprehensive medical and psychological evaluations both before and after surgery
5. Agree to avoid pregnancy for at least 1 year postoperatively
6. Be capable of and willing to adhere to nutritional guidelines postoperatively
7. Provide informed assent to surgical treatment
8. Demonstrate decisional capacity
9. Have a supportive family environmment

only 33 patients who underwent several different procedure, thus providing little overall guidance [22]. The review in Pediatrics suggests that at the present time the gastric bypass may be the most appropriate procedure.

4.   EFFECTIVENESS OF SURGICAL PROCEDURES

A number of studies have compared bariatric procedures against each other and against non-surgical techniques. These studies can be compared using several yardsticks. Actual weight loss may be reported and is one way of comparing treatments. However, because of differences in weight the loss of "excess" weight is a second way of comparing treatment groups that is often used in the surgical reports. This method calculates the excess weight above the weight at a BMI of 25 kg/m^2 (or some other standard) and expresses the weight loss as a percent of the excess weight. A third way that is used in comparing weight loss is as a percentage of those patients who lose a given amount of weight—say 5%, 10% or 20% from their initial or baseline weight.

Although the jejuno-ileal by-pass operation is no longer performed, there are 2 randomized and two prospective nonrandomized trials have been published between 1977 and 1981 using this technique [23–25]. The weight losses with the two procedures at 1 year were similar, but the complications observed with the jejunoileal bypass procedure over time were more significant. In a comparison of the jejunoileal bypass against the horizontal gastroplasty, weight loss of 33% favored the jejunoileal bypass compared to the 16% weight loss with the horizontal gastroplasty, but the side-effects were less severe with the gastroplasty [26].

Jejunoileal bypass has also been compared with dietary treatment in the Danish Obesity Project [27, 28]. There were 130 surgically treated patients and 66 patients treated medically. After 2 years, the weight loss was 42.9 kg in the surgical group and 5.9 kg in the diet group. The surgically operated patients had significant post-operative problems, but also had more improvement in blood pressure and quality of life.

The horizontal gastroplasty has been compared with the gastric bypass in several studies [29]. In the largest of these studies, 204 patients weighing 112 kg were included and followed for 3 years. The weight loss at 3 years was 39 kg in the group treated by gastric bypass compared to 17 kg in the group receiving the gastroplasty [30]. An additional problem with the horizontal gastroplasty operation is that more re-operations have been needed.

Horizontal gastroplasty has been compared with a very low calorie diet (VLCD) in a 2 year study with a follow-up for 5 years, but a drop-out rate in excess of 50%. After 2 years, the weight loss was only 8.2 kg in the VLCD group compared with a robust 30.6 kg in the surgically treated group [31, 32]. At 5 years successful weight loss was expressed as percentage losing more than 10% of initial body weight rather than actual weight loss. By this criterion there were 16% successes in the surgical group but only 3% in the VLCD group.

Vertical banded gastroplasty has been compared to gastric bypass in a number of trials ranging up to 10 years in length [1, 33, 34]. In the 10 year trial, individuals enrolled in the gastroplasty group lost about 16% of initial body weight compared to 24% for those in the gastric bypass group. Using different criteria, Howard et al. reported a loss of > 75% of excess weight after 1 year in 18% of the patients with vertical banded gastroplasty compared to 60% for those with gastric bypass. Using a criterion of a weight loss to a BMI of less than 35 kg/m^2, MacLean et al. [35] reported success rate of 83% for those with a gastric bypass and 43% for those with the vertical banded gastroplasty.

Two trials have compared gastric bypass against non-surgical treatment. In the first non-randomized trial, Martin et al. [36] compared gastric bypass in 201 patients against VLCD and diet in 161 patients. After 6 years of follow-up 34.5% of the gastric bypass group and 19.7% in the VLCD-diet group were available for evaluation. In the surgical BMI declined from 49.3 kg/m^2 at operation to a low of 31.8 kg/m^2 after 2 years and 33.7 kg/m^2 after 6 years. For the VLCD group, the corresponding data was a BMI of 41.2 kg/m^2 at baseline, 32.1 kg/m^2 after 2 years and 38.5 kg/m^2 after 6 years in those who returned for follow-up.

There is one trial comparing laparoscopic Roux-en-Y versus a mini-gastric bypass [37]. In this trial 40 subjects were randomized to each procedure and followed for a mean of 31.3 months. As expected, the operative time was shorter with the mini bypass procedure and the operative morbidity was higher in the Roux-en-Y procedure. Weight losses at 1 and 2 years were similar in the two groups. The authors conclude that the mini-gastric bypass is simpler and safer than the Roux-en-Y procedure.

The Swedish Obese Subjects (SOS) Trial is a second controlled, but non-randomized trial directly comparing surgical and non-surgical treatment for obesity, and is the largest trial comparing surgical versus medical treatment of morbid obesity [34, 38–40]. A total of 6328 obese (BMI > 34 kg/m^2 for men and > 38 kg/m^2 for women) subjects were recruited, of whom 2010 underwent surgery for obesity (gastric banding, gastroplasty or gastric bypass) while 2037 chose conventional treatment. Operated participants were matched on a number of criteria to a group of 6322 overweight men and women in the SOS registry who were not operated on. The SOS study began slowly in 1987 and has contributed significant new information about overweight individuals and the effects of surgical intervention. Prior to surgery there were an average of 7.6 kg weight loss attempts for the men and 18.2 kg for the women. The mean for the largest weight loss prior to surgery was 17.7 kg for the men and 18.2 kg for the women, but they were only able to maintain this for 7 to 10 months.

When the banding operation was compared with vertical banded gastroplasty and gastric bypass in the Swedish Obese Subjects study, Sjostrom et

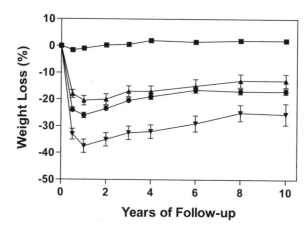

Figure 3. Weight loss following bariatric operations in the Swedish Obese Subjects Study.

al. reported similar weight losses out to 10 year in the lap-band and vertical banded gastroplasty that was significantly below that seen with the gastric by-pass [34] (Figure 3).

One randomized clinical trial compared intensive medical management versus laparoscopic insertion of an adjustable gastric band (LAP-BAND system). Included in the trial were individuals who had a BMI between 30 and 35 kg/m^2, who also had co-morbid conditions such as hypertension, dyslipidemia, diabetes obstructive sleep apnea, or gastroesophageal reflux disease, severe physical limitations or clinically significant psychosocial problems. The intensive medical program consisted of a very low calorie (energy) diet and behavior modification for 12 weeks followed by a transition phase over 4 weeks combining some VLCD meals with 120 mg of orlistat and then orlistat 120 mg before all meals. Surgery was performed by 2 surgeons. Of the 40 patients in each group, 1 withdrew before surgery leaving 39 at the end of 2 years and 7 dropped-out of the intensive intervention leaving 33 patients who completed treatment. Both groups had an identical 13.8% weight loss at 6 months. The surgical group continued to lose weight and were 21.6% below baseline at 2 years. The non-surgical group regained weight from 6 to 24 months at which time they were on average only 5.5% below baseline weight. At 2 years, the surgically treated group had significantly greater improvements in diastolic blood pressure, fasting plasma glucose level, insulin sensitivity index and HD-cholesterol level. Quality of life improved more in the surgical group. Physical function, vitality and mental health domains of the SF-36 were improved in the surgical group. Thus laparoscopic insertion of an adjustable gastric band may be beneficial to some patients with weights below those usually recommended for this procedure [20].

No randomized comparisons of the biliopancreatic diversion with other procedures have yet been published. However, there are two nonrandomized comparisons. When 142 patients with the biliopancreatic diversion were compared with 93 patients undergoing a lap-band procedure, excess weight loss was 60% with the diversion operation against 48% for the lap-band [41]. In a comparison of the diversion operation with a long-limb gastric bypass, BMI was reduced from 64 kg/m^2 to 37 kg/m^2 in the diversion group compared to a decrease from 67 kg/m^2 to 42 kg/m^2 [42]. The biliopancreatic diversion appears to have more side effects than other procedures. Scopinaro, who originated the procedure, reported a low mortality of 0.5% with an excess body weight loss of 75%. Anemia occurred in spite of iron and folate replacement in < 5%, stomach ulcer during H$_2$-blocker therapy in 3.2% and protein malnutrition in 3% [43].

5.   MECHANISMS FOR WEIGHT LOSS

There are at least 2 mechanisms that can account for the weight loss after bariatric surgery. The first of these is malabsorption. This was clearly an important component of the jejunoileal bypass [44], and is a prominent feature of the biliopancreatic diversion procedures. A second mechanism is altered hormonal secretion from the gastrointestinal track. Glucagon-like peptide-1 (GLP-1 or enteroglucagon) is secreted from the lower intestinal track and has effects on GI function and on food intake [45]. More interest has been sparked by ghrelin, a small peptide released from the stomach which stimulates food intake. Cummings et al. reported that after bariatric surgery the level of this peptide was significantly reduced [46, 47], but there have been contradictory reports since. The final mechanism is a decrease in food intake. This was also present in the patients with jejunoileal bypass [44]. In one report Lindroos et al. [48] found no different in energy intake between patients with a gastric bypass and those with a gastroplasty, although those with a gastroplasty lost less weight. In the Swedish Obese Subjects study food intake in the operated groups was less than in the control group at all time intervals (Figure 4).

The lap-band procedure also reduces food intake and feelings of satiety. In one trial Dixon et al. [49] gave a test meal to individuals with a lap-band on 2 occasions, one with optimal restriction, and one with reduced restriction. In the overweight control subjects with no bariatric procedure, the baseline levels of glucose, insulin and leptin were higher whereas the ghrelin level was lower. When they ate the test meal, the control subjects had a larger response of glucose and insulin, whereas the subjects with the lap-band had similar responses to both meals. Satiety, however, was less when the band was at the optimal restriction and there was less reduction in satiety when the band was not optimally inflated.

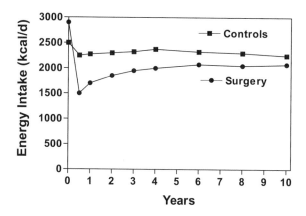

Figure 4. Food intake following bariatric operations in the Swedish Obese Subjects Study [34].

6.   BENEFITS FROM BARIATRIC SURGERY

Bariatric surgery produces more weight loss than conventional therapy for overweight, and the weight loss is more durable. After two years, weight reduction in the Swedish Obese Subjects study was 28 kg, which was significantly greater than the 0.5 kg in the matched registry patients [39]. After 10 years, control patients had gained an average of 1.4 kg compared with surgical patients who demonstrated persistent weight loss [34].

Although there is a small death rate resulting from bariatric surgery, data are beginning to accumulate that the long-term benefits weigh in on the side of reduced mortality after bariatric surgery. Christou et al. compared 1035 patients who had undergone bariatric surgery with an age- and gender-matched severely obese case-control population [50]. Patients who had bariatric surgery had a significantly lower rate of cardiovascular disease, cancer, and endocrine, infectious and psychiatric disorders than the case-controls. The overall mortality rate of 0.68% in the bariatric group was significantly lower than in the case-controls (6.17 percent, RR 0.11, 95% CI 0.04–0.27). Mortality rates are influenced by the amount of surgical experience [51, 52].

There are a number of reports showing improvement in the diseases associated with overweight. One of the most impressive has been sleep apnea. Even modest weight loss can benefit this disabling medical problem, and bariatric surgery has been particularly helpful [53].

Next to the effects on sleep apnea is improvement in the prospects for patient with diabetes or those at high risk for developing it. Pories et al. were the first to note the marked improvement of diabetes after surgery [54, 55]. Although there were design issues with these retrospective studies, they showed an annual incidence of 4.5% in the control group contrasted with only 1% in the surgically operated group. The Swedish Obese Subjects study has reported

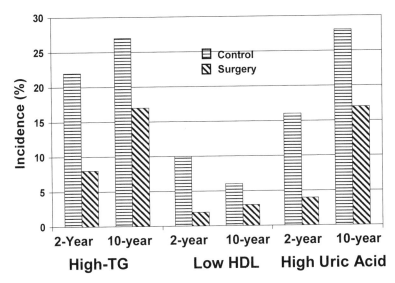

Figure 5. Incidence of diabetes mellitus, low HDL-cholesterol and high uric acid at 2 and 10 years following bariatric surgery for obesity in the Swedish Obese Subjects Study (from [34]).

similarly impressive data. After 2 years of follow-up the incidence of new-onset diabetes was 4.7% in the matched control group with no new cases in the surgical group. After 8 years the incidence of new-onset diabetes in the control group was 18.5% compared to only 3.6% in the operated group. The incidence rate was related to the amount of weight lost. In the subgroup losing more than 12% of their initial body weight, there were no new cases, in contrast to 7% in those losing 2% and 9% in those gaining 4% (Figure 5). This was reflected in the low odds ratio [OR] for diabetes (OR 0.10) and hyperinsulinemia (OR 0.1).

The incidence of other medical complications was also reduced. There was a linear reduction in the systolic and diastolic blood pressure with the degree of weight loss [56] and the odds ratio for incident hypertension was 0.38. Triglyceride and insulin levels also showed a linear decrease with weight loss (OR 0.28 for hypertriglyceridemia). The concentration of HDL-cholesterol increased linearly with weight loss (OR 0.28), but cholesterol did not decline significantly until weight loss had exceeded 25 kg (OR 1.24) [29].

Surgically treated patients required less medication for cardiovascular disease or diabetes than matched controls [57]. Among those not already requiring such medications, surgery reduced the proportion who required initiation of treatment, as well as the costs of medications [58]. Quality of life compared [38] was related primarily to the degree of weight-loss. Psychiatric dysfunction also improved [59], and patients become less depressed [60].

7.   COMPLICATIONS ASSOCIATED WITH BARIATRIC SURGERY

7.1.   Complications Following Lap-band Bariatric Surgery

Despite its relative technical ease, Laparoscopic Adjustable Gastric Band (LAGB) has been associated with several complications which are summarized in Table 3. Laparoscopic procedures have significantly reduced rates of wound infections. One advantage of the lap-band is that it eliminates leakage

Table 3. Complications from laparoscopic adjustable gastric band

- Revisional surgery up to 40%
- Acute stomal obstruction 2%
- Band erosion 0–3%
- Band slippage/prolapse up to 24%
- Port/tubing malfunction 0.4–7%
- Pouch/esophageal dilation up to 10%
- Infection at port site 0 to 9%

at staple lines. There is no significant difference in leak rates between the open versus laparoscopic approach. An initial trial of LAGB in the United States showed disappointing weight losses and high complication rates, associated with relatively high rates of revisional surgery (40 percent) [61]. However, complications following LAGB were described far less frequently in Europe, Australia, and in a more recent trial in the United States [62–64]. On average, approximately 13 to 15 percent of patients will require reoperation for various complications [65]. New standards for training and certification may ensure more standardized operative technique and optimal postoperative patient management, and thus may lead to improved outcomes [66]. Occasionally, the stomach wall prolapses upward or downward through the band leading to gastric obstruction. In the registration trials submitted to the Food and Drug Administration slippage occurred in 24% of patients but a lower incidence of 2 to 14% has been reported in subsequent studies [67, 68]. If the tube becomes disconnected from the subcutaneous port decompression of the band will occur. Port and tubing malfunction have occurred in 0.4 to 7.0% of patients [67, 69].

7.2.   Complications Following Restrictive Bariatric Surgery

A list of some of the complications following restrictive gastric operations is shown in Table 4. Mortality rate varies from one center to another. As noted

Table 4. Complications of gastric
restriction operations

- Disruption of staple line in VBG 27–31%
- Stomal stenosis 20–33%
- Band erosion 1–7%
- Gastroesophageal reflux
- Recurrent vomiting 8–21%

above, surgeons with more than 20 operations to their credit have significantly lower mortality. Wound infections were an important concern with the open procedures. Leaks around staple lines are a major life-threatening complication that can occur with vertically banded gastroplasty. Marginal (stomal) ulceration and stenosis, with band erosion at the end of the esophageal extension, gastro-esophageal reflux disease (GERD), nausea and vomiting, marginal ulcers are problems with the lap-band and with laparoscopic or open gastroplasty are examples. Regain of body weight is more common with gastroplasty than with gastric by-pass or biliopancreatic diversion [70, 71]. Gastroesophageal reflux after VBG presents with classic symptoms such as burning pain, heartburn, aspiration, and cough. It typically occurs as a late complication, as a result of stomal stenosis and pouch dilatation [72]. Wound infection of 10–15% are significantly greater with gastric bypass procedures than the 3–4% seen with laparoscopic procedures [73–75]. Perioperative use of antibiotics (usually cefazolin) can reduce this problem [76].

7.3. Complications with Malabsorptive Operations

Death following a Roux-en-Y gastric by-pass ranges from 0 to 1 percent or somewhat more [54, 77, 78]. In a recent assessment of deaths using the Medicare records, Flum et al. [79] noted that among 16,155 patients undergoing bariatric procedures between 1997 and 2002, the 30 day. 90 day and 1 year mortality rates were 2.0%, 2.8% and 4.6%, which are higher than the usual reported rates from surgical series. Men had higher early death rates than women. Death rates were also significantly higher among subjects over 65 years of age. After adjusting for sex and comorbidity index, the odds of death within 90 days were 5-fold higher in those over 75 years of age than in those 65 to 74 years old.

Leaks around staple lines are a major life-threatening complication of the gastric by-pass and the biliopancreatic diversion. Leaks from the staple lines are the most serious complication and require immediate surgical intervention. They may be responsible for up to 50% of deaths [46]. The quoted leak rate following gastric bypass is between 0 and 5.1 percent, with the average leak rate between 2 and 3 percent [52, 73, 74, 80]. Early symptoms of a suture line leak may be subtle, including a low-grade fever, respiratory distress, or an un-explained tachycardia [81]. Exploratory surgery should be performed without delay.

Hospitalization following Roux-en-Y gastric bypass is significantly in-creased. Between 1995 and 2004 there were 60,077 gastric bypass operations performed in California with 11,659 performed in 2004 alone [82]. The hos-pitalization rate was 7.9% in the year preceding the RYBGP and 19.3% in the year following. Among the 24,678 patients for whom 3 year of data were available, 8.4% were admitted in the year before surgery, 20.2% in the first year after bariatric surgery, 18.4% in the second year and 14.9% in the third year. The authors conclude that hospitalization in the years following gastric bypass is related to the surgery.

Another early post-operative risk common to all procedures is pulmonary embolus [83]. The incidence of deep vein thrombosis and pulmonary em-bolism varies between 0 and 3.3 percent with laparoscopic bypasses [52, 73, 74, 80] and 0.3 and 1.9 percent with open bypasses [30, 84, 85]. In an autopsy series [83] pulmonary embolism was the cause of death in 30% of patients. In addition 80% had silent pulmonary emboli despite prophylactic treatment with anti-coagulants. Risk factors associated with fatal PE include severe venous stasis disease, BMI > 60 kg/m^2, truncal adiposity, and obesity-hypoventilation syndrome [86]. Use of heparin prophylactically would appear to be a desirable post-operative procedure in obese patients having this operation.

Ventral hernias occur in up to 24% of patients who have open operations but with laparoscopic surgery it is reduced to an incidence of 0 to 1.8% [52, 54, 74, 75, 87]. The Roux-en-Y procedure also carries a risk of internal hernias, since the anatomical changes provide new holes through which bowel can be squeezed [88]. These internal hernias have been described in 0 to 5 percent of patients undergoing laparoscopic bariatric surgery [74, 75].

Development of gall stones is a common problem with rapid weight loss and thus cholelithiasis is to be expected follow surgical procedures for overweight. Gall stone disease has been reported to develop in as many as 38 percent of patients within six months of surgery [89]. The risk of gall stones can be re-duced to as low as 2 percent by using the bile salt (ursodeoxycholic acid) for 6 months following surgery [90].

Metabolic and nutritional derangements can pose significant problems fol-lowing after malabsorptive procedures. Life-long use of vitamins and minerals are important. Malabsorption of iron, vitamin B_{12}, and folate are the most likely problems. Malabsorption of fat soluble vitamins, protein, and thiamine may also occur and can manifest itself clinically.

8. OTHER OPERATIVE PROCEDURES FOR THE OVERWEIGHT PATIENT

8.1. Intragastric Balloon

The intragastric balloon (Bioenterics Intragastric Balloon, Inamed) is a temporary alternative for weight loss in moderately obese individuals. It consists of a soft, saline-filled balloon placed endoscopically that promotes a feeling of satiety and restriction. It is currently not available for use in the United States, but is undergoing extensive testing in Europe and Brazil. Mean excess weight loss is reported to be 38 percent and 48 percent for 500 and 600 mL balloons, respectively [91]. However, the results of a Brazilian multi-center study indicate weight loss is transient, with only 26 percent of patients maintaining over 90 percent of the excess weight loss to one year [92]. Side-effects include nausea, vomiting, abdominal pain, ulceration, and balloon migration.

8.2. Gastric Stimulation or Gastric Pacing

Gastric pacing as a technique for weight loss was pioneered in pigs where repeat stimulation produced significant weight loss [93]. The first clinical trial included 24 overweight human beings with a BMI > 40 kg/m^2. Over the 9 months of the trial the BMI was reduced 4.7 kg/m^2 with no significant side effects [93]. In a follow-up study of 11 patients with an initial BMI of 46.0 kg/m^2 who lost 3.6 kg in the 2 months after implantation of the pace maker, but before it was turned on, there was a further 6.8 kg weight loss after 6 months of electrical stimulation. Following a test meal there was a smaller rise in cholecystokininn, and lower levels of somatostatin, GLP-1 and leptin, although it is unclear whether this was secondary to the stimulation or weight loss. In a summary of experience on more than 200 patients who have had gastric implantation, Shikora [94] noted that some patients responded well whereas others did not. An algorithm was developed based on baseline age, gender, body weight, BMI and response to preoperative questionnaires. With this algorithm the selection rate for the procedure was 18% to 33%. When this algorithm is applied, excess weight loss is up to 40% in 12 months, compared to a 4% excess weight gain in the control group. More data is needed.

8.3. Liposuction and Omentectomy

Liposuction which is also known as lipoplasty or suction-assisted lipectomy is the most common esthetic procedure performed in the US with over 400,000 cases performed annually [95]. Although not generally considered to be a bariatric procedure, removal of fat by aspiration after injection of physiologic saline has been used to remove and contour subcutaneous fat. As the techniques have improved it is now possible to remove significant amounts of subcutaneous adipose tissue without affecting the amount of visceral fat. In a study to examine the effects of this procedure, Klein et al. [95] studied 7 overweight diabetic women and 8 overweight non-diabetic women with normal glucose tolerance before and after liposuction. One week after assessing insulin sensitivity, the subjects underwent large volume tumescent liposuction which consists of removing more than 4 liters of aspirate injected into the fat beneath the skin. There was a significant loss of subcutaneous fat as expected, but no change in the visceral fat. Subjects were reassessed 10–12 weeks after the surgery when the non-diabetic women had lost −6.3 kg of body weight and −9.1 kg of body fat which reduced body fat by −6.3%. The diabetic women had a similar response with a weight loss of −7.9 kg, a reduction in body fat of −10.5 kg and reduction in percent fat of −6.7%. Waist circumference was also significantly reduced. In spite of these significant reductions in body fat, there were no changes in blood pressure, lipids or cytokines (tumor necrosis factor-α, interleukin-6, or C-reactive protein). There was also no improvement in insulin sensitivity suggesting that removal of subcutaneous adipose tissue without reducing visceral fat has little influence on the risk factors related to being overweight.

   Omentectomy is the direct removal of the intra-abdominal fat by surgical means. One randomized controlled trial in 50 overweight subjects compared the effect of an adjustable lap-band alone with a lap-band plus removal of the omentum [96]. Of the original 50 operated patients, 37 were re-evaluated at the end of 2 years after the surgery. The reduction in body weight was 27 kg in the lap-band group and 36 kg in the lap-band + omentectomy group ($p = 0.07$). Glucose and insulin improved more in the subjects with omentectomy than in those without it. This study complements the one by Klein described above by showing that removal of extra visceral fat can have a small but significant effect, while decreasing subcutaneous fat alone has little impact.

9.   SUMMARY

   We are now at the end of this monograph written some 30 years after my first full length book about the Obese Patient. The survey began with definitions of overweight and how the problem has developed into the current epidemic. This was followed by a discussion of the hazards to health of excess weight, which set the stage for what we can do about the problem. Clearly the most effective long-term weight loss solution is bariatric surgery. However, from a societal perspective, we need to develop strategies that will help people avoid the problem so we can reduce the use of these drastic techniques to only a handful of people. Otherwise we may bankrupt the health care system.

The road toward prevention of overweight will be long and hard. The first law of thermodynamics which describes the fact that we gain weight from eating more than our bodies need has lulled us into the uncomfortable place of believing that through "will-power", increased food choices or more places to exercise we can overcome the current epidemic of obesity. At least that is the current approach of the Calories Count Program of the Department of Health and Human Services and the direction toward personal responsibility for being overweight that the food industry would like to have us take. However, I think this is an inadequate approach. Until we recognize that low food prices, driven in part by farm subsidies, drive food choices, that there is a hedonic override to our regulatory system for controlling body weight, and until we develop newer strategies to prevent the problem, I fear that overweight will remain a major problem well into the future. This will mean that the demand for bariatric surgery will continue. This conclusion brings us to a good place to end our adventure into the problems and solutions for overweight.

REFERENCES

[1] Sjostrom L. Surgical treatment of obesity: An overview and results from the SOS Study. In: Bray G, Bouchard C, eds. Handbook of Obesity: Clinical Applications. New York: Marcel Dekker, 2004;359–389.

[2] Buchwald H, et al. Bariatric surgery: A systematic review and meta-analysis. JAMA 2004;292(14):1724–1737.

[3] Shekelle PG, et al. Pharmacological and surgical treatment of obesity. Evid Rep Technol Assess (Summ) 2004;103:1–6.

[4] Inge TH, et al. Bariatric surgery for severely overweight adolescents: Concerns and recommendations. Pediatrics 2004;114(1):217–223.

[5] Bray G. Bariatric Surgery. UpToDate [Compact disc] 2006 [cited 2006 2 March 2006].

[6] Colquitt J, et al. Surgery for morbid obesity. Cochrane Database Syst Rev 2005;4: CD003641.

[7] Payne JH, Dewind LT, Commons RR. Metabolic observations in patients with jejunocolic shunts. Am J Surg 1963;106:273–289.

[8] DeWind LT, Payne JH. Intestinal bypass surgery for morbid obesity. Long-term results. JAMA 1976;236(20):2298–2301.

[9] Pace WG, et al. Gastric partitioning for morbid obesity. Ann Surg 1979;190(3):392–400.

[10] Gomez CA. Gastroplasty in morbid obesity. Surg Clin North Am 1979;59(6):1113–1120.

[11] Mason EE. Vertical banded gastroplasty for obesity. Arch Surg 1982;117(5):701–706.

[12] Bo O, Modalsli O. Gastric banding, a surgical method of treating morbid obesity: Preliminary report. Int J Obes 1983;7(5):493–499.

[13] Mason EE, Ito C. Gastric bypass in obesity. Surg Clin North Am 1967;47(6):1345–1351.

[14] Mason EE, Ito C. Gastric bypass. Ann Surg 1969;170(3):329–339.

[15] Marceau P, et al. Biliopancreatic diversion with a new type of gastrectomy. Obes Surg 1993;3(1):29–35.

[16] Fried M, Peskova M. Gastric banding in the treatment of morbid obesity. Hepatogastroenterology 1997;44(14):582–587.

[17] Belachew M, et al. Laparoscopic placement of adjustable silicone gastric band in the treatment of morbid obesity: How to do it. Obes Surg 1995;5(1):66–70.

[18] Gastrointestinal surgery for severe obesity: National Institutes of Health Consensus Development Conference Statement. Am J Clin Nutr 1992;55(Suppl 2):615S–619S.

[19] NIH conference. Gastrointestinal surgery for severe obesity. Consensus Development Conference Panel. Ann Intern Med 1991;115(12):956–961.

[20] O'Brien PE, et al. Treatment of mild to moderate obesity with laparoscopic adjustable gastric banding or an intensive medical program: A randomized trial. Ann Intern Med 2006;144(9):625–633.

[21] Bariatric Centers of Excellence. ASBS Newsletter 2003:4.

[22] Sugerman HJ, et al. Bariatric surgery for severely obese adolescents. J Gastrointest Surg 2003;7(1):102–107; discussion 107–108.

[23] Alden JF. Gastric and jejunoileal bypass. A comparison in the treatment of morbid obesity. Arch Surg 1977;112(7):799–806.

[24] Griffen WO Jr, Young VL, Stevenson CC. A prospective comparison of gastric and jejunoileal bypass procedures for morbid obesity. Ann Surg 1977;186(4):500–509.

[25] Buckwalter JA. A prospective comparison of the jejunoileal and gastric bypass operations for morbid obesity. World J Surg 1977;1(6):757–768.

[26] Deitel M, et al. Intestinal bypass and gastric partitioning for morbid obesity: A comparison. Can J Surg 1982;25(3):283–289.

[27] Randomised trial of jejunoileal bypass versus medical treatment in morbid obesity. The Danish Obesity Project. Lancet 1979;2(8155):1255–1258.

[28] Stokholm KH, Nielsen PE, Quaade F. Correlation between initial blood pressure and blood pressure decrease after weight loss: A study in patients with jejunoileal bypass versus medical treatment for morbid obesity. Int J Obes 1982;6(3):307–312.

[29] Sjostrom CD, et al. Reduction in incidence of diabetes, hypertension and lipid disturbances after intentional weight loss induced by bariatric surgery: The SOS Intervention Study. Obes Res 1999;7(5):477–484.

[30] Hall JC, et al. Gastric surgery for morbid obesity. The Adelaide Study. Ann Surg 1990;211(4):419–427.

[31] Andersen T, et al. Randomized trial of diet and gastroplasty compared with diet alone in morbid obesity. N Engl J Med 1984;310(6):352–356.

[32] Andersen T, et al. Long-term (5-year) results after either horizontal gastroplasty or very-low-calorie diet for morbid obesity. Int J Obes 1988;12(4):277–284.

[33] Howard L, et al. Gastric bypass and vertical banded gastroplasty—a prospective randomized comparison and 5-year follow-up. Obes Surg 1995;5(1):55–60.

[34] Sjostrom L, et al. Lifestyle, diabetes, and cardiovascular risk factors 10 years after bariatric surgery. N Engl J Med 2004;351(26):2683–2693.

[35] MacLean LD, et al. Results of the surgical treatment of obesity. Am J Surg 1993;165(1):155–160; discussion 160–162.

[36] Martin LF, et al. Comparison of the costs associated with medical and surgical treatment of obesity. Surgery 1995;118(4):599–606; discussion 606–607.

[37] Lee WJ et al. Laparoscopic Roux-en-Y versus mini-gastric bypass for the treatment of morbid obesity: A prospective randomized controlled clinical trial. Ann Surg 2005;242(1):20–28.

[38] Karlsson J, Sjostrom L, Sullivan M. Swedish obese subjects (SOS)—an intervention study of obesity. Two-year follow-up of health-related quality of life (HRQL) and eating behavior after gastric surgery for severe obesity. Int J Obes Relat Metab Disord 1998;22(2):113–126.

[39] Torgerson JS, Sjostrom L. The Swedish Obese Subjects (SOS) study—rationale and results. Int J Obes Relat Metab Disord 2001;25(Suppl 1):S2–S4.

[40] Sjostrom L, et al. Swedish obese subjects (SOS). Recruitment for an intervention study and a selected description of the obese state. Int J Obes Relat Metab Disord 1992;16(6):465–479.

[41] Bajardi G, et al. Surgical treatment of morbid obesity with biliopancreatic diversion and gastric banding: Report on an 8-year experience involving 235 cases. Ann Chir 2000; 125(2):155–162.

[42] Murr MM, et al. Malabsorptive procedures for severe obesity: Comparison of pancreati-cobiliary bypass and very very long limb Roux-en-Y gastric bypass. J Gastrointest Surg 1999;3(6):607–612.

[43] Scopinaro N, et al. Biliopancreatic diversion for obesity at eighteen years. Surgery 1996; 119(3):261–268.

[44] Bray GA. The Obese Patient: Major Problems in Internal Medicine, 9th edn. Philadelphia: WB Saunders, 1976.

[45] Kellum JM, et al. Gastrointestinal hormone responses to meals before and after gastric bypass and vertical banded gastroplasty. Ann Surg 1990;211(6):763–770; discussion 770–771.

[46] Cummings DE, et al. Plasma ghrelin levels after diet-induced weight loss or gastric bypass surgery. N Engl J Med 2002;346(21):1623–1630.

[47] Tritos NA, et al. Serum ghrelin levels in response to glucose load in obese subjects post-gastric bypass surgery. Obes Res 2003;11(8):919–924.

[48] Lindroos AK, Lissner L, Sjostrom L. Weight change in relation to intake of sugar and sweet foods before and after weight reducing gastric surgery. Int J Obes Relat Metab Disord 1996;20(7):634–643.

[49] Dixon AF, Dixon JB, O'Brien PE. Laparoscopic adjustable gastric banding induces pro-longed satiety: A randomized blind crossover study. J Clin Endocrinol Metab 2005; 90(2):813–819.

[50] Christou NV, et al. Surgery decreases long-term mortality, morbidity, and health care use in morbidly obese patients. Ann Surg 2004;240(3):416–423; discussion 423–424.

[51] Schauer P, et al. The learning curve for laparoscopic Roux-en-Y gastric bypass is 100 cases. Surg Endosc 2003;17(2):212–215.

[52] Wittgrove AC, Clark GW. Laparoscopic gastric bypass, Roux-en-Y- 500 patients: Tech-nique and results, with 3–60 month follow-up. Obes Surg 2000;10(3):233–239.

[53] Dixon JB, Schachter LM, O'Brien PE. Sleep disturbance and obesity: Changes following surgically induced weight loss. Arch Intern Med 2001;161(1):102–106.

[54] Pories WJ, et al. Who would have thought it? An operation proves to be the most effective therapy for adult-onset diabetes mellitus. Ann Surg 1995;222(3):339–350; discussion 350–352.

[55] Pories WJ, et al. Is type II diabetes mellitus (NIDDM) a surgical disease? Ann Surg 1992; 215(6):633–642; discussion 643.

[56] Sjostrom CD, Lissner L, Sjostrom L. Relationships between changes in body composition and changes in cardiovascular risk factors: The SOS Intervention Study. Swedish Obese Subjects. Obes Res 1997;5(6):519–530.

[57] Agren G, et al. Long-term effects of weight loss on pharmaceutical costs in obese subjects. A report from the SOS intervention study. Int J Obes Relat Metab Disord 2002;26(2):184–192.

[58] Narbro K, et al. Pharmaceutical costs in obese individuals: Comparison with a randomly selected population sample and long-term changes after conventional and surgical treat-ment: The SOS intervention study. Arch Intern Med 2002;162(18):2061–2069.

[59] Ryden A, et al. A comparative controlled study of personality in severe obesity: A 2-y follow-up after intervention. Int J Obes Relat Metab Disord 2004;28(11):1485–1493.

[60] Dixon JB, Dixon ME, O'Brien PE. Depression in association with severe obesity: Changes with weight loss. Arch Intern Med 2003;163(17):2058–2065.

[61] DeMaria EJ, et al. High failure rate after laparoscopic adjustable silicone gastric banding for treatment of morbid obesity. Ann Surg 2001;233(6):809–818.

[62] O'Brien PE, Dixon JB. Lap-band: Outcomes and results. J Laparoendosc Adv Surg Tech A 2003;13(4):265–270.

[63] FDA Trial Summary of Safety and Effectiveness Data: The Lap-Band Adjustable Gastric Banding System [website; cited 2006 2 March]; available from: http://www.fda.gov/cdrh/pdf/p000008.htm.

[64] Angrisani L, et al. Lap band adjustable gastric banding system: The Italian experience with 1863 patients operated on 6 years. Surg Endosc 2003;17(3):409–412.

[65] Kothari SN, et al. Lap-band failures: Conversion to gastric bypass and their preliminary outcomes. Surgery 2002;131(6):625–629.

[66] Schneider BE, Sanchez VM, Jones DB. How to implant the laparoscopic adjustable gastric band for morbid obesity. Contemporary Surgery 2004;60(6):256–264.

[67] Ren CJ, Horgan S, Ponce J. US experience with the LAP-BAND system. Am J Surg 2002;184(6B):46S–50S.

[68] Rubenstein RB. Laparoscopic adjustable gastric banding at a U.S. center with up to 3-year follow-up. Obes Surg 2002;12(3):380–384.

[69] Dargent J. Laparoscopic adjustable gastric banding: Lessons from the first 500 patients in a single institution. Obes Surg 1999;9(5):446–452.

[70] Balsiger BM, et al. Bariatric surgery. Surgery for weight control in patients with morbid obesity. Med Clin North Am 2000;84(2):477–489.

[71] Nightengale ML, et al. Prospective evaluation of vertical banded gastroplasty as the primary operation for morbid obesity. Mayo Clin Proc 1991;66(8):773–782.

[72] Balsiger BM, et al. Gastroesophageal reflux after intact vertical banded gastroplasty: Correction by conversion to Roux-en-Y gastric bypass. J Gastrointest Surg 2000;4(3):276–281.

[73] Schauer PR, et al. Outcomes after laparoscopic Roux-en-Y gastric bypass for morbid obesity. Ann Surg 2000;232(4):515–529.

[74] Nguyen NT, et al. Laparoscopic versus open gastric bypass: A randomized study of outcomes, quality of life, and costs. Ann Surg 2001;234(3):279–289; discussion 289–291.

[75] Higa KD, Boone KB, Ho T. Complications of the laparoscopic Roux-en-Y gastric bypass: 1,040 patients—what have we learned? Obes Surg 2000;10(6):509–513.

[76] Pories WJ, et al. Prophylactic cefazolin in gastric bypass surgery. Surgery 1981;90(2):426–432.

[77] Schneider BE, et al. Laparoscopic gastric bypass surgery: Outcomes. J Laparoendosc Adv Surg Tech A 2003;13(4): 247–255.

[78] Sugerman HJ, et al. Weight loss with vertical banded gastroplasty and Roux-Y gastric bypass for morbid obesity with selective versus random assignment. Am J Surg 1989; 157(1):93–102.

[79] Flum DR, et al. Early mortality among medicare beneficiaries undergoing bariatric surgical procedures. JAMA 2005;294(15):1903–1908.

[80] Westling A, Gustavsson S. Laparoscopic vs open Roux-en-Y gastric bypass: A prospective, randomized trial. Obes Surg 2001;11(3):284–292.

[81] Hamilton EC, et al. Clinical predictors of leak after laparoscopic Roux-en-Y gastric bypass for morbid obesity. Surg Endosc 2003;17(5):679–684.

[82] Zingmond DS, McGory ML, Ko CY. Hospitalization before and after gastric bypass surgery. JAMA 2005;294(15):1918–1924.

[83] Melinek J, et al. Autopsy findings following gastric bypass surgery for morbid obesity. Arch Pathol Lab Med 2002;126(9):1091–1095.

[84] Griffen WO Jr. Gastric bypass for morbid obesity. Surg Clin North Am 1979;59(6):1103–1112.

[85] Fobi MA, et al. Gastric bypass operation for obesity. World J Surg 1998;22(9):925–935.

[86] Sapala JA, et al. Fatal pulmonary embolism after bariatric operations for morbid obesity: A 24-year retrospective analysis. Obes Surg 2003;13(6):819–825.

[87] Nguyen NT, et al. A comparison study of laparoscopic versus open gastric bypass for morbid obesity. J Am Coll Surg 2000;191(2):149–155; discussion 155–157.

[88] Champion JK, Williams M. Small bowel obstruction and internal hernias after laparoscopic Roux-en-Y gastric bypass. Obes Surg 2003;13(4):596–600.

[89] Shiffman ML, et al. Gallstone formation after rapid weight loss: A prospective study in patients undergoing gastric bypass surgery for treatment of morbid obesity. Am J Gastroenterol 1991;86(8):1000–1005.

[90] Sugerman HJ, et al. A multicenter, placebo-controlled, randomized, double-blind, prospective trial of prophylactic ursodiol for the prevention of gallstone formation following gastric-bypass-induced rapid weight loss. Am J Surg 1995;169(1):91–96; discussion 96–97.

[91] Roman S, et al. Intragastric balloon for "non-morbid" obesity: A retrospective evaluation of tolerance and efficacy. Obes Surg 2004;14(4):539–544.

[92] Sallet JA, et al. Brazilian multicenter study of the intragastric balloon. Obes Surg 2004;14(7):991–998.

[93] Cigaina VV, et al. Long-term effects of gastric pacing to reduce feed intake in swine. Obes Surg 1996;6(3):250–253.

[94] Shikora SA. Implantable gastric stimulation for the treatment of severe obesity. Obes Surg 2004;14(4):545–548.

[95] Klein S, et al. Absence of an effect of liposuction on insulin action and risk factors for coronary heart disease. N Engl J Med 2004;350(25):2549–2557.

[96] Thorne A, et al. A pilot study of long-term effects of a novel obesity treatment: Omentectomy in connection with adjustable gastric banding. Int J Obes Relat Metab Disord 2002;26(2):193–199.

Index

Printed in the United States